Seventh Edition

Drugs in Perspective:

Causes, assessment, family, prevention, intervention, and treatment

Richard Fields, Ph.D.

Director/Owner, Faces Conferences
Private Counseling Practice
Bellevue, WA

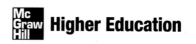 **Higher Education**

Boston   Burr Ridge, IL   Dubuque, IA   New York   San Francisco   St. Louis
Bangkok   Bogotá   Caracas   Kuala Lumpur   Lisbon   London   Madrid   Mexico City
Milan   Montreal   New Delhi   Santiago   Seoul   Singapore   Sydney   Taipei   Toronto

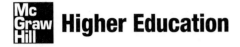

The McGraw·Hill Companies

Higher Education

Published by McGraw-Hill, an imprint of The McGraw-Hill Companies, Inc., 1221 Avenue of the Americas, New York, NY 10020. Copyright © 2010, 2007, 2004, 2001, 1998, 1995, 1992, All rights reserved. No part of this publication may be reproduced or distributed in any form or by any means, or stored in a database or retrieval system, without the prior written consent of The McGraw-Hill Companies, Inc., including, but not limited to, in any network or other electronic storage or transmission, or broadcast for distance learning.

This book is printed on acid-free paper.

1 2 3 4 5 6 7 8 9 0 DOC/DOC 0 9

ISBN: 978-0-07-338075-9
MHID: 0-07-338075-X

Editor in Chief: *Michael Ryan*
Publisher: *William Glass*
Sponsoring Editor: *Joe Diggins*
Marketing Manager: *Pamela Cooper*
Developmental Editor: *Phillip Butcher*
Production Editor: *Regina Ernst*
Manuscript Editor: *Leslie Ann Weber*
Cover Designer: *Allister Fein*
Photo Research: *Brian Pecko*
Production Supervisor: *Louis Swaim*
Composition: *10/12 Times Roman by Laserwords Private Limited*
Printing: *PMS 200, 45# New Era Matte Plus, R. R. Donnelley & Sons/Crawfordsville, IN*

Cover: Woman with glass: © Dynamic Graphics/JupiterImages; Therapist and Patient: © David Buffington/Getty Images; Man in flowers: © Royalty-Free/Corbis

Credits: The credits section for this book appears on page C-1 and is considered an extension of the copyright page.

Library of Congress Cataloging-in-Publication Data

Fields, Richard.
Drugs in perspective / Richard Fields.—7th ed.
      p. ; cm.
Includes bibliographical references and index.
ISBN-13: 978-0-07-338075-9 (alk. paper)
ISBN-10: 0-07-338075-X (alk. paper)
  1. Drug abuse. 2. Alcoholism. 3. Drug abuse—Prevention. 4. Alcoholism—Prevention. 5. Drug abuse—Treatment.
6. Alcoholism—Treatment. I. Title.
  [DNLM: 1. Substance-Related Disorders. WM 270 F462d 2010]
HV5801.F42 2010
362.29'17—dc22

                                                                                              2008049103

The Internet addresses listed in the text were accurate at the time of publication. The inclusion of a Web site does not indicate an endorsement by the authors or McGraw-Hill, and McGraw-Hill does not guarantee the accuracy of the information presented at these sites.

www.mhhe.com

I dedicate this book to my wife Deborah and my son Matthew.

Brief Contents

Contents

Preface

⋇ Purpose

The primary purpose of this text is to provide a relatively unbiased view or reporting of the literature on alcohol/drug prevention, intervention, and treatment. It is biased in that it is influenced by more than 30 years of clinical work with substance abusers, addicts/alcoholics, and, importantly, their families. The text has been updated and revised.

This book can help you better understand the confounding variables of substance abuse and dependence. I hope it will help you explore your own personal perspective about drugs. It will not give you a "simple solution."

This seventh edition of *Drugs in Perspective* has:

- Updated information
- Reorganized and new information in Chapter 2: Why Do People Abuse Drugs?
- New contemporary case studies throughout the text
- Chapter pedagogy: chapter objectives, in review section, case studies with discussion questions, information on co-occurring disorders, mindfulness and recovery, trauma, and sexual violation
- A revised and updated post-test

Website

The website for *Drugs in Perspective,* 7/e, www.mhhe.com/fields/7e, contains a number of useful tools for the instructor:

- **Test Bank** This resource includes a test bank of multiple choice, true/false, matching, and critical thinking questions.
- **Instructor's Manual** This manual provides valuable resources to help effectively present the text in a classroom setting.
- **PowerPoint** A complete set of PowerPoint slides prepared by the author for the course is included on the Instructor's Resource CD.

Acknowledgments

I would also like to thank the instructors who reviewed the previous edition and helped lay the groundwork for the improvements and changes needed in the seventh edition:

John Bourdette

Western New Mexico University

John Bureman

Oklahoma State University

Lori Meier

University of Idaho

Daryl Pitts

Liberty University

Richard Fields

Understanding Substance Abuse

Putting Drugs in Perspective

Objectives

1. Clarify and identify your personal biases, experiences, viewpoints, opinions, and perspectives on drug abuse and dependence.
2. List some simple solutions to the drug problem that have not worked and explain why.
3. List some scare tactics that did not work in preventing drug use and abuse.
4. Identify the various ways alcohol abuse and alcoholism-related problems have been minimized and explain why.
5. List several ways binge drinking on college campuses has created problems.
6. Identify and classify what role alcohol plays in
   - sexual assault and rape on college campuses,
   - intimate partner violence (IPV),
   - driving under the influence, and
   - intentional and unintentional deaths.
7. Identify some problems related to tobacco, the most deadly drug.
8. Describe the impact of a drug policy that focuses on the supply side and ignores the demand side.
9. List some racist policies related to drug use over the last 200 years and some that exist today.
10. Describe the scope of socioeconomic inequities that contribute to the drug problem in America.
11. Explain the role of academic failure and adolescent drug use and abuse.
12. Describe the denial of the addict/alcoholic and family members.
13. Identify and describe the kinds of adolescent co-occurring disorders.
14. Describe the primary goal of each of the five perspectives—moral-legal, medical-health, psychosocial, social-cultural, and spiritual.

⚹ Introduction

Exploring Your Own Perspective

This textbook is designed to help you clarify and understand the many confounding variables that influence substance use, abuse, and dependence. Chapter 1 emphasizes the problems in perception that have misdirected efforts toward effective drug/alcohol prevention, intervention, and treatment efforts. The chapter is designed to stimulate both classroom discussion and the exploration of your own biases, viewpoints, experiences, and personal opinions—to help you put **"drugs in perspective."**

I recommend keeping notes and answering the questions at the end of this chapter (Sixth Perspective) to help you understand your personal perspective. I also suggest keeping a journal after each chapter listing information, ideas, and thoughts and anything of special interest to you. When you finish reading the textbook, see if your perspective has changed in any way.

The Myth of the Simple, Magical Solution

During the Reagan administration, First Lady Nancy Reagan was influential in shaping the U.S. approach to the "drug problem." Although her intentions were noble and well intended, the "Just Say No" approach illustrates a simplistic view to a complicated problem. Suggesting that adolescents and young adults can overcome the drive to alter consciousness, peer influence, the disease of alcoholism/addiction, and the many factors that influence alcohol/drug abuse by "just saying no" minimizes the obstacles to be overcome.

Often a complicated, emotionally laden problem elicits a simple solution. A simple solution is easily understood and immediately reduces anxiety, shame, and emotional discomfort. However, a simple solution will not resolve the insidious, multifaceted problems of substance abuse and addiction. Drug use, abuse, and dependence are not easily understood. Mrs. Reagan made the same mistake that many people make. Too often, people search for that simple solution to an epidemic problem. Philosopher H. L. Mencken remarked that "any solution to a complex problem that is simple, is usually wrong."

Having spent more than 25 years working with individuals and their families, I still struggle case by case to try to find some common patterns and new insights into what works in treatment. I am constantly questioning what may have caused alcohol/drug problems and how best to engage, motivate, and approach clients with drug abuse and dependence. For some, the solution is abstinence and strong involvement in self-help groups; for others, it is a different path. For many, it is the acceptance of the "disease," while others label their alcohol/drug use as an "allergy" or a problem with tolerance. Some individuals can stay sober for a month or two and then experience a "binge relapse," while others can abstain for several years. Many, through the help of Alcoholics Anonymous, Narcotics Anonymous, a sponsor, and a recovery support group, can maintain sobriety as a life choice.

Failed Approaches to Alcohol/Drug Abuse

Historically, we have failed dramatically in our responses to the alcohol/drug problem in the United States. From the 1930s to the 1960s, public and private responses to alcohol/drug abuse caused tremendous damage, which we are still trying to overcome. These approaches were riddled with emotional and political biases, which denied the real dimensions of the problem. Scare tactics—a politically biased approach that alienated young people—began in 1937 and continued for the next 30 years in a variety of forms. For example, the following marijuana scare story appeared in the July 1937 issue of *American* magazine:

> An entire family was murdered by a youthful marijuana addict in Florida. When officers arrived at the home, they found the youth staggering about in a human slaughterhouse. He had ax murdered his father, mother, two brothers, and a sister. He seemed to be in a daze. He had no recollections of having committed the multiple murders. The officers knew him ordinarily as a sane, rather quiet young man; now he was pitifully crazed. They sought the reason. The boy said he had been in the habit of smoking something with youthful friends called "muggles," a childish name for marijuana.

The co-author of this article was Henry J. Anslinger, then commissioner of the Federal Bureau of Narcotics and Dangerous Drugs. After reviewing this single case and a study of the paranoid schizophrenic reactions of heavy hashish smokers in India, Anslinger expounded on the evils of marijuana. He described marijuana as a drug that would consistently result in violent, aggressive, paranoid behavior, as evidenced in the Florida case.

Another scare tactic example is the 1936 movie *Reefer Madness*. This movie's serious intent to discourage marijuana use backfired because the situations were so absurd that audiences viewed it as a humorous farce.

Those using scare tactics assumed that if young people were frightened by adverse reactions to drug use, they would be too frightened to use the drug. For the young people who perceived drug use as incongruent with their values, goals, and lifestyle, scare tactics were effective. For most young people, however, scare tactics proved to be an ineffective approach because much of the information was exaggerated, overgeneralized, or sensationalized. As a result, young people did not perceive the source of such information as credible. What young people heard did not bear any resemblance to what most users experienced. All in all, scare tactics alienated young people, heightened their curiosity, and increased rather than decreased their experimentation with drugs.

In the late 1960s and early 1970s, President Richard Nixon declared his famous war on drugs. Even though an all-out warlike effort was needed and money was readily available to fight drug addiction, no one knew how to tactically fight this war on drugs. Drug use had spread to epidemic proportions. Also, President Nixon was not the ideal general for this war, having already alienated young people during another war, in Vietnam.

During this same time period, the government was also duped by treatment programs that mismanaged funds for treatment. There were few experts and little, if any, clear direction to the battle. The failure of Nixon's war on drugs left a bitter taste in the mouths of government funding sources. Money for treatment programs was cut each year thereafter, and the focus shifted to prevention. Realizing that the war was being lost, the government developed a new, more positive approach: If we can reach the kids before they become dependent on drugs, we will prevent a future generation of drug casualties.

These early prevention efforts emphasized drug-specific information. The assumption was that if young people were to receive credible drug-specific information, they would then wisely decide not to use drugs. Unfortunately, the reverse held true. Drug-specific approaches heightened curiosity and alleviated the fears associated with drug use, resulting in increases of drug use by young people.

Throughout the ensuing years, U.S. administrations continued to fail to develop a comprehensive and cohesive drug policy. Most of the administrations put a major emphasis on the supply side of the drug problem and significantly neglected the demand side. Emotional and political biases of these administrations caused them to be blind to the many causes of drug dependence and resulted in an adherence to "a simple, magical solution" that was politically advantageous. Administration after administration adhered to a strong supply-side approach, without addressing the reasons for the demand that perpetuated the problem. The Clinton administration repeated this cycle, and the George W. Bush administration has been distracted by international issues. All these administrations have focused on the politically expedient supply-side approach of trying to stop drug trafficking, with little effort toward the demand side of the problem.

Major Problems in Perception
Minimizing Alcohol Abuse and Alcoholism

Alcohol abuse and alcoholism are major problems that are often minimized or overlooked as not being a part of the "war on drugs." Administrations have been distracted, focusing on drugs, often forgetting to include alcohol as a drug.

> Excessive alcohol consumption is the third leading preventable cause of death in the United States and is associated with multiple adverse health consequences, including liver cirrhosis, various cancers, unintentional injuries, and violence. (Centers for Disease Control 2004)

Alcohol is the most devastating drug we know of today in terms of the sheer numbers of people it affects. Estimates indicate that there are more than 12 million alcoholics in the United States and that a significant number of other people meet the criteria for alcohol abuse and alcohol dependence. (See Chapter 4 for diagnostic criteria for substance abuse and substance dependence.)

Alcohol is integrated into the fabric of the mainstream American lifestyle, causing many people to minimize its impact and cost to our society. It has been estimated that business and industry lose more than $136 billion each year for alcohol-related reasons: time lost at work because of absenteeism, illness, and/or personal problems, and reduced productivity, and health care costs.

However, the production, distribution, and sale of alcohol are also very big business in the United States. This side of the economics of America's developed taste for alcohol often deters our legislators from supporting new and creative ways to address the problems related to alcohol abuse and addiction. The tendency has been to emphasize the "war on drugs" and to exclude alcohol as a target of that war. Many established institutions in the United States agree that we must do something about the "drug" problem, yet they deny, ignore, or neglect addressing the larger problems related to the abuse of alcohol. The following section identifies major problems related to alcohol abuse and addiction.

Alcohol-Related Problems
Binge Drinking on College Campuses

> Binge drinking is at once the most important public health problem on our
> campuses and a critical challenge to institutional mission. (Keeling 2002)

Binge drinking is a significant problem on college campuses. Research indicates that 40 to 45 percent of college students binge drink; the significant negative consequences include academic problems, property damage, sexual assault, personal injury, and death. At least half of the sexual assaults on college campuses involve alcohol consumption by the perpetrator, the victim, or both.

In the 1990s, binge drinking by college students gained national publicity because of significant problems it was causing on campuses. Unfortunately, this trend still continues into the new millennium: Binge-drinking college students continue to cause property damage, personal injury, and deaths.

Alcohol use on college campuses was first reported to be a problem on college campuses a half century ago (Straus and Bacon 1953). Today, studies clarify the extent of the problems of binge alcohol use on college campuses. The Harvard School of Public Health's College Alcohol Study (CAS) (O'Malley and Johnston 2001) found that 40 to 45 percent of college students binge drink. They also found an alarming increase in the prevalence of frequent binge drinking among women— from 5.3 percent in 1993 to 11.9 percent in 2001 for women enrolled in all-women colleges, with a smaller increase in coed colleges. More underage students on college campuses reported having been drunk on three or more occasions in the past 30 days.

In his article "The Time to Purge Binge Drinking Is Now" (2004/2005), Dwayne Proctor, Ph.D., personalizes the epidemic of binge alcohol use by highlighting 3 of the estimated 1,400 college students who will die of alcohol-related incidents during the 2004–2005 school year:

> At Colorado State University, 19-year-old Samantha Spady died after downing
> between 30 and 40 drinks. At nearby University of Colorado, 18-year-old
> freshman Lynn Gordon Bailey died in what was reported to be a hazing incident
> involving alcohol. And at the University of Oklahoma, 19-year-old Blake
> Hammontree was found dead with a blood alcohol level more than five times
> the state's legal driving limit.

The first 6 weeks of the school year are certainly "party time" as the freshman class is inaugurated into the ritual of fraternity and sorority life, which often involve binge alcohol abuse. Many parents send their children off to college proud of this important rite of passage but fearful of how their 18-year-old daughters and sons will cope with the freedom, the peer influence, the availability of alcohol and drugs, the party atmosphere, and sexuality, let alone the classes and schoolwork.

> The first 6 weeks of the school year have been cited as the most dangerous with
> respect to drinking behavior due to the increased stress levels associated with a
> new environment and the pressure to be accepted by a peer group. (Bonnie and
> O'Connell 2004)

The rates of self-reported "heavy" drinking over the last decade have remained at approximately 44 percent (Wechsler et al. 2002). Frequent heavy drinking, which is defined as three or more times in the past 2 weeks, has increased according to Harvard School of Public Health Surveys (Wechsler et al. 2002).

Of the emergency room visits by college students at a large university medical center, 13 percent were alcohol related. Injuries accounted for 53 percent of emergency room visits, and acute intoxication accounted for 34 percent (Turner and Shu 2004). Accidental injury is the leading cause of death among older adolescents and young adults, and binge drinking is involved in many of these accidents.

Schools with patterns of heavy or binge drinking have more incidents of verbal, physical, and sexual assaults and property damage.

There is general agreement that programs aimed at preventing binge drinking need to address both the students and the kind of institutions they are attending. The prevention program should address the college environment, student campus culture, and individual factors to reduce high-risk alcohol use (Presley, Meilman, and Leichliter 2002). The key elements for successful prevention programs on campus involve "changing the campus social environment by encouraging student participation and involvement, using educational and informational processes, and engaging in campus regulatory and physical change efforts" (Ziemelis, Bucknam, and Elfessi 2002).

Other Alcohol-Related Problems on College Campuses

Some other problems related to alcohol use and abuse on campus include

- academic difficulties
- problems in attending class and completing assignments
- property damage
- accidents and injuries
- anger, fights, violence, road rage
- interpersonal and social problems
- psychological issues and problems (e.g., depression)
- high-risk sexual behaviors
- other high-risk behaviors (e.g., drinking and driving) (see Table 1.1)

Sexual Assault and Rape on College Campuses

The prevalence of sexual assault before and since entering college was more than one in four women (28.5 percent of the 5,446 women in The Campus Sexual Assault Study [January 2005–December 2007]). The frequencies with which women reported getting drunk since entering college increase the odds of being incapacitated sexual assault victims, and are positively associated with being a victim of both physically forced and incapacitated assault. However, voluntary use of other illicit drugs (other than marijuana) was not associated with experiencing incapacitated sexual assault since entering college.

Another factor, the frequency with which women attended fraternity parties since entering college, was positively associated with being a victim of incapacitated

TABLE 1.1

Potential Negative Consequences of College Student Drinking

Damage to Self

Academic impairment
Blackouts
Personal injuries and death
Short- and longer-term physical illnesses
Unintended and unprotected sexual activity
Suicide
Sexual coercion/rape victimization
Impaired driving
Legal repercussions
Impaired athletic performance

Damage to Other People

Property damage and vandalism
Fights and interpersonal violence
Sexual violence
Hate-related incidents
Noise disturbances

Institutional costs

Property Damage
Student attrition
Loss of perceived academic rigor
Poor "town-gown" relations
Added time demands and emotional strain on staff
Legal costs

SOURCE: Perkins 2002.

sexual assault (The Campus Sexual Assault Study, 2008). At least half of the sexual assaults on college campuses involve alcohol consumption by the perpetrator, the victim, or both (Abbey 2002).

Sexual assault is defined as any act that includes forced touching or kissing, verbally coerced intercourse, or physically forced vaginal, oral, or anal penetration. Rape is any behavior that involves some type of vaginal, oral, or anal penetration due to force or threat of force, a lack of consent, or an inability to give consent due to age, intoxication, or mental status (Abbey 2002).

A Harvard School of Public Health Alcohol Survey of randomly selected women in 119 colleges found that approximately one in twenty (4.7 percent) women reported being raped. Even more astounding is that almost three-quarters of these women (72 percent) were intoxicated at the time of the rape.

Women who were under 21, were white, resided in sorority houses, used illicit drugs, drank heavily in high school and attended colleges with rates of heavy episodic drinking were at higher risk of rape while intoxicated. (Mohler-Kuo et al. 2004)

Male college students who are intoxicated at high levels exhibit impaired sexual function but have increased physical aggression. Female college student (victim) intoxication increases vulnerability to penetration but does not reduce odds of injury (Testa et al. 2004). This stresses how intoxication by male and/or female college students increases vulnerability to rape, physical aggression, and/or sexual assault.

Alcohol and Violence

Many problems associated with alcohol use involve violence (see Figure 1.1).

Intimate Partner Violence It is estimated that alcohol is involved in 25 to 50 percent of cases of intimate partner violence (IPV). The psychophysiological effects of alcohol use can lead directly or indirectly to IPV. Alcohol consumption can result in impaired judgment, cognitive impairment, loosened inhibitions, and numerous physical effects that can lead to violence. Alcohol abuse can also lead to exacerbation of already dysfunctional marital or partner relationships and have negative effects on family life, which increases the probability of violence.

Drinking by men seems to be a stronger predictor of IPV than does drinking by women. This suggests that prevention and treatment programs aimed at problem drinking among young men would reduce IPV (White and Chen 2002).

Many women entering substance-abuse treatment have a history of physical violence with a family member or significant other (Easton, Swan, and Sinha 2000).

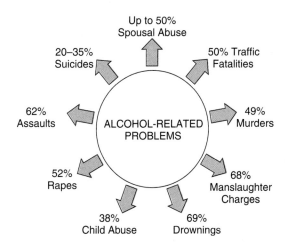

FIGURE 1.1 *Americans Have a Big Problem with Alcohol, the Number-One Drug of Abuse*
SOURCE: Office for Substance Abuse Prevention, modified. Data derived from the National Institute on Alcohol Abuse and Alcoholism. In Carroll, Charles R., *Drugs in Modern Society*, Brown & Benchmark, 1993.

Alcohol use by offenders and/or victims is found in approximately one-third to two-thirds of rape incidents (Abbey 2002).

Drug use also plays a major role in intimate partner violence.

Relative to the non-substance users, substance users scored significantly higher on all measures of perpetration and receipt of intimate partner violence after controlling for alcohol use.

Illicit substance users (ISU) had significantly greater perpetration and victimization of

- psychological abuse,
- physical assault,
- sexual coercion, and
- injury from violence

compared to the non-substance-abusing group (Moore and Stuart 2004).

Alcohol—Drinking and Driving—Young Drivers

Drinking alcohol and driving continues to be a major problem as evidenced by the many traffic fatalities while people are under the influence of alcohol. The relative risk of a fatal single-vehicle crash with blood alcohol (BAC) levels of 0.08 to 0.10 percent, varies from 11 percent (for drivers aged 35 and older) and 52 percent (for male drivers aged 16–20). The highest driver fatality rates where alcohol is involved are found among the youngest drivers. Among male drivers younger than 21, a BAC increase of just 0.02 percent more than doubles the relative risk for a single-vehicle fatal crash (National Institute for Alcohol Abuse and Alcoholism 2001).

Factors contributing to young drivers' greater crash risk include the following:

- A lack of driving experience
- Overconfidence
- The presence of other teenagers in the car (encouraging risky driving)

As a result, many states are instituting stricter guidelines for younger drivers–such as not allowing other young people in the car for the first year of driving, issuing provisional licenses that are suspended with any traffic violation, and increasing the age at which young people can get a driver's license.

In 2002 and 2003, 21 percent of persons aged 16 to 20 reported that they had driven in the past year while under the influence of alcohol or illicit drugs (National Survey on Drug Use and Health 2004).

The tragedy of young people driving under the influence (DUI) is dramatically etched in the fact that 29 percent of drivers aged 15 to 20 who were killed in motor vehicle crashes in 2002 had been drinking alcohol (National Highway Traffic Safety Administration 2003). In 2002 and 2003, more than 4 million drivers aged 16–20, or 21 percent of that age group, had reported driving under the influence in the last year (National Survey on Drug Use and Health 2004).

In addition, the severity of accidents while driving under the influence increases with alcohol involvement. In 2002, only 2 percent of the 15- to 20-year-old drivers involved in property-damage-only crashes had been drinking, 4 percent of those involved in crashes resulting in injury had been drinking, and 23 percent of those involved in fatal crashes had been drinking (National Center for Statistics & Analysis 2002).

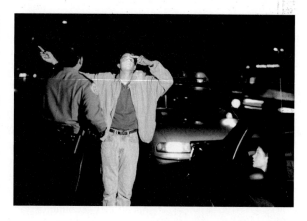

Alcohol-Related Intentional and Unintentional Deaths Other Than Traffic Fatalities—Under the Age of 21   There is a tendency to focus on traffic fatalities that are alcohol related, but many deaths are not related to drinking and driving. In 2002, there were 15,733 unintentional alcohol-related deaths of youths under the age of 21. The majority of those deaths, 8,707 (55 percent), were traffic deaths, but a significant number, 6,936 (45 percent), were from other causes (e.g., drowning, burns, falls) (National Center for Statistics & Analysis 2002).

Night DUI stop: Police officer testing driver.

Intentional injury deaths that are alcohol related include homicides and suicides. For young people under the age of 21, 36 percent of homicide deaths, 12 percent of male suicide deaths, and 8 percent of female suicide deaths were alcohol related (Levy, Miller, and Lox 1999). It is estimated that, in 2000, persons under the age of 21 committed more than 1,500 homicides and 300 suicides that were alcohol related (Bonnie and O'Connell 2003).

This is remarkable considering the difficulty in determining if a traffic fatality is actually a suicide attempt and not just a traffic accident. It also points to the importance of early intervention and education in preventing homicide and suicide in young people and of creating awareness of the very strong influence alcohol plays in intentional and unintentional deaths for young people under the age of 21.

Drugged Driving

A frequently overlooked reality is that many young and older people drive under the influence of illicit drugs mainly marijuana and cannabis products. In 2002, almost 11 million people aged 12 or older drove under the influence of illegal drugs, and drugged driving peaked at 18 percent among 21-year-olds (National Survey on Drug Use and Health, 2003). Drugged driving is often viewed not as a risky behavior but just the opposite. Many who drive under the influence of marijuana see drug use as enhancing their driving skills. A motor vehicle is thought by many to be a safe place to use drugs, and some see the likelihood of being apprehended for drugged driving by police as minimal (Davey et al. 2005).

Tobacco: The Most Deadly Drug

Tobacco is responsible for more than 400,000 deaths annually, mostly related to lung cancer and cardiovascular disease. Cigarettes kill more Americans than AIDS, accidents, fires, illegal drugs, and suicide combined. Smoking tobacco is the single most preventable cause of death.

Almost 35% of young people aged 12 to 17 reported smoking at least once during their lifetime. (National Institute on Drug Abuse 2002)

A study of children's beliefs about smoking (Gillmore et al. 2002) found that fourth graders held very negative beliefs about smoking and were strongly anti-smoking. Yet many children change their beliefs as they become adolescents. Young children have strong all-or-nothing, black-and-white, concrete beliefs about things. It appears that this is true of fourth graders. However, adolescents tend to the gray on issues, and their beliefs are less concrete and rigid. Although adolescents see smoking as being somewhat risky, they admire some aspects of smoking. Two primary aspects of cigarette smoking that adolescents viewed as favorable were solidarity with friends and providing relief from boredom (Loughlin et al. 2001).

Alcoholics account for 25 percent of the population of smokers, and many of those in recovery from alcoholism will die of smoking-related illnesses. This creates a challenge for most chemical dependency treatment programs: If they save their clients from alcoholism but don't get them to stop smoking, their clients can still die prematurely.

The risks of smoking are numerous. Prevention approaches with young people, education and treatment for those already addicted to smoking and nicotine, increasing the tax on cigarettes, and fighting the alcohol lobby when it misrepresents the harmful effects of cigarette smoking are just a few of the approaches to reduce adolescent cigarette smoking.

It seems ironic that recovering alcoholics and addicts will stay sober and maintain sobriety from alcohol/drugs but often fail to address the more frightening addiction to cigarettes. They will have escaped the ravages of alcoholism and drug addiction but not have avoided the many health consequences of smoking, suffering respiratory problems, potential lung disease, and death.

✴ Systemic Problems

Emphasis on the Supply Side and Neglect of the Demand Side of the Drug Problem in the United States

Approximately 70 percent or more of the federal money available to fight the drug problem is being spent on programs and agencies that focus on reducing the supply of drugs in the United States. Despite these efforts, there appears to be no real reduction in the availability of drugs. The lucrative profits are such a strong incentive at every level of the illegal drug trade that government efforts to decrease drug trafficking have not been successful.

As a result of this strong emphasis on the supply side, funding has been neglected for demand-side programs of drug prevention, intervention, and treatment. The problem has escalated to such levels that respected government officials and other prominent individuals are considering the legalization of illicit drugs. In 1988, Mayor Kurt Schmoke of Baltimore, Maryland, asked for a "national debate on the question of decriminalizing marijuana." Schmoke's suggestion was not well received by supply-siders in the war on drugs, because it dramatically highlighted the ineffectiveness of the supply-side approach. Even considering legalizing drugs clearly points to the frustration of a segment of the American society with the lack of progress being made by the supply-side approach.

Most publicly funded agencies are seeing their funding base diminishing, caseloads increasing, and severity of their patients' needs increasing. The March 1990 survey by the National Association of State Alcohol and Drug Abuse Directors indicated that publicly financed programs had long waiting lists for both inpatient and outpatient treatment services. The average waiting time for publicly funded outpatient alcohol/drug treatment was 22 days. The average waiting time for publicly funded inpatient alcohol/drug treatment was 45 days. Nationally, more than 65,000 people are waiting to enter public alcohol/drug treatment programs. Once the alcoholic/addict is ready for treatment and breaks through denial, there is such a long waiting list that relapse is inevitable. This costs taxpayers additional money in increased crime and public health care costs.

The same survey reported that, in 1988, states outspent the federal government in supporting chemical dependency treatment programs. Only 23 percent of the $2.1 billion spent on state-supported treatment programs comes from the federal government. In the 1991 federal budget, the $700 million in treatment grants represented only an 11 percent increase, despite backlogs in treatment services and dramatic funding needs to expand alcohol/drug treatment services.

There is a gap between the demand for substance-abuse treatment and its availability. The 1996 National Household Survey on Drug Abuse estimated that 5.3 million people, age 12 and over, needed drug treatment but only 37 percent of that number received it in the same year (NIDA 2002).

In 1997, the U.S. Bureau of the Census reported that 16 percent (43,448,000) of U.S. residents did not have health insurance, making it very difficult for large numbers of people who need alcohol/drug treatment to receive it because they lack the resources to pay for it.

Money alone cannot necessarily solve the problem. However, it can alleviate delays in providing treatment for those desperately seeking and needing treatment.

Funding for innovative programs addressing the needs of the inner-city crack addict and programs for the prevention of addiction in pregnant women are high priorities. Funding is also needed for alcohol/drug prevention programs for high-risk youth in their communities, with a special early focus on kindergarten to sixth grade. To make a major impact, longitudinal prevention projects with funding for several years are needed. Innovative yet realistic methods of funding are also necessary to attract the support of big business.

Racist Approach to the Drug Problem

Historically, there has been prejudice and oppression of people of color, a scapegoating of minorities, and a neglect of substance-abuse problems in the inner city. Legislation on drug policy was often based more on racial scapegoating prejudices than on a concern for the harmful impact of drugs on people. "People's attitudes toward a specific drug became inseparable from their feelings about that group of people with which the drug's use was associated" (White 1976). For instance, in 1875, the goal of suppressing opium smoking and opium dens had little to do with the control of opium but more to do with the fear of interracial contact and a fear of interracial mixing of the Chinese with American women and the white working class. The Chinese question dominated California politics in the 1870s. The tremendous racial and class conflicts resulted in many race riots, the lynching and killing of Chinese, and the burning of their dwellings in numerous West Coast cities. The California Working Man's Party was organized under the cry "The Chinese must go!"

The association between opium and the Chinese into the 1900s was part of the national legislation to prohibit opium smoking and opium dens, even though, at the time, opium was a primary ingredient in most over-the-counter medications and elixirs for physical ailments (White 1976).

The noted scholar Edward M. Brecher, in his classic book *Licit and Illicit Drugs* (1992), articulately describes various examples of government policies that were driven more by personal agendas and biases, and political reasons, than by the true dimensions of the problem.

Brecher accurately describes the United States of America during the nineteenth century as "a dope-fiend's paradise." That might be a rather strong description, but it is quite realistic. Opium was inexpensive, legal, and conveniently sold in not only the local drugstore but even the local grocery store. Physicians were quick to dispense opiate to their patients. Patent medicines, elixirs, and tonics that contained opium or morphine were marketed and sold as the rage for many ailments and conditions.

Opium Elixirs

- Ayer's Cherry Pectoral
- Mrs. Winslow's Soothing Syrup
- Darby's Carminiative
- Godfrey's Cordial
- McMunn's Elixir of Opium
- Dover's Powder

Brecher points out how drug ordinances were more about rascist fears than the drugs themselves. The most notable early examples were the ordinances adopted by the City of San Francisco in 1875 that prohibited the smoking of opium in smoking houses, or "dens." This was in contrast with the widespread use of opiates in other forms and venues described above.

"The roots of this ordinance were racist rather than health-oriented. . . ."

The San Francisco authorities, Brecher says, learned upon investigation that "many women and young girls, as well as young men of respectable family, were being induced to visit the (Chinese opium-smoking) dens, where they were ruined morally and otherwise." The Chinese were also a cheap, industrious, and large source of labor and were taking jobs away from the less competitive white population. The Chinese were hated by the white workers and labeled the "yellow peril."

The same held true for the association between cocaine and African Americans during the late 1800s and early 1900s. Hamilton Wright, a State Department official considered by many as the father of American narcotics laws, went before Congress in 1910 and gave the following warning about cocaine.

> It has been authoritatively stated that cocaine is often the direct incentive to the crime of rape by the Negroes of the South and other sections of the country.
>
> Once the Negro has reached the stage of being a "dope taker" [dope here referring to cocaine] . . . he is a constant menace to his community until he is eliminated. . . . Sexual desires are increased and perverted, peaceful Negroes become quarrelsome, and timid Negroes develop a degree of "Dutch courage." . . . Many of these officers in the South have increased the caliber of their guns for the express purpose of stopping the cocaine fiend when he runs amuck. (Williams 1914/1976)

These racial associations with drugs were documented in a *New York Times* article that reflected anti-Semitic feelings of the time: "There is little doubt that every Jew Peddler in the South carries the stuff [cocaine]."

This historical association of drugs with minority groups includes the following:

- Opium with the Chinese
- Cocaine with African Americans
- Alcohol with urban Catholic immigrants
- Heroin with urban immigrants, African Americans
- Marijuana and PCP with Latinos

The underlying assumption was that minorities were not able to control or tolerate the use of alcohol and drugs because they were inherently lazy and physically, emotionally, and morally/ethically weak. Of course, it was thought, most self-respecting white men could control their alcohol/drug use. This prejudice and association of drugs with minority subgroups caused politicians and others to stir up negative emotions to gain support for antidrug legislation.

Unfortunately, as long as drugs were confined to minority populations, funding and treatment resources were limited. It wasn't until the 1960s, when white middle- and upper-class young adults and college students were using marijuana, hallucinogens, and other drugs, that the modern drug war began.

Until we resolve the more dramatic issues of socioeconomic inequities, racial prejudice and the oppression of minorities, inequities in pay and occupational opportunities, and other related issues, the inner city will continue to be a breeding ground for the abuse of alcohol/drugs.

Socioeconomic Inequities That Undermine the American Dream

The inequities in socioeconomic opportunities have created bitterness, racial conflict, and a general rebelliousness and hopelessness, which fuel the desire to use alcohol/ drugs. The American Dream is a nightmare for those who are unable to develop feelings of competency and pride in their lives.

The reality is that hard work and dedication can be rewarded with the attainment of each person's American Dream. Many successful people have refused to be limited by the prejudice of others to the color of their skin, their sex, their religious or ethnic background, or their lack of membership in the inner circles of our society. Many individuals positively strive to reach their full potential by overcoming the prejudices of others and work to correct these inequities when they have an opportunity to change them. Other individuals become so embittered by socioeconomic injustices that they give up, become alienated from society, and lack a personal commitment to strive in life. They use alcohol/drugs to numb and shut down these feelings of embitterment, anger, and pain. Instead of working through these issues and resolving the conflict, they give in to a bitter hopelessness that makes their lives feel meaningless.

Lizbeth Schorr, in her book *Within Our Reach: Breaking the Cycle of Disadvantage* (1988), identifies poverty as the greatest risk factor for chemical dependency and other destructive behaviors. Violent crime, school-age childbearing, and school failure are outcomes that need "early interventions to prevent rotten outcomes," and "high-risk families need high-intensity services." Changes in economic policy, health care reform, and welfare reform can help in "breaking the cycle of disadvantage."

American society needs to acknowledge and address these issues of disparity in opportunity. Other factors contributing to the alcohol/drug problem are the breakdown of the neighborhood, changes in the traditional nuclear and extended family system, limited support systems, stress, and trauma.

Academic Failure and the Failure of the U.S. Educational System to Motivate and Educate Young People to Strive for Productive Lives

In 1959, the launching of the first manned spacecraft by the U.S.S.R. (now Russia) caught the United States by surprise. As a result, the United States took up the challenge for space by rededicating energy and resources to the study of science and math as well as the general education of our young people. Perhaps the current failure of the U.S. educational system and the high incidence of alcohol/drug use by young people will be the impetus to implement reform and innovation in school systems, much like that of the 1960s.

The U.S. educational system has become so neglected that the rates of academic failure and dropout are continually rising. The academic standards for students who do graduate are inferior. The ripple effect of this lowering of academic standards is also seen in colleges and education in general. Illiteracy has increased, and the quest for knowledge and general personal and intellectual improvement is not emphasized or valued by the average American citizen. This complacency in education affects standards in American business and industry. The worker who has no motivation for personal improvement also is not motivated to do high-quality, productive work on the job. The quality and pride in American workmanship are also decreased, resulting in inferior goods and services and a general public attitude that accepts these standards. The industries that employ individuals with good educational backgrounds and positive self-motivating attitudes tend to experience fewer of these problems.

The current failure of the U.S. educational system results from a variety of problems. The biggest problems are poor administration, teacher burnout, lack of adequate funding, and a bureaucratic system that promotes complacency.

The factor that contributes the most to teacher burnout is lack of support from the principal and school board. Innovation is threatening to some school administrations, and the fear of parents' complaints and litigation often results in a political administration that is more concerned with how parents and the school board may respond than the effective development and education of the child.

Another factor is the lack of incentives—other than the genuine desire to work with young people—for teachers to invest themselves in their profession. The teacher who repeats the same lesson plan over and over without making any investment in the job receives the same salary as the teacher who is attentive, is involved, and spends time and energy in educating students.

The combination of inadequate pay, lack of support from the administration, and no financial incentives or other motivations has resulted in dedicated and talented teachers leaving the educational system. This puts students in the hands of teachers who lack the talent or motivation to help them overcome academic failure and a poor sense of self.

Reforms such as site-based management, parent involvement, shared decision making, accountability, and alternative schools have been successful in turning school systems around. We need to apply these principles in educational reform to provide children with the opportunity for academic and personal success. The development of our children as a natural resource is essential in developing a future generation strong enough not to become dependent on or addicted to alcohol/drugs.

Denial of Substance Abuse, Addiction, and Alcoholism—A Problem in the Family

Denial is jokingly referred to as a river in Egypt (de-Nile), or denial can stand for I **D**on't **E**ven k**N**ow **I** **A**m **L**ying. Despite these jokes, denial is a problem that leads to the worsening of consequences over time, not only for the substance abuser and addict/alcoholic but also for family members and friends. The longer a family denies and enables the alcohol/drug problems, the more vulnerable the family members become to experiencing the destructive consequences of substance abuse and addiction.

Parental substance abuse, addiction, and alcoholism make the children in that family four to eight times more likely to develop problems with alcohol/drugs. Children who grow up in alcoholic, drug-dependent families exhibit far more problems than children from normal families. Emotional and physical abuse, sexual violation, and other traumas are at a greater risk of occurring when parents abuse alcohol and drugs.

Families and family members, including the addict/alcoholic, often resist admitting that they have a problem. They often feel so ashamed that they maintain their addiction and continue the negative consequences in a cascading, vicious cycle. Asking for help is often difficult for adult family members, for children of the addict/alcoholic, and for the addict/alcoholic.

Early assessment of alcohol/drug problems, related dysfunctional behaviors, and negative consequences of drinking/drugging may prevent a problem from getting out of control. Destigmatizing the dimensions of addiction that emphasize the "disease" and decrease shame while restoring dignity can help facilitate people admitting they have a problem, breaking through denial and helping them to "ask for help."

Public media can address the importance of asking for help and also bring to awareness the impact on the entire family.

Adolescent Co-occurring Disorders— Complicates Treatment

Co-occurring disorders in adolescents complicates the treatment for substance abuse. Many more issues need to be addressed in coordination with the treatment for substance use disorder (SUD). Estimates of rates of co-occurring conduct disorder with substance use disorder are 50–80 percent.

The disorders that co-occur with substance abuse can be classified as

- internalizing problems—depression, anxiety, or trauma disorders, suicidal thoughts
- externalizing problems—conduct disorders, ADHD, victimization, physical violence toward others, illegal activity (see Figure 1.2)

✴ The Major Perspectives on Alcohol/Drug Use

In *Drugs Demystified,* Helen Nowlis (1975) described four major perspectives on drug use: moral-legal, medical-health, psychosocial, and social-cultural. The fifth perspective is spirituality, and the sixth perspective is your perspective.

The Moral-Legal Perspective

The moral-legal perspective is primarily the viewpoint of law enforcement and the criminal justice system. The major focus of this perspective is to keep specific drugs away from people and people away from specific drugs. This approach reduces the availability of drugs and uses punishment as a deterrent in addressing the supply side of drugs, not the demand side.

The agencies in this perspective have not been able to significantly diminish the availability of drugs. Although they are doing their best with limited resources, these agencies are unable to substantially affect the price of drugs by reducing their availability. The criminal justice system is a deterrent for some people, but few people stop using or dealing drugs because they fear criminal-justice interventions. The antisocial personality of the people caught by the system makes rehabilitation difficult. The weak rehabilitative components of the criminal-justice system have resulted in minimal changes in the attitudes of those convicted or caught by the system.

The moral-legal perspective is the one emphasized by most politicians, yet this perspective alone cannot be effective. Unless we address the demand side, the moral-legal perspective is ineffective. With so many buyers in the marketplace, sellers are motivated to deal, despite the risks.

The moral-legal perspective also encodes specific value judgments about drugs and alcohol. These are often expressed in the licit-versus-illicit debate, personal biases about punishment for illegal use, and moral/ethical views regarding the use of alcohol and other drugs.

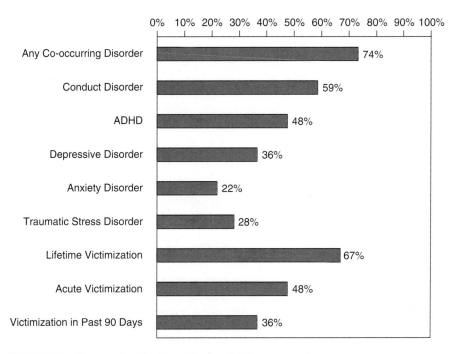

FIGURE 1.2   *Co-occurring Disorders at Intake: CSAT*
The chart represents the rates of co-occurring disorders drawn from GAIN assessments (N = 4,421) administered in CSAT-funded adolescent programs from 1998 to 2004. The chart clearly illustrates the high prevalence of co-occurring disorders for adolescents. The development tasks of adolescence include issues of identify, self-concept, social skills, academic skills, and many other issues. No wonder it is difficult for young people to work through these developmental issues when they have both psychiatric and substance problems to address.

The Medical-Health Perspective

The medical-health perspective is held by physicians, nurses, and the medical and health treatment fields. In this perspective, alcohol and drug use is a public health problem. Treatment focuses on the physical damage related to alcohol/drug use, abuse, and dependence.

The medical-health perspective assumes that people seek good health. The perspective is also based on the assumption that health information influences attitudes and behaviors. However, information alone does not change attitudes about the use of alcohol/drugs.

The Psychosocial Perspective

The psychosocial perspective is a common viewpoint shared by a variety of agencies that specialize in addressing the demand side of alcohol/drugs. The services these agencies provide include these:

- Recovery from substance dependence
- Intervention and treatment services

- Early intervention approaches with adolescents
- Prevention services for young children, adolescents, adults, and seniors

The goals of this perspective are to prevent, intervene in, and treat alcohol/drug problems. Inadequate funding for chemical dependency treatment programs and alcohol/drug prevention programs has made it difficult for many alcohol/drug users to obtain treatment services and for agencies to maintain prevention programs long enough to see conclusive results. (See Chapter 8.)

The Social-Cultural Perspective

The social-cultural perspective is held by most social agencies and institutions. The basic goal of this perspective is to adapt the environment to meet the individual's needs. The underlying assumption of this perspective is that alcohol/drug use is due to the frustration and hopelessness of people's lives. If users had any hope that they could attain the American Dream, they would be motivated to achieve and establish a constructive place in society.

Unfortunately, most social agencies are impersonal, bureaucratic, and rigid in dealing with their clients' needs. Such agencies are poorly funded and therefore poorly staffed; their employees are overworked, underappreciated, and underpaid. As a result, the agencies are reluctant to change, change too slowly, or may even lack a mechanism to change.

Edward Brecher (1992) believes we should "stop viewing the drug problem as primarily a national problem to be solved on a national scale. In fact, . . . the drug problem is a collection of local problems." By supporting neighborhood and community efforts, we could provide an environment that could prevent the development of alcohol/drug problems.

The Fifth Perspective—Spirituality
Spirituality and Recovery from Alcoholism/Drug Addiction

An important dimension of alcohol/drug recovery is "spirituality." Spirituality has so many different meanings and is defined differently by many individuals. In Alcoholics Anonymous spirituality is defined as "god," "a higher power," or belief in something greater than yourself.

George Valliant (1983) describes the symptoms of alcoholism as an emptiness and spiritual void that requires spiritual healing. A theme of spirituality is a growing sense of inner meaning, self-transcendence, and purpose.

> Persons with alcoholism often report a lack of purpose in life and a lack of spiritual well-being. In contrast, persons in recovery have reported a growing sense of purpose, which has been associated with increased length of sobriety, and spiritual well-being. (Piderman et al. 2007)

A study by Piderman and associate, exploring "Spirituality in Alcoholism during Treatment" (2007), found that:

- having conservative religious beliefs (i.e., being a member of a conservative religious group, attending religious services weekly,

and engaging in private prayer) was a protective factor against developing alcoholism
- evidence suggests that private prayer is positively associated with recovery
- on the other hand, factors associated with negative outcomes for those actively alcoholic are watching or listening to religious programming and others praying for them

The alcoholic/addict's source of spirituality can be found in a variety of ways. This could include both traditional religious practices and nontraditional practices. It is up to the individual to find and define their own sense of spirituality. The aggressive dogma of one way is counterproductive to helping the addict/alcoholic find their own definition and source of spirituality.

The Sixth Perspective—Your Perspective

What is your perspective on alcohol/drugs? Complete the following Sixth Perspective Worksheet to clarify your perspective on alcohol/drugs.

The Sixth Perspective—Worksheet
Moral-Legal Perspective

1. Should drugs be legalized? Explain.
2. Is the supply-side approach to the drug problem effective? Explain.
3. Is alcoholism/drug addiction a defense for irresponsible or criminal behavior? Explain.

Medical-Health Perspective

1. Is alcoholism/drug addiction a disease? Explain.
2. Describe the physician's role in making a patient aware of problems with alcohol/drugs.
3. Do people need more information about the health risks of alcohol/drug use? Does this information change attitudes? Explain.

Psychosocial Perspective

1. What role does parenting play in the development of alcohol/drug problems?
2. Is it important for the entire family system to be involved in alcohol/drug treatment? Explain.
3. How can alcohol/drug treatment be more effective?

Spiritual Perspective

1. What role does "religion" and "spirituality" play in recovery?
2. What roles do meaning and purpose play in recovery?
3. How do you define spirituality?

Personal Perspective

Circle *true* or *false* and explain the reasoning supporting your answer to each question.

1. Illicit drugs are not necessary, and drug use is harmful.
   True
   False
2. Illicit drugs can play a role in enhancing life experiences.
   True
   False
3. Alcohol is a drug with great potential for abuse.
   True
   False
4. My family history does not make me at risk for developing problems with alcohol/drugs.
   True
   False
5. If a family member or close friend had an alcohol/drug problem, I could suggest that the person either get help or participate in an intervention.
   True
   False
6. Persons with alcohol/drug problems have to break through their own denial.
   True
   False
7. Alcoholism and drug addiction are family diseases.
   True
   False
8. Parent modeling of alcohol/drug use is an important influence on a child's use of alcohol/drugs.
   True
   False
   Other personal views

A Perspective of Hope

Perhaps the problems that spawn alcohol/drug abuse and addiction seem too difficult to overcome. The negative impact of these problems frequently gives rise to feelings of hopelessness that we can never adequately resolve these issues. However, there has been positive and dramatic success: Millions of Americans are in recovery from alcoholism and drug addiction. Family members are changing their own codependent and enabling behavior in relationships. Adult children of alcoholics are overcoming the trauma of their childhoods. Most important, families are successfully developing more functional and healthy systems for the next generation of youngsters. Their children will be less vulnerable to the familial problems of alcohol/drug dependence and addiction.

There is something to be said for thinking small. Initially, this might sound like strange advice. We each must think about our own small contribution to solving problems that seem large and insurmountable. Each of us needs to first think about our own behavior and our own family and address growth and positive development in those areas. Then we can begin to address these issues in our neighborhoods, communities, workplaces, and other interpersonal interactions. My hope is that we can each, in our own small ways, address the issue of alcohol/drug dependence and other issues in our society by focusing on our own and our children's functional growth and development.

✄ In Review

- There are no "simple, magical solutions" (e.g., "Just Say No") to a complex problem like drug abuse and dependence.

    H. L. Mencken—"Any solution to a complex problem that is simple, is usually wrong."

- Scare tactics backfired in early prevention efforts. In 1937, Henry Anslinger saw marijuana as evil and feared that blacks would get violent and rape white women.

- Binge drinking is a significant problem on college campuses. Research indicates that 40 to 45 percent of college students binge drink; the significant negative consequences include academic problems, property damage, sexual assault, personal injury, and death. At least half of the sexual assaults on college campuses involve alcohol consumption by the perpetrator, the victim, or both.

- Alcohol is often involved in sexual assault and rape, both by the perpetrator and by the victim.

- Alcohol is estimated to be involved in 25 to 50 percent of intimate partner violence. Drinking by men seems to be a stronger predictor of such violence than does drinking by women.

- Alcohol is often involved in intentional and unintentional deaths. Intentional injury includes homicide and suicide.

    In young people aged 21 and older, alcohol was involved in

    36 percent of homicide deaths

    12 percent of male suicide

    8 percent of female suicide

- Drinking and driving is still a major problem but has decreased over the past decade, especially among young drivers.

- Tobacco is responsible for more than 400,000 deaths annually from lung cancer and cardiovascular disease. It is estimated that 40 million adults and 3 million adolescents are active smokers. Eight out of every ten alcoholics is a smoker.

- Denial of family problems (such as parental alcoholism and addiction), academic failure, and trauma, violence, and violation are some of the risk factors for problems with alcohol/drugs.

- The following systemic problems make it hard to address prevention of substance abuse:

    - An emphasis on the supply side and neglect of the demand side in the "war on drugs"

    - Academic failure, and schools' failure to address the learning and motivational needs of their students

- A long history of neglecting the treatment needs of people of color
- A breakdown in family, neighborhood, and community support
- Socioeconomic inequities
- The many perspectives on alcohol/drug use include the moral-legal perspective, which is primarily the viewpoint of law enforcement and the criminal justice system; the medical-health perspective of the medical and health fields; the psychosocial perspective of alcohol/drug and mental health treatment agencies; the social-cultural perspective, which is held by most social agencies and social institutions (e.g., regarding housing and employment); and the spiritual perspective.

⚹ Discussion Questions

1. Please rank and explain why you ranked the following problems as a result of binge drinking on campus, from most common to least common:
   Academic difficulties
   Problems in attending class and completing assignments
   Property damage
   Accidents and injuries
   Fights
   Interpersonal and social problems
   Problems with mood and/or psychological problems
   High-risk sexual behavior

2. Rank the problems in Question 1 in terms of seriousness.
3. What do you consider to be intimate partner violence? Who do you think is at fault most of the time? How would you define "date rape"?
4. What role do you think alcohol and drugs play in sexual violations? Explain.
5. What do you think the legal age should be to start driving?
6. What do you think the penalties should be for first-time driving under the influence (DUI)?
7. Would you consider someone who has two DUI convictions as being an alcoholic or having a drug problem? Explain.
8. Which of the five perspectives—moral-legal, medical-health, psychosocial, social-cultural, and spiritual—do you think is most effective? Why?

⚹ References

Abbey, Antonia. 2002. Alcohol-related sexual assault: A common problem among college students. *Journal of Studies on Alcohol* 14: 118–127.

Bonnie, Richard J., and Mary Ellen O'Connell, eds. 2004. *Reducing underage drinking: A collective responsibility.* Washington, D.C.: National Academy Press.

Brecher, Edward M. 1992. *Licit and illicit drugs.* Boston: Little, Brown.

Centers for Disease Control and Prevention [CDC]. 2004. Alcohol—Attributable deaths and years of potential life lost—United States, 2001. *Morbidity and Mortality Weekly Report* 53(37): 866–70.

Davey, J., et al. 2005. Drug driving from a user's perspective. *Drugs: Education, Prevention, and Policy* 12(1)(February): 61–70.

Easton, Caroline J., Suzanne Swan, and Rahita Sinha. 2000. Prevalence of family violence in clients entering substance abuse treatment. *Journal of Substance Abuse Treatment* 18: 23–28.

Gillmore, M. R., E. A., Wells, E. E., Simpson, D. M., Morrison, M. J., Hoppe, A. A. Wilsdon, and E. Murowchick. 2002 Children's beliefs about smoking. *Nicotine and Tobacco Research,* 4: 177–183.

Keeling, Richard. 2002. Binge drinking and the college environment. *Journal of American College Health* 50(5): 197–201.

Krebs, Christopher P., Christine H. Lindquist, Tara D. Warner, Bonnie S. Fisher, and Sandra L. Martin, 2008. *The Campus Sexual Assault (CSA) Study, Final Report, Performance Period January 2005—December 2007.* Washington, D.C.: National Institute of Justice.

Levy, D., T. Miller, and K. Cox, 1999. *Costs of Underage Drinking.* Calverton, Md.: prepared by Pacific Institute for Research and Evaluation for the Office of Juvenile Justice and Delinquency Prevention.

Mohler-Kuo, Meichun, et al. 2004. Correlates of rape while intoxicated in a national sample of college women. *Journal of Studies on Alcohol* 65(1): 37–40.

Moore, Todd M., and Gregory L. Stuart. 2004. Illicit substance use and intimate partner violence among men in batterers intervention. *Psychology of Addictive Behaviors* 18: 385–89.

National Center for Statistics & Analysis. 2002. Traffic safety facts, 2002—Young drivers.

National Highway Traffic Safety Administration [NHTSA]. 2003.

National Institute for Alcohol Abuse and Alcoholism [NIAAA]. 2001. *Alcohol Alert,* no. 52 (April).

National Institute on Drug Abuse [NIDA]. 2002. *NHSDA Report.* (May 31).

National Survey on Drug Use and Health. 2003. Drugged driving: 2002 Update. *NSDUH Report* (September).

National Survey on Drug Use and Health. 2004. Driving under the influence (DUI) among young persons. *NSDUH Report* (December 31).

Nowlis, Helen. 1975. *Drugs demystified.* Paris: UNESCO Press.

O'Malley, Patrick, and Lloyd Johnson. 2002. Epidemiology of alcohol and other drug use among American college students. *Journal of Studies on Alcohol* 14: 91–100.

Perkins, H. Wesley. 2002. Surveying the damage: A review of research on consequences of alcohol misuse in college populations. *Journal of Studies on Alcohol* Supplement (14): 91–100.

Piderman, Katherine M., et al. 2007. Spirituality in alcoholism during treatment. *The American Journal of Addictions* 16: 232–237.

Presley, Cheryl, Phillip Meilman, and Jami Leichliter. 2002. College factors that influence drinking. *Journal of Studies on Alcohol* 14: 82–89.

Proctor, Dwayne. 2004/2005. The time to purge binge drinking is now. *Washington FOCUS* 14(4)(Winter): 5.

Schorr, Lisbeth B., and Daniel Schorr. 1988. *Within our reach: Breaking the cycle of disadvantage.* New York: Anchor/Doubleday.

Straus, R., and S. D. Bacon. 1953. *Drinking in college.* New Haven, Conn.: Yale University Press.

Substance Abuse and Mental Health Services Administration [SAMHSA]. 2004. 4 Million have co-occurring serious mental illness, substance abuse. *SAMHSA News* 12(5)(Sept./Oct.): 16.

Testa, Maria, et al. 2004. The role of victim and perpetrator intoxication on sexual assault outcomes. *Journal of Studies on Alcohol* 65: 320–29.

Turner, James C., and Jianfeu Shu. 2004. Serious health consequences associated with alcohol use among college students: Demographic and clinical characteristics of patients seen in an emergency department. *Journal of Studies on Alcohol* 65(2).

U.S. Surgeon General. 1988. *The health consequences of smoking: Nicotine addiction.* Rockville, Md.: National Institute on Drug Abuse.

Vailiant, G.E. 1983. *The natural history of alcoholism: Causes, patterns and paths to recovery.* Cambridge, Mass.: Harvard University Press.

Washington FOCUS. 2004. Risk factors identified in inhalant abuse. *Washington FOCUS* 14(3)(Fall): 7.

Wechsler, H., et al. 2002. Trends in college binge drinking during a period of increased prevention efforts: Findings from four Harvard School of Public Health study surveys, 1993–2001. *Journal of American College Health* 30(5): 203–17.

White, H. R., and Ping-Hsiu Chen. 2002. Problem drinking and intimate partner violence. *Journal of Studies on Alcohol* 63(1–3): 205–14.

White, William. 1976. Chemical prohibition. In *Facts about drug abuse: Participant manual.* Rockville, Md.: National Institute on Drug Abuse.

Wiechelt, Shelly A. 2007. Trauma and substance misuse: Critical considerations in understanding the maelstrom. *Journal of Substance Use and Misuse* 42: 527–553.

Williams, Edward H. 1914/1976. [Editorial from *Medical Record Newspaper,* 1914.] In *Facts about drug abuse: Participant manual.* Rockville, Md.: National Institute on Drug Abuse.

Ziemelis, Andris, Ronald Bucknam, and Abdulaziz Elfessi. 2002. Prevention efforts underlying decreases in binge drinking at institutions of higher learning. *Journal of American College Health* 50(5): 238–52.

Why Do People Abuse Drugs?

A Better Understanding of Models and Theories of Drug Dependence and Addiction

Objectives

1. Explain the relationship between "the drive to alter consciousness" and alcohol/drug abuse.
2. Identify the three criteria in defining a "disease" and explain alcoholism as a disease.
3. Describe the key elements of the following models and theories of substance abuse disorders (SUD):
   - Disease model of alcoholism
   - Genetic model of alcoholism
   - Personality and substance abuse
   - Tension reduction models
   - Family models
   - Trauma and SUD
   - Depression, mood, and feelings
   - Boredom—an emerging need for research
   - Self-medication motive for drug use
   - Personality theories
   - Personality disorders
   - Psychosocial models—social learning theory (SLT)
   - Sociocultural models
   - Psychoanalytic models and meanings
   - Existential issues
   - Conditioning and substance abuse

❉ Introduction

This chapter explores the various models and theories of substance abuse. It is important for you to be able to identify the many and varied factors that contribute to substance abuse. The models provide a framework for the development of an integrated treatment approach. The theories help the clinician to better understand the specific treatment strategies that may be implemented. This chapter lays the foundation for later chapters that focus on assessment, prevention, intervention, and treatment of substance abuse.

I recommend that you complete the worksheet at the end of this chapter to help you explore your own model and theoretical orientation to substance abuse.

❧ Why Do People Abuse Alcohol/Drugs?

It's peer pressure. . . . No, it's poor self-concept. . . . It's just because it's fun and pleasurable. . . . It's the hopelessness of our society. . . . It's due to the dishonesty and hypocrisy of our institutions. . . . No, it's our inability to connect with each other and establish effective relationships. . . . It's the parents. . . . It's the media that promote instant pleasure, short-term goals, and alcohol use. . . . It's the ineffectiveness of the school system and other institutions. . . . It's the avoidance of pain and hedonism of modern society. . . . It's the lack of caring for our fellow humans. . . . It's stress, pressure, and the breakdown of the family. . . . It's socioeconomic inequities. . . . It's just available. . . . Why not?

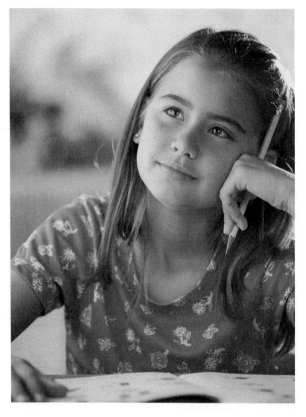

All people consciously or subconsciously alter their states of consciousness. Some common ways children achieve this are through daydreaming, rolling downhill, tumbling, and spinning.

Our Innate Drive to Alter Consciousness

It has been said that there are four primary drives: hunger, thirst, sex, and our desire to alter our consciousness. Drugs have been used throughout history to alter consciousness and will continue to be used in this way in the future.

Some people believe drugs open avenues to unconscious issues, conflicts, and possibly an awareness or perception new to the user's life. On the downside, drugs can easily become traps that keep us from using our minds in positive ways. Drug use becomes unrealistic and neurotic when it becomes an addiction. People who are addicted to drugs tend to be passively dependent and destructive. The nervous system becomes less functional, and the addicted person is less able to function in active, constructive, and interesting ways. Our society is becoming more aware of positive ways to alter consciousness while avoiding addictions to alcohol/drugs, food, gambling, television, work, and many other activities.

Drug Use as a Passive Activity

Many people are passive procrastinators and conflict avoiders. In my private counseling practice, I often see clients who deny the painful issues that initially brought them to counseling. Once they get some immediate relief, they avoid the real issues. Nonetheless, growth involves working through painful conflicts. Our search for the magic pill or cure for the pain of the human condition has created a modern marketplace for alcohol and drug elixirs.

Using alcohol or other drugs is a passive activity; individuals take pills, powders, or liquids and wait for the desired effect—an alteration of their consciousness. In some cases, such as freebasing cocaine or injecting drugs (e.g., heroin), the desired effect is almost instantaneous. Instead of facing and working through feelings of boredom, sadness, stress, and loneliness, the individual passively changes what he or she feels by using alcohol/drugs. Changing your mood by more active approaches involves more effort and motivation. This is frequently a learning process, especially if the individual has a lifelong pattern of either avoiding feelings or self-medicating feelings with alcohol/drugs. We explore such proactive approaches in Chapter 11.

⋇ Models of Alcohol/Drug Dependence and Addiction

We cannot isolate one specific cause of alcoholism and other drug addictions. There are often multiple, confounding reasons for addiction, just as there are numerous causes for cancer and other medical diseases. Many theories and models of causality exist. Early models of alcoholism labeled alcoholics as inherently weak or unable to control or tolerate their consumption of alcohol. One test of manliness was the ability to "really hold his liquor." Other early models focused on individual psychopathology, arguing that alcoholics used alcohol in a pathological manner to block out memories of unpleasant, traumatic personal experiences that brought with them unmanageable feelings. Over time, a physiological model of alcoholism developed as scientists searched for a biochemical link to, or a genetic marker of, alcoholism.

Today, those of us in the alcohol/drug field generally accept the fact that alcoholism and drug addiction have multiple causes, or etiologies. Clearly, a matrix of both genetic and environmental factors can cause an individual to develop problems with alcohol and drugs. "Evidence has accumulated to indicate that alcoholism is a heterogenous entity arising from multiple etiologies" (Tabakoff and Hoffman 1988).

The models described in this chapter present an overview of prevailing theories, research, and clinical observations in the field of alcohol and drug use and abuse. The models are intended to help individuals who are entering or already working in the field gain a better understanding of substance abuse.

I encourage you to study and explore all of these models. Don't discount any of them due to your current biases—try applying each model in your work in the field. In the classroom, discuss the application and validity of these models, taking into account each student's individual experiences.

Unfortunately, no one model explains all substance abuse or fits all users' reasons for using. In the spirit of the old adage "If you are a hammer, everything else is a nail," many people want to find a single variable, approach, or model that will predict all cases of substance abuse—when the reality is that there are many confounding variables. Clients/patients are all different, with different coping skills, family histories, physical traits, affective temperaments, personality traits, and developmental histories. Studying the models will make you aware that factors that play a major role in one individual's substance abuse might play no role at all in another person's drug problems—one size does not fit all.

We might someday have medical tests that accurately predict substance abuse—a simple blood test, or a test for patterns of neurotransmitter activity that correlate with risk, for instance. Or maybe one of the models you're going to study in this book will prove to be more correct than the others. For now, our best resource is to study the available models and understand how each can be used to prevent, intervene in, and treat substance abuse.

Disease Model of Alcoholism

In 1957, the American Medical Association declared alcoholism a disease on the basis of three criteria: (1) Alcoholism has a known etiology (cause), (2) the symptoms get worse over time, and (3) alcoholism has known outcomes. The outcomes of alcoholism are dependence, physical symptoms, and eventual death. For more than thirty years, research has indicated an increasingly strong case for a genetic component of alcoholism; this validates the disease model.

The disease model is the foundation of Alcoholics Anonymous and many other self-help programs. The increased acceptance of this disease model is due to continuing research linking alcoholism to genetic markers.

The 12-step approach (see Table 2.1) is based on the disease model. It has been described as an informal biopsychosocial spiritual model. The disease model assumes alcoholics/addicts were predisposed to addiction by genetically transmitted biological risk factors.

Another model is the genetic influence disease model. This model does not emphasize genes or specific disorders but instead assumes that multiple biological risk factors interact with psychosocial environmental factors. It also assumes that addiction is influenced by interpersonal relationships, including family, community, and culture.

> In effect, neither genetic nor environmental operating alone is sufficient to produce alcoholism or drug addiction; alcoholism and drug addiction require the joint presence of both biological and psychosocial environmental factors. (Tarter and Edwards 1985)

The 12-step program helps the addict/alcoholic overcome the terrible sense of isolation and aloneness that occurs as a result of the many negative consequences of use.

> . . . for many people, heavy drinking and drug use culminate in intense feelings of alienation, apartness, emptiness, meaninglessness, and lack of purpose in living. Moral values may have been compromised in the erratic acting out of intoxicated behaviors, urges, cognitions and motivations. (Rotgers et al. 2003)

The shame-based stigma of addiction, along with the guilt, negative feelings, and spiritual bancruptcy, makes the 12-step approach of Alcoholics Anonymous an effective recovery tool for addicts/alcoholics.

Genetic Model of Alcoholism

In January 1990, researchers at the University of California, Los Angeles, and the University of Texas, San Antonio, identified a link between the receptor gene for the neurotransmitter dopamine and alcoholism (Blum et al. 1990). Although these

TABLE 2.1

The Twelve Steps

1. We admitted we were powerless over alcohol—that our lives had become unmanageable.
2. Came to believe that a Power greater than ourselves could restore us to sanity.
3. Made a decision to turn our will and our lives over to the care of God as we understood Him.
4. Made a searching and fearless moral inventory of ourselves.
5. Admitted to God, to ourselves, and to another human being the exact nature of our wrongs.
6. Were entirely ready to have God remove all these defects of character.
7. Humbly asked Him to remove our shortcomings.
8. Made a list of all persons we had harmed and became willing to make amends to them.
9. Made direct amends to such people wherever possible, except when to do so would injure them or others.
10. Continued to take personal inventory and, when we were wrong, promptly admitted to it.
11. Sought through prayer and meditation to improve our conscious contact with God as we understand Him, praying only for knowledge of His will for us and the power to carry that out.
12. Having had a spiritual awakening as the result of these steps, we tried to carry this message to alcoholics and practice these principles in all our affairs.

SOURCE: The Twelve Steps are reprinted with permission of Alcoholics Anonymous World Services, Inc. Permission to reprint the Twelve Steps does not mean that AA agrees with the views expressed herein. AA is a program of recovery from alcoholism—use of the Twelve Steps in connection with programs and activities that are patterned after AA but that address other problems does not imply otherwise.

findings need to be replicated with a larger sample, they establish more clearly the significance of a genetic factor predisposing people to alcoholism. Ernest Noble of UCLA said that this research "more firmly establishes alcoholism as a disease, and adds to evidence that genetic factors are as important as environmental factors in predisposing people to the disease." The general opinion is that alcoholism is related to several genes, however, and that no one gene can be a genetic marker to identify individuals at risk for alcoholism.

Devor (1994) describes a developmental-genetic model of alcoholism. He proposes that "alcoholism must no longer be thought of as a single disease with a cause that is either genetic or environmental but as a group of illnesses in which the influences of genes and the environment ebb and flow over the course of the at-risk lifetime." The logical conclusion is that treatment for alcoholism would be individually designed and fine-tuned to consider both pharmacological and behavioral therapies.

Adoption Studies

Donald W. Goodwin (1971) conducted a series of adoption studies in Denmark, indicating that sons of alcoholics are four times more likely to become alcoholics than are sons of nonalcoholics. In the study, the results held true whether the sons were raised by nonalcoholic foster parents or their own biological parents, thus supporting the genetic component of alcoholism. Cloninger, Bohman, and Sigvardsson (1981) conducted detailed and extensive adoption studies that confirmed the earlier work of Goodwin in demonstrating the following:

1. Adopted sons of alcoholic biological parents are four times more likely to become alcoholics than adoptees whose biological parents are not alcoholics.
2. Sons of alcoholic biological parents are more likely to be classified as alcoholics at an earlier age than their peers.
3. Daughters of alcoholic fathers, although not demonstrating a greater incidence of alcoholism, exhibit a high incidence of somatic anxiety and frequent physical complaints.

Twin Studies

Studies of identical (monozygotic, or MZ) and fraternal (dizygotic, or DZ) twins have supported a genetic factor. Because identical twins are genetically identical but fraternal twins have no more genes in common than nontwin siblings, research should show a higher rate of alcoholism in MZ twins than in DZ twins. Kaij (1960) examined 174 sets of twins and demonstrated that, indeed, the MZ twins had a 71 percent concordance rate, and the DZ twins had only a 32 percent concordance rate. In 1981, Hrubec and Omenn again demonstrated a higher concordance rate in MZ twins (26 percent) than in DZ twins (12 percent). A 1984 study by Gurling and associates, however, did not support the previous studies' results.

Currently, no significant genetic research is exploring drug abuse due to the many research design problems with illicit drugs. The assumption is that the genetic factors for drug addiction are comparable with the genetic research findings on alcoholism.

⋊ Personality and Substance Abuse

> It's my personality. . . . I'm compulsive. . . . I drink/drug to quiet my temper. . . . It quiets my moodiness. . . . I use because I'm bored.

Addictive Personality

For quite some time, the media have emphasized the concept of an **addictive personality.** This simplistic approach makes the mistake of labeling all alcoholics and other addicts as possessing a particular personality that leads to addictive and compulsive behavior. It is more accurate to recognize that many personality traits can make an individual vulnerable to the diseases of alcoholism and drug addiction, but to conclude that there is a particular addictive personality is beyond the scope of modern medicine. It is more accurate to say that such individuals have **psychological vulnerability:** a prior psychological factor that makes a pattern of substance dependence more likely to develop (Jellinek 1960).

It is difficult to identify the relationship of alcoholism and drug addiction to particular dimensions of personality, because many personality traits overlap. Cloninger's (1987) three-dimensional model of personality has been applied to the research literature on alcohol-use disorders. Cloninger identifies three temperament constructs that correlate with alcohol-use disorders:

1. Harm avoidant—cautious, apprehensive, fatigable, inhibited
2. Reward dependent—ambitious, sympathetic, warm, industrious, sentimental, persistent, moody
3. Novelty seeking—impulsive, excitable, exploratory, quick-tempered, fickle, extravagant

Tension-Reduction Models

> It's stress. . . . I just drink to calm down. . . . I need to relax. . . . I'm so tense. . . . It lets me worry less. . . . I can avoid the conflicts. . . . It makes decisions easier. . . . I can do the tedious work easier. . . . I can summon energy. . . . It reduces the tension. . . . It allows me not to think so much. . . . It makes me feel better. . . . It is pleasurable.

These are common rationalizations people give for using drugs—whether with a martini at the end of a busy workday, or marijuana, cocaine, or another drug.

The tension-reduction theory (TRT) is one of the most widely researched theories of drug use. Early research focused on tension reduction and relief from stress as a primary reason for alcohol and drug use. Today, the tension-reduction theory is considered one aspect of drug use. Individuals consume drugs for a variety of reasons, including the sheer pleasurable feelings that accompany drug use.

The tension-reduction model involves the concept of homeostasis, or balance. The individual will use alcohol/drugs to counteract (or balance out) stress, anxiety, emotional tension, and conflict—any aversive emotional state. Alcohol/drugs are therefore used as tension reducers.

Tension has been defined as any state that is an aversive source of motivation, causing feelings of fear, anxiety (vague fear), conflict, and frustration due to blocked goals. Stress is just a modern version of tension. Here is one definition of stress, from *Merriam-Webster's Collegiate Dictionary* (11th edition, 2003): "a physical, chemical, or emotional factor that causes bodily or mental tension and may be a factor in disease causation." The tension-reduction theory of alcohol use has two major assumptions: alcohol reduces tension, and individuals drink alcohol for its tension-reducing properties (Blane and Leonard 1988). Genetically predisposed individuals may find that alcohol or other drugs have effects that buffer, or reduce, stress for them.

A noted authority on alcohol and drugs, Stanley Gitlow, emphasizes an etiological model that focuses on discomfort and tolerance to stress as a major factor in the decision to use alcohol/drugs. Gitlow believes that we have biological variations in our levels of tolerance to stress and stimulation. "The initiating stimulus could well be perceived by one individual as minimally inconvenient, while another individual would perceive that same stimulus as agonizingly urgent. The overriding determinant and major variable of appetite regulation is most likely the intensity of the individual's perception of need for relief" (Gitlow 1985). Petrie (1960) identified three basic classifications in dealing with stimuli: (1) *stimulus reducers* perceive and react to a stimulus as if that stimulus were less than it is; (2) *stimulus moderators* perceive and react to the stimulus as it is; (3) and *stimulus augmenters* perceive and react as if that stimulus were more than it is. "A perceptual characteristic, such as stimulus augmenting, leading to an overly sensitive need for relief from any discomfort, appeared to be a possible and intriguing genetically determined CNS factor" (Gitlow 1985). In 1984, Lynne Hennecke reported a significantly higher incidence of stimulus augmenters in the sons of alcoholic fathers than in the sons of nonalcoholic fathers. Hennecke suggests that, in stimulus augmenters, alcohol is used to shut down the stimulation overload from the environment.

Gitlow (1972) describes alcoholism as a biochemical defect. The individual possessing this defect is easily agitated by stimuli, becomes uncomfortable, and uses alcohol for its sedating effect. Unfortunately, withdrawal from alcohol creates an agitating effect, and the individual must drink again to relieve this discomfort.

Family Model

> I drink/drug because I come from a "dysfunctional family.". . . My mom drank a lot . . . . I felt neglected . . . . I was abandoned . . . . I was abused . . . . I was shamed, violated, and traumatized.

The family model is the model most emphasized throughout this book; it includes all aspects of family life. Factors contributing to alcohol/drug use in the family include the following:

- Imbalance in parenting
- Marital discord
- Alcoholic/addict behavior
- Imbalanced and dysfunctional family interaction
- Significant trauma and stress in the family
- Physical, emotional, sexual, and psychological violation
- Inappropriate boundaries
- Shame, abandonment, rejection

The family model of chemical dependency is developed in more detail throughout this book.

According to the family model of alcohol/drug use, alcohol and drug addiction and dependence are **family diseases.** The genetic predisposition to alcoholism is well documented. The probability of developing the disease of alcoholism and drug addiction is four times higher for those individuals who have one alcoholic or drug-addicted parent. The probability increases to eight times higher if both parents are alcoholics or addicts.

Children from alcoholic, dysfunctional, and shame-based family systems are at greater risk for developing problems with alcohol/drugs. The modeling of family members who use alcohol/drugs also greatly influences the development of alcohol/drug dependence. Exhibiting poor communication, the alcoholic/addict family has specific "no talk, no feel, no trust" rules (see Chapter 7). Such a family system breeds childhood traumas of fear, rejection, abandonment, and sometimes violation (see Chapters 5 and 6).

Parents with substance-abuse problems have extreme difficulty in being effective parents. "Parenting is a difficult, time-consuming, complicated task. Staying on top of the situation requires quick, sensitive, and intuitive judgment of that which works best" (Kempher 1987). Parents with alcohol/drug problems are ill-equipped to provide the kind of patient, dedicated care necessary for children to develop and grow. Their parenting styles tend to be rigid and insensitive to the needs of children. These parents tend not to be nurturing and available. They often use coercive or abusive parenting techniques they learned from their own parents.

Adolescence

As children enter adolescence, they are at risk for alcohol/drug problems. (See Case Study 2.1 and 2.2.) In *Drugs and Drinking* (1985), Jay Strack classifies five major factors in adolescent abuse of drugs, using the mnemonic *PEACE:*

P—pressure (peer pressure)
E—escape
A—availability (of alcohol/drugs)
C—curiosity
E—emptiness

Poor Self-Concept

The most frequently generalized risk factor for problems with alcohol/drugs is a poor self-concept. Parents and schools talk about children's general under-achievement, shyness, and aggressive or antisocial behavior as being a result of this lack of a good self-concept. Report cards and progress reports include comments such as "does not work up to his/her potential," "has difficulty finishing assignments and staying on task," "fails to participate in class, daydreams," and "more concerned with peers than teacher." It should be no surprise that the same evaluations occur for adults who have difficulty with work relationships and general achievement.

There are so many definitions of self-concept that isolating this variable as a causative factor for alcohol/drug problems is impossible. While exploring all of these definitions of self-concept, I developed a more workable behavioral definition that better explains what we are talking about. Instead of using the label *self-concept,* which implies something one gets from outside of oneself and is, therefore, beyond one's internal ability to develop, I relabeled it **sense of self.** A sense of self is less static than self-concept, involves more choices by the individual, and is active rather than passive. A sense of self comes from within to the outside world, rather than the outside world's defining who the individual is. This important point has implications

Case Study 2.1

Adolescents and Alcohol/Drugs

After her birth, Joan was adopted into a wealthy family. Her birth mother had a history of emotional problems, and it is unknown whether she had problems with alcohol/drugs.

Joan, now 16 years old, was coming to counseling for an alcohol/drug evaluation. She was drunk at a party at her private high school. The parents described Joan's behavior as erratic, sometimes very loving and sensitive, and at other times explosively angry and out of control.

Joan was not adhering to simple boundaries that her parents had established (e.g., ignoring curfew, not calling if she is going to be late). They knew Joan was smoking marijuana but were unable to prevent her from using it.

The evaluation revealed that Joan is out of control. She blatantly told her parents that they were awful, and she was not going to listen to anything they said. Joan had a new older boyfriend (a 20-year-old) and she was staying out overnight with him, doing cocaine and drinking alcohol. She had told her parents she was staying with friends.

Joan told the counselor her parents can't do anything. Joan did not see herself as having a drug problem, but did admit that she frequently lost her temper. Her grades in school were very good (3.8 GPA). She stated: "I just want to do what I want to do, and I am tired of my parents nagging all the time."

Discussion Questions

1. What role do you think being adopted plays in Joan's behavior and alcohol/drug use? Explain.
2. Do you think Joan has personality traits that are problematic? Explain.
3. Do you think Joan has an alcohol/drug problem? If so, explain with examples.
4. What kind of treatment counseling would you recommend for Joan and her family?

for individuals who develop codependent relationships with addicts and alcoholics. (See Chapter 7.) Under this definition, a person with a sense of self is

1. A unique, worthwhile individual with emerging talents and skills.
2. An individual who can accomplish things (e.g., develop, prioritize, and achieve goals; solve problems; resolve conflicts; accept and carry out responsibilities; and have the maturity to develop and grow).
3. An individual who can trust and be trusted, one who sets appropriate boundaries for intimacy in relationships.

In his article "Beyond Drug Education," Paul Robinson (1975) argued that the goal is "not to convince people not to do drugs" but to empower them to enhance their development of self. Robinson suggests that we need to emphasize educational programs that help students acquire this sense of self, by helping students develop the skills to

- Control their destructive impulses.
- Understand their values, needs, and desires.

> ## Case Study 2.2
> ### *Debra*
>
> Debra, 16 years old, is very bright, attractive, precocious, and looks like she is 18 or older. All her friends are older, and she prefers to spend time with college students. She has frequently attended fraternity parties.
>
> Her parents are concerned because there is a family history of alcohol/drug addiction (i.e., her mother is a recovering alcoholic).
>
> Recently, she confided to her parents that she drank too much and was date-raped by a boy she met at a college fraternity party.
>
> Despite her parents' concerns about alcoholism, Debra believes she has no problem.
>
> ### *Discussion Questions*
>
> 1. Do you think Debra has an alcohol problem? Explain why or why not.
> 2. What impact do you think the "date rape" had on Debra?
> 3. What developmental issues do you think need to be addressed?
> 4. If you were Debra's counselor, what would you want to work on?

- Make wise decisions.
- Resist peer pressure when it endangers their welfare or inhibits their growth.
- Find nonchemical means of fulfillment and satisfaction.
- Think intelligently and rationally.

By focusing on programs that teach children and adults to develop and enhance a sense of self, we make them less at risk for alcohol and drug problems.

The more time I spend working in the fields of alcohol/drug recovery and mental health, the more clearly I see that a poor sense of self is a strong predictor of problems with alcohol/drugs. Families that do not promote the child's sense of self cause those children to be emotionally disabled (i.e., they develop a poor sense of self). In later chapters, I discuss these specific family issues in more detail.

Encouraging potential alcoholics and addicts to develop a sense of self is just one aspect of the problem; other factors must also be addressed. Even children and adults who possess a wonderful and creative sense of self can be at risk. Improving the sense of self is a preventive inoculation but is neither a cure nor a guarantee against having alcohol/drug problems. (See Chapter 10.)

Adolescence, in itself, is a time of risk for substance abuse. The developmental tasks of identify, self-worth, sexual and interpersonal identity, independence, school path toward career, achievement, motivation and direction, and other developmental issues are exacerbated by hormonal change, growth spurts, physical image and changes, peer identity and acceptance, and values clarification. Combine that with puberty, mood changes, conflicts with parents, school, driving, and other issues. It is no wonder that adolescents are at risk for substance abuse.

Hawkins, Catalono, and Miller (1992) have identified seventeen risk factors for adolescent substance abuse of alcohol and other drugs and listed corresponding ways in which to prevent or address these factors. This comprehensive study, presented in

Appendix D (available for download at www.mhhe.com/fields7e), is an invaluable resource for helping you explore adolescent substance abuse.

⋇ Trauma and Substance Use Disorders (SUD)

The American Psychological Association defines "trauma" as directly experiencing or witnessing an event that "involves actual or threatened death, or serious injury, or other threat to physical integrity, or learning that a family member or close associate has experienced such events, and have a response that involves intense fear, helplessness, or horror."

Traumatic stressors that fit this definition include disasters, motor vehicle accidents, emergency worker exposed to trauma, war, rape and sexual assault, intimate partner violence (IPV), stalking, torture, prostitution and sex-trafficking, life threatening illness, child abuse.

There are two major hypotheses regarding trauma and substance use disorders (SUDs). The existing research tends to support the first theory: Substance use and abuse is an attempt by the individual to assuage feelings related to traumatic experiences. The individual self-medicates by trying to "numb out," soothe, or escape the overwhelming feelings of pain, hopelessness, and shame associated with trauma.

The second theory is that substance use and abuse contribute to the development of post-traumatic stress disorder (PTSD). The use and misuse of alcohol/drugs can affect the individual in a number of ways making them more susceptible and "in harms way" for trauma.

Chronic substance abuse can change neurochemistry, making the individual more susceptible to PTSD. The lifestyle of substance abuse and alcoholism/addiction puts the individual in situations that are traumatic (e.g., intimate partner violence). The risk behaviors that are associated with substance abuse put the individual in situations that have significant and traumatic negative consequences (e.g., driving under the influence, drug dealing, violence, stealing, medical problems, problems in judgment, criminal and civil issues resulting from financial, interpersonal, work/school problems).

The research tends to view the self-medication theory of trauma and substance use disorders as more likely than the high-risk hypothesis. It is important to realize that the risks of substance use disorders confound the problems of trauma. In addition, these individuals often experience strong feelings of "shame" and self-deprecation that further escalate negative feelings about self.

Individuals who have both trauma and substance use disorders often do better in inpatient/residential treatment programs that specialize in the treatment of both trauma and substance use disorders, as well as the feelings of shame and self-doubt. Treatment programs that do not have this sensitivity or expertise will often result in the client having multiple relapses and further shame.

Traumatized Youth and Substance Dependence

Upon treatment intake, traumatized youth report higher substance frequency and substance problems than nontraumatized youth. Even though youth with high traumatic stress (HTS) respond to treatment, on average, they have higher substance use frequency and problems over time. This suggests that HTS youth may struggle more with substance recovery than nontraumatized youth, and require additional support and more specialized treatment. (Williams 2008). (See Case Study 2.3 and 2.4.)

Depression, Mood, and Feelings
Mood and Affect (Feeling) Disorders

> Drugs quiet the pain of my depression. . . . Drugs are catalysts to my mania.

Disturbances in affect, mood, and depression are common causes of substance abuse and addiction to medical and nonmedical psychoactive substances, especially in women (Whitlock et al. 1967).

Individuals who are experiencing problems in regulating their affect and mood may self-medicate with alcohol/drugs. Alcohol/drugs may be used to alleviate and self-medicate feelings of anxiety or panic, as well as other negative emotional states, including melancholia, depression, and even mania. Major depression, dysthymic disorder, cyclothymic disorder, atypical depression, and bipolar disorder (manicdepressive illness) are the primary affective, or feeling, disorders associated with self-medicating with alcohol/drugs (for more information on these disorders, see Chapter 10).

Major depression and dysthymia occur one and a half to two times more commonly in alcoholics (Helzer and Pryzbeck 1988). Female alcoholics have a tenfold increased incidence of mania, and male alcoholics have a threefold increased incidence of mania (Hesselbrock, Meyer, and Keener 1985).

Patients with major depression who experience intermittent or chronic dysphoria may come to value the powerful, though brief, euphorigenic effects of opioids or cocaine. Patients with bipolar or cyclothymic disorder who use cocaine may discover that the drug not only can bring them out of their depressive episodes but also can enhance their endogenously produced highs (Marin and Weiss 1986). Seasonal affective disorder (SAD) is another form of depression that leads to increased alcohol/drug use, especially during the "sunless" winter months in certain environments.

The person who starts taking alcohol or other drugs to assuage the negative effects of a mood or affect disorder can be led by those drugs into a spiraling pattern of isolation and interpersonal distancing. This isolation exacerbates the affective disorder. The pattern can lead to social phobia and paranoid ideations.

Some Feelings That Contribute to Drug Abuse

Feelings of Hopelessness It is hard to identify a single factor that leads to feeling hopeless, so hopeless that the person gives up (even if only temporarily) and stops trying to grow, achieve, and develop. Many clients feel as if they are getting nowhere, despite their continued efforts. It could be the hopelessness of poverty or financial disaster or of other socioeconomic loss. It could be the shattering of idealism in one's work or relationships. It could be the frustration of blocked goals and aspirations

Case Study 2.3

Trauma and Addiction

Daniel was traumatized throughout his life. As a young child he could do very little to help his mother escape beatings from his father. He hated his father, not only for beating him and his mother, but also because his father sexually violated him. His father had a negative attitude about everyone. He frequently blamed others for his own misfortune. He then had an excuse to hit the bottle. His father would create conflicts at home so he could leave the house, hit the bars, and get drunk.

At an early age, Daniel learned to be hypervigilant (i.e., watching every move his father made when he was at home) to avoid being the object of his father's wrath.

As an adolescent Daniel was jumping off a cliff with some friends into a swimming hole, when one of the boys drowned. While Daniel was always an outsider with his peer group, when the accident occurred, it pushed him further from his peers. This perpetuated Daniel's feelings of isolation and depression.

Many years later Daniel had a back injury and was introduced to morphine following surgery. He described it (morphine) as the first time he felt good in his life. The morphine not only numbed the physical pain but also quieted the pain of the trauma, the shame, and blotted out the world. It did not take very long before Daniel was in a cycle of heroin addiction that lasted several years.

Attempts at recovery were difficult. Daniel could stay sober for five to six days, and then would lapse back to heroin use. His back problems combined with emotional and interpersonal issues, plus the unresolved trauma, continued to push Daniel back to regular heroin use.

Despite inpatient/residential alcohol/drug treatment, Daniel continued to relapse. After several years of intensive outpatient treatment (i.e., individual and group treatment) Daniel was able to maintain sobriety. He became very active studying Buddhism, and found the teachings both intellectually stimulating and spiritually fulfilling. The combination of a strong therapeutic program, a solid relationship with his partner, and a spiritual and intellectual foundation in Buddhist teachings all helped him maintain recovery, sobriety, and a solid sense of self.

Discussion Questions

1. Explain the confounding problems of trauma and addiction as they relate to this case study.
2. Explain why traditional alcohol/drug treatment was not effective with Daniel.
3. Do you think Daniel would have embraced Alcoholics Anonymous or Narcotics Anonymous? Explain.
4. What role did Buddhist teachings and mindfulness play in Daniel's recovery?

in employment, career, or interpersonal relationships. It could be the devastation of physical health, disease, physical injury, or the loss of a loved one. It could be the hopelessness of not knowing how to read or other blocks in learning or achievement. It could be the continual shame and loss of pride from emotional, physical, or sexual violation. It could be a single or continued exposure to a traumatic event or great loss

Case Study 2.4
Sexual Violation and Addiction

Regina was repeatedly sexually violated by her uncle when she was 5 to 8 years old. Her parents divorced when Regina was 10, because of her father's physical abuse of her mother and Regina. Her mother, an alcoholic with periods of sobriety, had a succession of boyfriends, and one of those boyfriends raped Regina when she was 12.

Regina left her mother and lived with her aunt after the rape. Her mother stayed with the boyfriend and claimed Regina was lying about the rape. When Regina was 18, she left her aunt and lived with an older man (32 year old). Although they lived together, she rarely had sex with him. It was a few years later that Regina began dancing at strip clubs. She said she enjoyed the attention. She also was prostituting. This coincided with her increased use of alcohol and marijuana, which then led to cocaine and cocaine freebase.

For several years Regina was still living with her same boyfriend (a drug dealer) and dancing and prostituting. Her cocaine use had escalated to the point where she was frequently on the street, smoking crack, and doing whatever it took to get it.

Regina was found dead in an alley in a drug dealing section of the city.

Discussion Questions

1. What do you think could have been done to stop this tragic story?
2. Can you explain the relationship between sexual violation and drugs?

---

that leads to feelings of hopelessness. One or all of these can lead to hopelessness, which can lead to increased drug use, alcohol/drug problems, and addiction.

Pessimism Many of my clients recovering from alcohol/drugs described their fathers as "pessimists." Their fathers (and sometimes their mothers) were extremely negative, sarcastic, shaming, critical of others, judgmental of their spouses and other family members, and pessimistic about the world in general. This pessimistic attitude was not limited to the fathers. Some family members were fearful and worried, expressing the philosophy that others would take advantage of people and "rip you off," either financially or emotionally. They viewed the world as hostile. As a result, they approached the world defensively, expecting to get hurt, looking for the negative. Some of these parents were alcoholics/addicts; some led lives that were limited, isolated in social and emotional connection, not trusting or getting close to others.

Unfortunately, this pessimistic attitude contributes to alcoholism/addiction and is detrimental to recovery. Pessimistic individuals can maintain abstinence from alcohol/drugs, but they have difficulty trusting others or being vulnerable and real enough to get close to others, and they struggle with giving to others or attaining a spiritual sense of self. Developing and maintaining a support system for alcoholism/drug addiction is an integral element of recovery. However, developing the skills to overcome pessimism, and the mistrust of others and the world in general, is an ongoing developmental process.

Pessimism and Learned Optimism   Martin Seligman, in his book *Learned Optimism* (1991), describes pessimists as having a very negative view of the world and interpreting events as being **permanent, pervasive, and personalized.** These three *P*s of pessimism color the individuals' thoughts, beliefs, and attitudes about themselves and the world. Pessimists have these distorted thoughts about the world and over time continually approach situations with this distorted thinking process. They interpret a loss as permanent, verbalizing the all-or-none perception that "it will never get better, it will always be this way," making shaming self-statements, and seeing the world as hard, cruel, and uncaring. The pessimist takes one negative incident or a few negative situations or encounters and generalizes that they are pervasive (e.g., one or a few rejections lead to "No one loves me, there is nothing lovable about me, all of me is ugly"). Of course, the pessimist personalizes everything ("It was my fault," "If only I were . . ."). Most cognitive-behavioral therapists encourage their clients to take up these distorted thoughts by *disputing* the distorted reality and by *distracting* themselves from the incessant cycle or focus of these thoughts. This process of disputing and distracting from the distorted thoughts is a common strategy for cognitive-behavioral change.

> Distorted thought—"I can never be loved or find love."
> Dispute—"Love is precious but rare."
> Distorted thought—"No matter how hard I try, I can't ever be successful."
> Dispute—"Success is doing my best."

Seligman defines success as "talent/skill + drive + optimism." In his book, he has a test on optimism. I was very proud of how well I did on the test, soon to find out as I read the next page that even a little bit of pessimism can sabotage all the optimism you have.

TABLE 2.2

Optimism and Pessimism

Dr. Seligman describes pessimists as thinking that a "negative event or interaction" is **permanent, pervasive** (in all parts of one's life), **and personalized** (caused by your own inadequacy).

Whereas, an **optimist's** reaction to a negative event or interaction is very **temporary, specific** (related to this one event), and **external** (does not reflect the internal self).

Pessimism and Optimism	
Pessimism	**Optimism**
Permanent	Very temporary
Pervasive	Specific
Personalized	External

SOURCE: *Learned Optimism* by Martin Seligman, Pocket Press, 1991.

Seligman says that an optimistic individual views setbacks, mistakes, and failure as *very temporary,* often confined to a *specific* situation, and *external,* or outside of oneself (i.e., not an internal personalized flaw). Another term that many prevention specialists use to describe the optimistic personality is *resiliency.* Despite negative situations, resilient individuals challenge themselves to improve and don't think of themselves as victims. Optimists develop a plan to overcome the negative obstacles in their lives. They persevere through adversity (see Table 2.2).

You can certainly see how pessimism is a major characteristic of and contributing factor to alcoholism/addiction. The alcoholic/addict's sarcasm and sarcastic sense of humor underlie a **negative worldview.** Procrastination about organizing, cleaning up, or dealing with one's life is an ongoing aspect of this pessimistic view.

⁕ Boredom—An Emerging Need for Research

Boredom is often cited as a major factor in alcohol/drug abuse by adolescents as well as adults. As previously described, the drive to alter one's consciousness is directly related to using alcohol/drugs to counter uncomfortable feelings of boredom.

Surprisingly there has been very little research to date into the nature of the relationship between boredom and alcohol/drug problems, alcoholism/addiction. Nor have there been concerted efforts to help addicts/alcoholics deal with boredom as a relapse dynamic.

McWelling Todman, PhD, an expert on the topic of boredom and psychiatric disorders, states:

> Despite its prominence in studies of human performance in industrial settings . . .
> the construct of boredom continues to be ignored by most clinicians. Even in the
> field of substance abuse, a field for which there has been no shortage of anecdotal
> and speculative commentary on boredom's motivational role in the addictive cycle,
> there has been surprisingly little in the way of empirical scrutiny. (Todman 2003)

The recent emphasis in the alcohol/drug recovery field of using meditation practices and mindfulness training is directly related to teaching people how to be more present and aware, and to be able to deal more effectively with boredom by "showing up and being present" (see Chapter 11 on treatment and relapse prevention).

Boredom can involve many different issues. Early research on boredom and alcohol use (Orcutt 1984) identified two different types of boredom. Existential boredom, which is defined as a lack of purpose in life, was found to have a strong, positive relationship to frequency of alcohol use among males. Another kind of boredom, interpersonal boredom, is defined as being bored with "small talk" versus having feelings of "happiness with people." Orcutt found that the more you are interpersonally bored, the more the quantity of alcohol consumed by males and females.

Items in Existential Boredom Survey
1. In general, how often do you feel bored?
   a. Very often
   b. Often

    c. Occasionally

    d. Very rarely

    e. Never

2. I'm always too busy to be bored.
3. I am bored more often than most other people my age.
4. I feel that my life has a clear direction and purpose.

Items in Interpersonal Boredom Survey

1. I find most of my happiness in being with other people.
2. It bores me to engage in small talk with other people.
3. I get very restless if I have to stay around home for any length of time.
   (from Orcutt 1984)

There are many things you can do to overcome boredom. Here are a few:

- Train yourself to enjoy life, your environment, and the richness of life and relationships
- Be more mindful and practice mindfulness: "the awareness that emerges through paying attention on purpose, in the present moment, and nonjudgmentally to the unfolding experience, moment by moment" (Kabat-Zinn, 2003)
- Show up and be present
- Be creative
- Have many interests, hobbies, and relationships
- Have regular physical activity and exercise
- Have challenges and goals
- Have the ability to get into "flow" states—concentration, attention, and focus
- Have a spiritual sense of self
- Deal with depression, anxiety, and anger in healthy ways
- Keep busy and active
- Stay open and flexible, young at heart
- Be less critical of self and others
- Have compassion for self and others
- Pursue your talents and skills
- challenge yourself within your skill level
- Be artistic
- Be active and involved
- Select and explore entertainment and learning
- Be active versus passive
- Have the ability to enjoy yourself
- Have fun
- Learn how to relax
- Learn how to rest when needed
- Get good rejuvenating sleep
- Tak care of yourself: physically, emotionally, and spiritually
- Remember that moods change—boredom will pass in time, especially if you implement these outlined strategies

Kinds of Boredom

Interpersonal Boredom

Being bored with "small talk" versus having feelings of "happiness with people"

Existential Boredom

Having difficulty with meaning or purpose in life

An inability to know what will make you happy leading to a pervasive sense of meaninglessness

Abandoning important life goals and dreams because of practical concerns or other pressures

Leisure Time Boredom

Not being able to find rewarding things to do during leisure time

Life Boredom

Neglect of life goals leading to a state of emotional ambivalence

✄ Theories of Drug Use

Self-Medication Motive for Drug Use

People use drugs to get a variety of desired effects, such as pleasure, relaxation, excitation, relief from negative emotional states, and enhancement of positive emotional states (Table 2.3). For example, opiates (narcotic analgesics—e.g., heroin, morphine) are used to kill pain, numb, shut down, or shut out the world. In contrast, stimulants (e.g., cocaine, amphetamines) are used to increase stimulation, activity, and action. Unfortunately, continued drug use creates a negative cycle of abuse, dependence, and addiction.

Edward Khantzian (1985) makes the case that drug use is not a random phenomenon. Instead, he says, it is a purposeful attempt by the user to assuage painful affective states and manage psychological problems and disorders:

> Rather than simply seeking escape, euphoria, or self-destruction, addicts are attempting to medicate themselves for a range of psychiatric problems and painful emotional states. Although most such efforts at self-treatment are eventually doomed, given the hazards and complications of long-term, unstatble drug use patterns.

Khantzian observed more than 200 narcotics addicts with lifelong problems of rage and violent behavior, and concluded that these addicts used opiates primarily for the drugs' anti-aggression and anti-rage action. In his work with cocaine addicts,

TABLE 2.3	
Drugs and Their Effects	
Drugs	**Effects**
Narcotic analgesics	Kill pain, numb, shut out, slow down
CNS depressants (e.g., alcohol)	Decrease activity, relaxation
CNS stimulants	Increase activity, excitation
Hallucinogens	Change the user's view of the world
Marijuana	Relaxation, stimulation of senses, stimulation of thought

he found that these addicts tended to take cocaine to medicate themselves against chronic depression, hyperactivity, restless syndrome, attention deficit hyperactivity disorder (ADHD), and two mood (affective) disorders—cyclothymic disorder and bipolar disorder (see definitions of these disorders in Chapter 10).

Clearly, the importance in exploring the self-medication motive is to help users identify why they are taking drugs and then learn how to better cope with the affective states and psychological problems they find so unbearable. The ability to identify and label emotional states, and then to "work through" these feelings, is a foundation of drug prevention with young people and of treatment for those who are experiencing drug abuse, dependence, and addiction.

An example of the self-medication motive for marijuana is listed in Table 2.4. These adult daily users had a variety of reasons for using marijuana. The table highlights the many self-medication reasons for smoking marijuana.

Personality Theories
Personality Traits of Addicts/Alcoholics

Many researchers and clinicians have described various personality traits of alcoholics/addicts, including the following:

- High emotionality
- Anxiety and overreactivity
- Immaturity in interpersonal relationships
- Low frustration tolerance
- Inability to express anger adequately
- Anger over dependence and ambivalence to authority
- Low self-esteem with grandiose behavior
- Perfectionism
- Compulsiveness
- Feelings of isolation
- Sex role confusion
- Depression
- Dependence in interpersonal relationships

T A B L E 2 . 4

Aspects of Life Experience Adult Daily Users Most Frequently Described as Positively Affected by Marijuana

- Ability to relax and enjoy life
- Enjoyment of food
- Ability to overcome worry and anxiety
- Ability to sleep well
- Ability to avoid feeling bored
- Enjoyment of sex
- Understanding of others
- Creativity
- Ability to avoid feeling angry
- Ability to enjoy varied activities
- Self-understanding
- Overall happiness
- Ability to avoid feeling depressed
- Ability to be tolerant and considerate of others

SOURCE: Herbert Hendin et al., *Living High: Daily Marijuana Use by Adults,* Copyright © 1987 Human Sciences Press. Reprinted by permission of Insight Books, New York, NY.

- Hostility
- Sexual immaturity
- Rigidity and inability to adapt to changing circumstances
- Simplistic, black-and-white thinking

Impulsivity/Disinhibition—Risk-Taking Behavior

It seemed like a good idea at the time.

Impulsivity/disinhibition includes personality traits such as sensation seeking and aggressiveness. I refer to some substance abusers as "edgewalkers"—people who are living on the edge of danger or risk. Impulsive/disinhibited individuals are at increased risk for alcohol-related problems (Caspi et al. 1997; Schukit 1998), and the traits of impulsivity/disinhibition are elevated in the children of alcoholics (Alterman et al. 1998; Scher 1991).

Alcohol/drug use involves taking the risks involved in using. There have always been individuals who, when told no, are curious and perhaps contrary and translate that no into yes. This is especially true of adolescents. Alcohol/drug use affects each individual's physical and emotional balance; for some, that balance is very delicate, even before they start to use alcohol/drugs. Individuals who have a need to be in control usually have a negative reaction when they use alcohol/drugs. People who enjoy losing control and are looking for an altered state of consciousness that approaches their outer limits of effective functioning become more involved in alcohol/drug use. Some thrill seekers may go further, to substance dependence and addiction.

The alcoholic/drug addict lifestyle, subculture, and environment are the most alluring features of addiction for some. Scoring drugs, hanging out in bars, associating with users, stealing, and engaging in other antisocial behaviors all reinforce the actual use of alcohol/drugs. The risk-taking behavior itself creates feelings of rebellion, aggression, rage, self-destructiveness, and "aliveness" (i.e., the adrenaline rush accompanying danger and fear).

The problems that result from these risk-taking behaviors lead to a vicious cycle of taking more alcohol/drugs to alleviate the feelings of pain, anxiety, and depression. This debilitating cycle continues until users recognize their own powerlessness and destructive behavior, or until they are in jail or dead.

Personality Disorders

> I'm angry and drugs quiet me. . . . It's hard for me to get close to others without drugs. . . . I feel anxious and fearful, so drugs relax me. . . . I am bored and isolated, so drugs soothe that. . . .

Of all the personality disorders, the one with the strongest relationship to substance abuse is narcissism. The personality disorder with the second highest correlation to substance abuse is borderline personality disorder (for more information on these disorders, see Chapter 10). (See Case Study 2.5.)

Psychosocial Models—Social Learning Theory (SLT)

> It's fun to use and be with friends. . . . It's peer pressure. . . . It's cool to use and chill out. . . . I can use drugs and belong. . . . I can connect with others when we are together. . . . Sex is better. . . .

A variety of models can be considered psychosocial or social learning models. The key element of these models is the social learning aspect of alcohol/drug use. Social learning theory also incorporates other models, such as the tension-reduction model. For example, the young child who sees Dad drink his martini at the end of the day and witnesses the relief of tension may come to see drinking alcohol as an extremely positive experience. Children often experience their parents as more approachable and positive after they have used drugs or alcohol. Nathan (1983) describes alcohol use as a socially acquired, learned behavior pattern, maintained by antecedent cues (classical conditioning and expectancies), consequent reinforcements (operant conditioning and tension reduction), cognitive factors, modeling influences, and the interaction of behavioral and genetic mechanisms.

Marlatt and Gordon (1985) emphasize certain social learning and cognitive-behavioral points about addiction:

- Addictive behaviors are a category of "bad habits" (or learned maladaptive behaviors). Biological factors may contribute to predisposing an individual to alcohol problems, but specific patterns of use are learned.

Case Study 2.5

Borderline and Narcissistic Personality Disorders with Substance Use Disorders (SUD)

Diane, an extremely attractive 39-year-old woman, has been in residential treatment twice for alcoholism. Upon returning home, she relapsed within two weeks.

The pattern of relapse is related to escalated conflicts with her boyfriend. Despite strong suggestions from the treatment program and her outpatient therapist, Diane continues to battle over issues with her boyfriend. She exhibits a jealous rage and escalated conflicts that get physical. There is a pattern of extreme closeness that they engage in, followed by strong conflicts when she gets disgusted with the way he treats her. This back and forth, in and out of the relationship, high drama is enervating and distracts them from working on their own issues.

Rusty, Diane's 42-year-old boyfriend, is a wealthy accountant and has started dating a very attractive 27-year-old attorney. This occurred after Diane and Rusty's last big conflict. When Diane found out about the dating, she relapsed and showed up at Rusty's house drunk. Rusty apologized and told her that he loved her (Diane), and they reconnected.

Rusty has been diagnosed as narcissistic with a mood cycling disorder. A few weeks after he and Diane reunited, he went on a cocaine binge and told Diane that he was still dating the young attorney. This started another cycle of escalated conflicts. They disengaged, and a few weeks later, Rusty called her and told her the relationship with the young female attorney was over.

Discussion Questions

1. Can you explain this dramatic and chaotic cycle in terms of their personality traits and their substance abuse disorder?
2. What treatment recommendations would you make for Diane? And for Rusty?

- Addictive behaviors occur on a continuum of use—that is, behavior such as alcohol abuse is not categorical (e.g., present or absent) but instead varies in quantity and frequency of occurrence.
- All points along the continuum of addictive behavior are influenced by the same principles of learning. Therefore, the same mechanism that may be applied to explaining alcohol use can be invoked to explain alcohol-use disorder.
- Addictive behaviors are learned habits that can be analyzed in the same way as any other habit.
- The determinants of addictive behaviors are situational and environmental factors, beliefs and expectations, and family history and prior learning experiences with the substance or activity. Emphasis is also placed on the

consequences of addictive behavior to understand its reinforcement and punishing features.

- Besides the effects of alcohol (or another substance or activity in question), it is also important to discern the social interpersonal reactions that the individual experiences before, during, and after engaging in the addictive behavior. Social factors are important in both the acquisition and later performance of the addictive behavior.
- Frequently, addictive behaviors are exhibited under conditions that are perceived as stressful. To that degree, they represent maladaptive coping behaviors.
- Addictive behaviors are strongly affected by the individual's expectations of achieving desired effects of engaging in the addictive behavior. Furthermore, self-efficacy expectancies (i.e., expectations of being able to use behavioral skills to cope with a situation without engaging in the addictive behavior) are important. If self-efficacy in a situation is low, and the individual believes (expects) that engaging in the addictive behavior would help him or her cope with it, then the likelihood of engaging in the behavior increases.
- The acquisition of new skills and cognitive strategies in a self-management program can result in changes in addictive behavior to new, more adaptive behaviors, which come under control of cognitive processes of awareness and decision making. Accordingly, the individual can assume and accept a greater degree of responsibility for changing the addictive behavior.

Sociocultural Models

In his review of cultural and cross-cultural studies, Bales (1946) identified factors in the influence of a culture or sociological organization on rates of alcoholism:

1. The degree to which a culture causes acute needs for adjustment of inner tension in its members
2. The attitudes toward drinking that the culture produces in its members
3. The degree to which the culture provides substitute means of satisfaction

Societies, cultures, communities, socioeconomic groups, and even neighborhoods offering few or limited alternatives to drinking and drugging as tension relievers are more susceptible to addiction. The more these groups produce acute inner tensions (shame), suppressed or acted-out aggression, extreme conflict, dilemmas, mixed messages, sexual tensions, and the condoning of attitudes about alcohol/drugs as the normal, accepted way of relieving these tensions, the more prone individuals are to develop alcohol/drug dependence. When there is no limit on supply and distribution, attitudes are liberal, and cost is relative, the incidence of alcohol and drug abuse is high.

The attitude of the culture and ethnic customs may also facilitate patterns of alcohol/drug use. "The Irish and the American Indian groups positively sanction men's drinking to intoxication away from home; in these cultures the rates of alcoholism are high. Drug/alcohol dependence and addiction are influenced by sociological factors such as age, occupation, social class and subculture, and religious affiliation. In the United States, for example, young, single, unemployed urban men have a high incidence of abuse" (Donovan 1986).

Individuals who feel alienated from a larger society and who have no sense of belonging may feel that the society's rules and values about alcohol and drugs don't apply to them. This feeling of alienation from a larger social body may result in more favorable attitudes about alcohol/drugs. The application of this social model of alcohol/drug use is evidenced by the crack cocaine epidemic.

The lack of opportunity or hope that one can achieve the American Dream can contribute to feelings of despair that lead to alcoholism and/or drug addiction. This despair is most prevalent in the ghettos in America's inner cities. However, this sense of despair can occur in any locale, in any socioeconomic setting. From the blue-collar bars, to the shooting galleries in abandoned buildings, to middle-class suburban high schools, to the plush boardrooms of major corporations, drugs and alcohol infest our society.

Psychoanalytic Models

The traditional psychoanalytic view of alcohol/drug dependence focused on a fixation at the oral stage of development, resulting in an oral and narcissistic premorbid personality. Otto Fenichel (1945) theorized that individuals use psychoactive drugs "to satisfy the archaic oral longing which is a sexual longing, a need for security, and need for the maintenance of self-esteem simultaneously." Menninger (1963) believed that alcohol may function as a coping device to alleviate stress and that the primary psychoanalytic root is a mother's denial of milk (security) in infancy. Other psychoanalytic theories suggest drinking as a strategy for allaying anxiety over masculine inadequacy (Machover et al. 1959). Analytical theories also suggest that abusers use alcohol/drugs to suppress latent homosexuality and ego-dystonic feelings of homosexuality (i.e., the person's ego is not compatible with the possibility of being homosexual).

The dominant psychoanalytic explanation of alcohol/drug use today is that it is caused by "a structural deficit in object relations." This means that individuals have a hard time establishing effective interpersonal relationships due to their difficulty in managing their affect (feeling) and impulse controls. They often establish their defense mechanism of denial by defensive grandiosity. In 1986, James Donovan outlined psychoanalytic descriptions used by various researchers in identifying this difficulty in object relations:

H. Krystal and H. A. Raskin (1970) indicated a defective stimulus barrier and an inability to desomatize emotions.

Chein et al. (1964) described drug use to cope with painful feelings and overwhelming responsibilities in the outside world.

L. Wursmer (1974) emphasized the maladaptive narcissism of the addict, a defensive stance against the potentially overwhelming feelings of rage and loneliness.

E. J. Khantzian (1978) pointed to the impoverished self-esteem, the lack of capacity for self-care, and the poor emotional regulation of the alcoholic.

Khantzian (1982) and Khantzian, Halliday, and McAuliffe (1990) described an inability to handle emotions and behavior characterized by swings from overcontrol to undercontrol. Feelings are often vague, ill defined, and confusing when expressed.

Wursmer (1987) suggested drugs may be used to deny or "overthrow" a particularly burdensome and chafing inner authority figure.

Psychoanalytic Meaning

Sometimes the choice of a particular drug is related to the meaning that drug has, both consciously and subconsciously, for that person.

Alcohol/Drugs as Power

Alcohol/drugs frequently denote power or feeling powerful to users. The expression *getting high* symbolizes feeling above others or above one's usual sense of self. Ironically, despite the original reason for using drugs to feel powerful, the ultimate state in the cycle of addiction makes the individual powerless. Cocaine is a drug that has a symbolic meaning of power. As a power drug, cocaine is attractive because of its status as well as its physical and psychological effects. An energizing stimulant, cocaine produces a sublime feeling of well-being; users describe being on top of the world, in control, able to accomplish a great deal, able to have tremendous

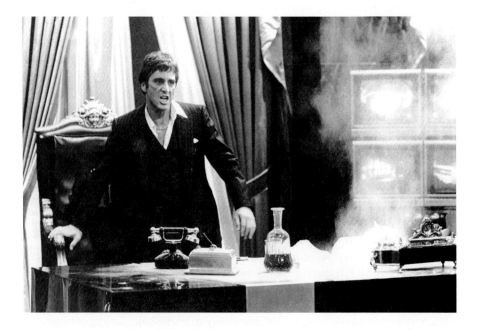

Although cocaine may give users feelings of power, cocaine use can actually have many negative effects on personality and can quickly lead to addiction for some people.

capabilities and insights, and able to stimulate sexual arousal and performance. However, the reality today is that cocaine is one of the most addicting drugs, and one of the fastest addicting drugs, and it ultimately renders users powerless.

Alcohol and other drugs symbolize power in the forms of sensuality and sexuality; potency; the feelings of being supernatural, of pleasure, sensitivity, insensitivity, or not feeling pain; productivity; rebelliousness; high energy; and so forth. Our review of the research on why adolescents initially used marijuana indicated the following reasons: for pleasure, contentment, the joy of being high, relaxation, and recreation; to facilitate social interactions; to achieve status in one's peer group; to achieve friendship leading to better understanding; to defy authority, seek thrills, and flirt with danger; for curiosity and excitement, escapism, and enhancement of activity; to enhance aesthetic appreciation or sexual stimulation; to alleviate a sense of alienation; to make life better and more tolerable; to understand or find oneself; to expand one's mind for religious insights; to improve oneself.

Alcohol/Drugs as Self-Destruction

Alcohol/drugs can also have a powerful meaning as weapons of self-destruction and ultimately death. In *Family Therapy of Drug Abuse and Addiction,* M. Duncan Stanton and associates (1982) describe the addict as "part of a continuum of self-destruction." Stanton et al. report that, compared with the general public, addicts have a higher death rate, a shorter than average life expectancy, and a greater than normal incidence of sudden death. Compared to nonaddicts, addicts also have a more positive and potent view of death and are more likely to express a wish for death.

A number of clinicians have described alcoholism and drug addiction as an unconscious death wish. Self-destructiveness is the failure of ego functions involving self-care and self-protection. "We are all subject to our instincts, drives, and impulses, and if they are expressed indiscriminately, we are subject to hazard and danger" (Gottheil 1983).

Alcohol/Drugs in Seduction and Sexuality

Alcohol/drugs have important symbolic seduction and sexuality meanings. Practically all drugs and alcohol have been described at some time as aphrodisiacs. Unfortunately, no drug is truly an aphrodisiac. Alcohol/drugs may reduce inhibitions and stimulate sexual arousal at low doses; however, alcohol and other drugs impair sexual performance, especially with prolonged use.

The symbolic seduction and sexuality meanings of alcohol/drugs are exploited in advertisements for tobacco and alcohol products. If such advertising were legal, it would probably be used to advertise illicit drugs, too.

Whether celebrating an important event with a traditional toast of wine, champagne, or alcohol; passing around a pipe filled with marijuana; or sharing cocaine, heroin, or other drugs, the symbolic meaning is a shared altered state of consciousness (see Case Study 2.6).

Case Study 2.6

Lyn: Marijuana and Seduction

Lyn is a female client in outpatient therapy who successfully stopped smoking marijuana 10 months ago. At a party, a male acquaintance flirts with Lyn from across the room. She is very interested, so she returns the seductive eye contact. When they eventually make it to the same part of the room, they begin a conversation. He asks her out to the balcony where it is quieter. Even though Lyn has not smoked marijuana in 10 months and has a history of marijuana dependence, she accepts and smokes the marijuana he offers her, without much thought.

Discussion

Drugs are often linked to seduction and sexuality. For Lyn, the seductive nature and excitation of this new relationship was too powerful a draw for her to refuse the marijuana. She knew that marijuana had had significant negative consequences in her life, but the trigger of seduction overcame this awareness. Often people will say, "It seemed like a good idea at the time," rather than recognize the long-term consequences.

Discussion Questions

1. What role do alcohol/drugs play in seduction and sexuality?
2. Do you think alcohol/drugs can be cross-addicting with sexuality?
3. Explain the interaction dynamic of alcohol/drugs and sexuality (i.e., "Drugs, Sex, and Rock 'n' Roll").
4. What developmental problems can occur when alcohol/drugs are used to facilitate sexuality and intimacy?

Existential Issues

Existential issues have to do with the limitations of existence. These can include the limitations of life itself or how long we live, the unknowns related to death and dying, the pain of poor health, health-related problems and illness, the traumatic and untimely death of those close to us, ultimately being alone, the feelings of helplessness in not being in control, the dysphoria of life, boredom and ennui, the unknown, the betrayals, the loss or lack of spirituality, chronic long-lasting problems, even the eventual destruction of the planet Earth.

Drugs are a way to quiet, distract, or escape these existential issues and to gain a temporary relief and change in focus or perspective. However, it is a temporary and passive approach that doesn't resolve any issues but often leads to more drug use, and perhaps to a vicious pattern of substance abuse and/or addiction.

Poor Future Orientation

Michael Yapko, in his book *Breaking the Patterns of Depression* (1997), describes depression as having its roots in a "poor future orientation." Individuals who see their future as negative might abuse drugs, having a short-range view. Many addicts/alcoholics report that they don't expect to live very long. Thinking that their life span is limited, they are not concerned about having good physical health. As one client put it, "I might as well party hearty, since I will die young, anyway."

Many adolescents have a poor future orientation because of a continued pattern of academic failure or a difficult family situation. Academic failure, especially in the late elementary grades, highly correlates with early antisocial behavior and alcohol/drug abuse (Johnston et al. 1978; Kandel, Kessler, and Margulies 1978; Robins 1978). Many of these children fail to develop the skills necessary to learn, integrate concepts, and succeed in school. Many exhibit learning disabilities, emotional problems, and attention deficit disorder. These children's parents are frequently in denial of these emotional and learning disabilities, and the school system may not adequately address these problems, resulting in educational failure for the children. Some of these children do well during adolescence, some barely escape alcohol/drug problems, some develop addictions, and some die in alcohol/drug–related accidents and overdoses.

Some young adults might be frustrated that their careers are not developing. Middle-aged persons may be realizing that they face limitations and may not accomplish what they had intended. Older adults may have the existential despair about aging, future health problems, or death itself (see Case Study 2.7).

All of these issues may cause a person to have a poor future orientation. The adolescent, the young adult, the middle-aged person, and the elder may choose to abuse alcohol/drugs to cope with these discouraging issues. The obvious goal, whether the difficulty is poor future orientation, pessimism, or hopelessness, is to address these issues and to find new ways to enjoy life and relationships.

Conditioning and Substance Abuse

> I use drugs because it feels good. . . . Drugs make for a good time. . . .
> I expect to feel good under the influence. . . . There is no "guesswork"
> here—take the drug for the desired effect. . . . It's modern chemistry. . . .

A strong reinforcing factor in alcohol/drug use is the memorable feeling attached to the first use. A first-time experience with a drug- or alcohol-induced altered state of consciousness is a new and unforgettable awareness. This first or early experience with alcohol/drugs is so reinforcing that time after time the individual attempts to reproduce or recapture that original memorable experience. Heroin smokers call it "chasing the dragon." This can be similar to one's first romantic involvement or to the extremely pleasurable yet painful romantic associations of unrequited love. Alcohol/drugs can become that first love, like no other experience ever felt before. Unfortunately, it is impossible to duplicate that feeling. The cycle of addiction has begun: the individual tries to repeat an experience that cannot be recaptured because by definition it was the first. This is the reason addicts continue using alcohol/drugs even though the feeling and behavioral experiences clearly have become negative and unpleasant. They hope that somehow the next time will be different.

Frequently, alcoholics and addicts have **euphoric recall** of the pleasant experiences they had during earlier, excessive uses of alcohol/drugs. They forget the

Case Study 2.7

Poor Future Orientation

George: Recovering from Alcohol but Dying from Cigarettes

George had been in recovery from alcoholism for more than 2 years and recognized the benefits of sobriety. His financial situation was manageable and improving, he was losing weight gradually, he had a better relationship with his daughter, and even got along with his ex-wife.

When confronted in group therapy about his continued habit of smoking cigarettes, George maintained that he was going to smoke for one more year and then quit. His father had died of a heart attack at age 50, and George was now 49. He espoused a distorted belief that he had held for most of his life—that he was going to die by age 50. He rationalized that if he made it to 50, he would then stop smoking.

Discussion

Poor future orientation often involves limitations in one's view of future events and possibilities, whether financial, interpersonal, employment-related, or health-related. Poor future orientation is a major factor that exacerbates mood, often leading to depression.

This case illustrates George's pessimism about his own future health and his expectation and fear that he will (as his father did) die at age 50. George is living his life based on this belief, which is a distortion of reality. Although George is in recovery from alcohol and sees the benefits of his sobriety and working a recovery program, he is not committed to quitting smoking. Exploring his belief that it may not be worth working on smoking cessation is an integral element to his taking action.

Discussion Questions

1. Do you think the addiction to "cigarettes" should be addressed when the person is in alcohol/drug treatment?
2. Do you think self-help meetings (e.g., Alcoholics Anonymous and Narcotics Anonymous) should be smoke-free?
3. How hard do you think nicotine addiction is to overcome, compared to other drugs?
4. Do you think people are still not in recovery if they are smoking cigarettes compulsively? Explain.

negative consequences and dangerous situations that they barely escaped. The human mind defends against the overwhelming fear and shock of these negative experiences and instead recalls the good times. Thus, alcoholics and addicts forget how destructive and dangerous their experiences with alcohol/drugs can be.

If illicit drugs were legal, imagine the unlimited advertising campaigns that could be developed for their sale, based on these characteristics:

Feeling down and depressed? Lack the energy to do even the most basic things? Suffer from lowered sex drive, sleep disturbances, or have difficulty with interpersonal relationships? Not making the kind of money you would like to, need a vacation, a general lift? Wondering what life is all about or if it is even worth it? Try Zippy, the new non-narcotic wonder medication brought to you by the What's Happening Now, Don't Worry, Be Happy Institute of Living Life.

Expectancy and cognitive models assert that alcohol/drug use is an anticipatory response to a pleasure state, conditioned by previous use. This may describe the obsessive-compulsive aspect of chemical dependency.

Biobehavioral models focus on the conditioning, reinforcement, stimulus situations (triggers), and pleasure and withdrawal states associated with alcohol/drugs.

A good example of positive conditioning is a recent study that explored the association of positive responses to marijuana to later addiction. It was found that the more positive the responses of early use, the more likely that addiction would occur. Of those with five or more positive responses, 39.1 percent became addicted. On the other hand, only 5.2 percent of those with no positive responses became addicted, and of those with one positive response, only 8.5 percent became addicted.

Individuals who have an initial negative reaction to drug use or don't actually experience getting high are often likely to stop trying the drug. Many individuals who are concerned with security and safety and like to be in control have negative reactions to drug use. Those who are fearful or have negative attitudes about drug use will either refrain from drug use or have negative reactions because of the negative "set and setting" (see Chapter 3).

✘ Some Other Theories of Drug Abuse

In this section, I highlight some of the many theories of drug abuse to help give you an orientation that will help you explore your own perspective of drug abuse.

- **Personality-Deficiency Theory—David P. Ausubel, M.D., Ph.D.**
  Describes narcotic addicts as having developmental personality traits of motivational immaturity, lacking in ego maturity of long-range goals, responsibility, self-reliance and initiative, volitional and executive independence, and the ability to defer the gratification of immediate hedonistic needs for the sake of achieving long-term goals.
- **The CAP Theory—Steven R. Gold, Ph.D.** The **cognitive-affective-pharmacogenic** (CAP) theory believes the cognitive style of the drug abuser is viewed as the pivotal factor in an individual's moving from drug experimentation to drug abuse. The abuse process begins with conflict, having difficulty meeting society's demands or expectations, which leads to anxiety. The individual's interpretation of that anxiety is crucial. If he or she feels unable to alter or control the situation, the person feels powerless and is prone to using drugs to alter the anxiety and related feelings.
- **Existential Theory—George B. Greaves, Ph.D.** Individuals use drugs as a passive means of euphoria, or at least as a means of removing some of the pain and anxiety attending a humorless, dysphoric lifestyle.

- **An Ego-Self Theory of Substance Dependence—Edward J. Khantzian**
  Individuals are predisposed to drug use and dependence, as a result of severe
  ego impairments and disturbances in the sense of self, involving difficulties
  with drive and affecting defense, self-care, dependency, and the need for
  satisfaction.
- **An Availability-Proneness Theory of Illicit Drug Abuse—Reginald G.
  Smart, Ph.D.** Availability refers to the set of physical, social, and economic
  circumstances surrounding the ease or difficulty of obtaining drugs,
  especially the cost and the physical effort required to obtain them. The
  theory also looks at psychological problems as making individuals "prone"
  to certain drugs and drug abuse.
- **Drug Use as a Protective Defense—Leon Wurmser, M.D.** Drug use as a
  pharmacologically reinforced denial—an attempt to get rid of the feeling import
  of more or less extensive portions of undesirable inner and outer reality.
- **Problem-Behavior Theory—Richard Jessor, Ph.D., and Shirley Jessor,
  Ph.D.** In problem-behavior theory, the personality system is represented by
  a number of specific variables belonging to three component structures—a
  motivational-instigation structure, a personal belief structure, and a personal
  control structure.
- **Drug Subculture Theories—Bruce D. Johnson, Ph.D.** Explores the
  linkages between the parent subcultures, peer cultures, and drug subcultures.
- **Self-Esteem and Self-Derogation Theory of Drug Abuse—Howard
  B. Kaplan, Ph.D.** Adoption of the deviant response (drug abuse) has
  self-enhancing consequences if it facilitates intrapsychic or interpersonal
  avoidance of self-devaluing experiences associated with the traditional
  values of the culture.
- **The Iowa Theory of Substance Abuse Among Hyperactive Adolescents—
  Jan Loney, Ph.D.** Diagnostic evidence has centered upon the four *As*—activity
  (hyperkinetic reaction of childhood), attention (attention deficit disorder),
  aggression (conduct disorder), and/or achievement (learning disability).
- **A Family Theory of Drug Abuse—M. Duncan Stanton, Ph.D.** Symptoms
  occur and serve functions within a context (the family), both for the symptom-
  bearer and for the other family members. Accumulated data indicate that a
  high percentage of drug abusers' families have experienced premature loss or
  separation during the family's life cycle. Families of drug abusers show a high
  proportion of traumatic, untimely, or unexpected loss of a family member.
- **Self-Esteem Theory of Drug Abuse—R. A. Steffenhagen, Ph.D.** This
  theory is a developmental one emanating from an Adlerian approach in
  which self-esteem is seen as the main psychodynamic mechanism underlying
  all drug use and abuse, including inferiority-superiority, social interest, goal
  orientation, and lifestyle.
- **Psychosocial Theory of Drug Abuse: A Psychodynamic Approach—
  Herbert Hendin, M.D.** In the case of the drug problem, social variables
  ranging from sexual activity to association with fiends who use drugs have
  been shown to be related to drug use. There is a need for a psychodynamic
  approach to psychosocial problems.

- **Toward a Sociology of Drug Use—Irving F. Lukoff, Ph.D.** The view that it is less useful to speak of drug use alone, because those who are heavily invested in drug use are also part of more integrated lifestyles, different in the ghettos than on the campuses, but at variance with many aspects of conventional adult culture.
- **Achievement, Anxiety, and Addiction—Rajendra K. Misra, D.Phil.** Drug use is initiated as a time-saving device to cope with the stress of achieving. Drugs are used to relieve anxiety, to induce relaxation, and overcome boredom.
- **Addiction to Pleasure—Nils Bejerot, M.D.** Describes drug addiction as a chemical love. The pleasure mechanism may be stimulated in a number of ways and give rise to a strong fixation on repetitive behavior.
- **Brain and Neurotransmitters: Pharmacological Approach—William R. Martin, M.D.** The brain has a variety of receptors and several neurotransmitters that are involved in feelings of well-being. Further, many addicts and alcoholics have an affective disorder that appears to be the polar opposite of feelings of well-being produced by drugs of abuse.

SOURCE: Adapted from "Theories of Drug Abuse," National Institute on Drug Abuse *Research Monograph 30,* 1960.

⊰ In Review

- Drugs will always be used for a variety of purposes, including altering consciousness; regulating mood (affective states); relieving stress, negative feelings, and boredom; stimulating thought or action; and disconnecting or connecting.
- Drug abuse is a passive activity, whereas "flow" requires active consciousness, focus, involvement, and concentration. Csikszentmihalyi (1992) defines flow as "When consciousness is harmoniously ordered, you pursue what you are doing for the sheer sake of doing it."
- In 1957 the American Medical Association declared alcoholism a disease, based on three criteria: (1) There is a known etiology (cause), (2) the symptoms get worse over time, and (3) alcoholism has known outcomes.
- Devor (1994) describes alcoholism in terms of a developmental-genetic model. He proposes that "alcoholism no longer be thought of as a single disease, but as a group of illnesses in which the influences of genes and environment ebb and flow over the course of the at-risk lifetime."
- Adoption studies and twin studies support the view that there is a genetic predisposition to alcoholism.
- Various personality traits are more pronounced in addicts/alcoholics (e.g., risk-taking behaviors, impulsivity). The two primary personality disorders related to substance abuse are narcissistic and/or borderline personality disorder.
- Drugs are used to regulate mood and affect (feeling). Feelings of depression, isolation, and emotional pain are often temporarily sedated by drugs. Ironically, patterns of substance dependence and addiction lead to a spiraling pattern of depression, interpersonal problems, feelings of isolation, and developmental problems.

Individuals who are experiencing problems in regulating their affect and mood may self-medicate with alcohol/drugs. Alcohol/drugs may be used to alleviate and self-medicate feelings of anxiety or panic, as well as other negative emotional states, including melancholia, depression, and even mania. Major depression, dysthymic disorder, cyclothymic disorder, atypical depression, and bipolar disorder (manic-depressive illness) are the primary affective, or feeling, disorders associated with self-medicating with alcohol/drugs.

- The dominant psychoanalytic explanation of alcohol/drug use today is that it is caused by "a structural deficit in object relations." This means that individuals have a hard time establishing effective interpersonal relationships due to their difficulty in managing their affect (feeling) and impulse controls.
- Tension-reduction models are the most highly researched models and are the foundation for a number of treatment approaches. According to this model, drugs are used to counter tension, stress, anxiety, conflict—any aversive emotional state.
- The family model is strongly emphasized in this textbook. According to this model, dependence on alcohol or other drugs is a "family disease" and family plays a major role in how family members deal with drugs.
- As children enter adolescence, they are at risk for alcohol/drug problems. The most frequently generalized risk factor for problems with alcohol/drugs is a poor self-concept. A good self-concept is defined as

    a.   A unique, worthwhile individual with emerging talents and skills
    b.   An individual who can accomplish things (e.g., develop, prioritize, and achieve goals; solve problems; resolve conflicts; accept and carry out responsibilities; and have the maturity to develop and grow)
    c.   An individual who can trust and be trusted, one who sets appropriate boundaries for intimacy in relationships

---

✳ Discussion Questions

1. Describe and discuss some positive ways you alter consciousness and get into "flow states."
2. Do you think you can have positive addictions? If yes, what would the negative consequences be?
3. In Worksheet 2.1, describe your rationale for ranking the models and theories of addiction.
4. How would you counsel a client who had an addiction and/or alcoholism and who, after his 30-day residential program, decided to stop attending AA, and told you this in his outpatient counseling session?
5. Do you think antidepressants might help an individual who has depression and substance abuse? Explain why or why not.
6. Give some examples of family denial and explain the possible impact on the family.
7. Describe why adolescents are at risk for substance-abuse problems. What at-risk factors most impacted you during adolescence?

W O R K S H E E T   2 . 1

Exploring Your Own Perspective
Models and Theories of Substance Abuse

Please rate the following models and theories

0—No Impact
3–5—Medium Impact
7—Extremely Strong Impact

Base your rating on your personal experiences, clinical or otherwise, and your personal and family experiences. Please feel free to write reasons for your ratings.

Models	0	1	2	3	4	5	6	7
Disease								
Genetic								
Personality								
Tension Reduction								
Psychoanalytic								
Family								
Psychosocial								
Sociocultural								
Spiritual								

Theories	0	1	2	3	4	5	6	7
Self-Medication								
Personality Traits								
Personality Disorders								
Mood/Affect Disorders								
Existential Issues								
Conditioning								
Adolescence								

❧ References

Alterman, A. I., et al. 1998. Personality pathology and drinking in young men at high and low familial risk for alcoholism. *Journal of Studies on Alcohol* 59:495–502.

Bales, R. 1946. Cultural differences in rates of alcoholism. *Quarterly Journal of Studies of Alcohol* 6:480–99.

Benward, J., and J. Densen-Gerber. 1975. Incest as a causative factor in antisocial behavior: An exploratory study. *Contemporary Drug Problems* 4:323–40.

Blane, Howard T., and Kenneth E. Leonard, eds. 1988. *Psychological theories of drinking and alcoholism.* New York: Guilford Press.

Blum, Kenneth, et al. 1990. Allelic association of human dopamine D2 receptor gene in alcoholism. *Journal of the American Medical Association* 263(15):2055–60.

Brown, Kirk Warren, and Norman C.D. Sundberg. 1986. Boredom proness—the development and correlates of a new scale. *Journal of Personality Assessment* 50: 4–17.

Caspi, A., et al. 1997. Personality differences predict health-risk behaviors in adulthood: Evidence from a longitudinal study. *Journal of Personality and Social Psychology* 73:1052–63.

Chein, I., et al. 1964. *The road to H.* New York: Basic Books.

Cloninger, C. R. 1987. A systematic method for clinical description and classification of personality variants. *Archives of General Psychiatry* 44:573–88.

Cloninger, C. R., M. Bohman, and S. Sigvardsson. 1981. Inheritance of alcohol abuse. *Archives of General Psychiatry* 38:861–68.

Csikszentmihalyi, Mihalyi. 1992. *Flow: The psychology of optimal experience.* New York: Tarcher/Putnam.

Devor, Eric. 1994. A developmental-genetic model of alcoholism: Implications for genetic research. *Journal of Consulting and Clinical Psychology* 62(6): 1108–15.

Donovan, James M. 1986. Etiological model of alcoholism. *American Journal of Psychiatry* 143:1–11.

Eisner, Robert. 2005. Marijuana abuse and the age of initiation: Pleasure of response foreshadows adult outcomes. *NIDA Notes* 19 (January): 1.

Fenichel, Otto. 1945. *The psychoanalytic theory of neurosis.* New York: W. W. Norton.

Gitlow, S. E. 1972. The pharmacological approach to alcoholism. *Journal of Drug Issues* 2(3): 32–41.

Gitlow, S. E. 1985. Considerations on the evaluation and treatment of substance dependency. *Journal of Substance Abuse Treatment* 2: 175–79.

Gitlow, S. E., and Herbert S. Peyser. 1988. *Alcoholism: A practical treatment guide.* Philadelphia: Grune & Stratton.

Goodwin, D. W. 1971. Is alcoholism hereditary? A review and critique. *Archives of General Psychiatry* 25:545–49.

Gosline, Anna. 2007/2008. Bored? *Scientific American Mind* (December/January): 20–27.

Gottheil, Edward, ed. 1983. *Etiological aspects of alcohol/drug abuse.* Springfield, Ill.: Charles C. Thomas.

Gurling, H. M., et al. 1984. Genetic epidemiology in medicine: Recent twin research. *British Medical Journal* 288:3–5.

Hammond, D. C., G. Q. Jorgenson, and D. M. Ridgeway. 1979. *Sexual adjustment of female alcoholics.* Salt Lake City: University of Utah.

Hawkins, David, R. Catalono, and J. Miller. 1992. Risk and protective factors for alcohol and other drug problems in adolescence and early childhood: Implications for substance abuse prevention. *Psychological Bulletin* 112(1): 64–105.

Helzer, J. E., and T. R. Pryzbeck. 1988. The co-occurrence of alcoholism with other psychiatric disorders in the general population and its impact in treatment. *Journal of Studies on Alcohol* 49:219–24.

Hennecke, Lynne. 1984. Stimulus augmenting and field dependence in children of alcoholic fathers. *Journal of Studies on Alcoholism* 45:486–92.

Hesselbrock, M. N., R. E. Meyer, and J. J. Keener. 1985. Psychopathology in hospitalized alcoholics. *Archives of General Psychiatry* 42:219–24.

Hrubec, Z., and G. S. Omenn. 1981. Evidence of genetic predisposition to alcoholic cirrhosis and psychosis: Twin concordance for alcoholism and its end points by zygosity among male veterans. *Alcoholism* 5:207–15.

Jellinek, E. M. 1960. *The disease concept of alcoholism.* New Haven, Conn.: Hillhouse Press.

Johnston, L. O., et al. 1978. Drugs and delinquency: A search for causal connections. In *Longitudinal research on drug use,* edited by D. B. Kandel. Washington, D.C.: Hemisphere.

Kabet-Zinn, John. 2003. Mindfulness-based interventions in context: Past, present and future. *Clinical Psychology: Science and Practice:* 145–146.

Kaij, L. 1960. *Alcoholism in twins: Studies in the etiology and sequelae of abuse of alcohol.* Stockholm: Alonquist & Winkell.

Kandel, D. B., R. Kessler, and R. Margulies. 1978. Antecedents of adolescent initiation into stages of drug use: A developmental analysis. In *Longitudinal research on drug use,* edited by D. B. Kandel. Washington, D.C.: Hemisphere.

Kempher, Carol. 1987. Special populations: Etiology and prevention of vulnerability to chemical dependence in children of substance abusers. In *Youth at high risk for substance abuse.* Washington, D.C.: U.S. Department of Human Services.

Khantzian, E. J. 1978. The ego, the self, and opiate addiction: Theoretical and treatment considerations. *International Review of Psychoanalysis* 5: 189–98.

Khantzian, E. J. 1982. Psychopathology, psychodynamics, and alcoholism. In *Encyclopedia handbook of psychiatry,* edited by E. M. Pattison and E. Kaufman. New York: Gardner Press.

Khantzian, E. J. 1985. The self-medication hypothesis of addictive disorders: Focus on heroin and cocaine dependence. *Journal of Psychiatry* 142(11): 1–39.

Khantzian, E. J., K. S. Halliday, and W. E. McAuliffe. 1990. *Addiction and the vulnerable self.* New York: Guilford Press.

Krystal, H., and H. A. Raskin. 1970. *Drug dependence: Aspects of ego functions.* Detroit: Wayne State University Press.

Machover, S., et al. 1959. Clinical and objective studies of personality variables in alcoholism: An objective study of homosexuality in alcoholics. *Quarterly Journal of Studies in Alcohol* 20: 528–42.

Marin, Steven, and Roger D. Weiss. 1986. Psychiatric comorbidity in drug and alcohol addiction. *Journal of Drug Education.*

Marlatt, A., and J. Gordon. 1985. *Relapse prevention: Maintenance strategies in the treatment of addictive behaviors.* New York: Guilford Press.

Menninger, K. 1963. *The vital balance.* New York: Viking Press.

Miczek, K., Elise M. Weerts, and Joseph F. Debold. 1992. Alcohol, aggression, and violence: Biobehavioral determinants. In *Alcohol and interpersonal violence: Fostering multidisciplinary perspectives,* edited by Susan E. Martin. NIAA Research Monograph 24. Washington, D.C.: U.S. Dept. Health and Human Services.

Nathan, P. E. 1983. A behavioral overview of alcohol abuse and alcoholism. In *Etiological aspects of alcohol and drug abuse,* edited by E. Gottheil, K. A. Druley, T. E. Skoloda, and H. M. Waxman, pp. 141–58. Springfield: C. C. Thomas.

National Institute on Drug Abuse. 1960. Theories of drug abuse. Research Monograph 30.

Orcutt, J. D. 1984. Contrasting effects of two kinds of boredom on alcohol use. *Journal of Drug Issues* 14(1): 161–173.

Petrie, A. 1960. Some psychological aspects of pain and the relief of suffering. *Annals of the New York Academy of Sciences* 86: 13–27.

Robins, L. W. 1978. Sturdy childhood predictors of adult antisocial behavior: Replication from longitudinal studies. *Psychology Medicine* 8: 617–22.

Robinson, Paul E. 1975. Beyond drug education. *Journal of Drug Education* 5(1): 183–91.

Rotgers, Frederick, et al. 2003. *Treating Substance Abuse: Theory & Technique.* New York: Guilford Press.

Scher, K. J. 1991. *Children of alcoholics: A critical appraisal of theory and research.* Chicago: University of Chicago Press.

Scher, K. J., and T. H. Trull. 1994. Personality and disinhibitory psychopathology: Alcoholism and anti-social personality disorder. *Journal of Abnormal Psychology* 103: 92–102.

Schukit, M. A. 1998. Biological, psychological, and environmental predictors of alcoholism risk: A longitudinal study. *Journal of Studies in Alcohol* 59: 485–94.

Seligman, Martin E. P. 1991. *Learned optimism: How to change your mind and your life.* New York: Pocket Books.

Stanton, M. Duncan, et al. 1982. *The family therapy of drug abuse and addiction.* New York: Guilford Press.

Strack, Jay. 1985. *Drugs and drinking: What every teen and parent should know.* Nashville: Nelson.

Tabakoff, Boris, and Paula L. Hoffman. 1988. Genetics and biological markers of risk for alcoholism. *Public Health Report* 103(6): 690–98.

Tarter, R., and K. Edwards. 1985. Neuropsychology of alcoholism. In *Alcohol and the brain,* edited by R. Tarter and Van Thiel, pp. 217–42. New York: Plenum.

Todman, McWelling. Summer 2003. Boredom and psychotic disorders: Cognitive and motivational issues. *Journal of Psychiatry* 66(2).

Turner, S., and F. Colao. 1985. Alcoholism and sexual assault: A treatment approach for women exploring both issues. *Alcoholism Treatment Quarterly* 2(1): 91–101.

Varley, Christopher. 1995. Hyperactive adults. *Professional Counselor.* December.

Whitlock, F. A., et al. 1967. Drug dependence in psychiatric patients. *Medical Journal of Australia* 1: 11–57.

Williams, Julie K., Douglas C. Smith, Hyonggin An, and James A. Hall. March 2008. Clinical outcomes of traumatized youth in adolescent substance abuse treatment: A longitudinal multisite study. *Journal of Psychoactive Drugs* 40(1).

Wursmer, L. 1974. Psychoanalytic considerations of the etiology of compulsive drug use. *Journal of the American Psychoanalytic Association* 22: 820–43.

Wursmer, L. 1987. Flight from conscience: Experience with the psychoanalytic treatment of the compulsive drug abuser. *Journal of Substance Abuse Treatment* 4: 169–79.

Yapko, Michael D. 1997. *Breaking the patterns of depression.* New York: Doubleday.

Drug-Specific Information
Drugs on the Street Where You Live

Objectives

1. Identify drug problems in the new millennium (e.g., crystal methamphetamine) and the populations that are impacted.
2. Define terms used in describing drug dependence and addiction.
3. Define and describe addiction, routes of administration, set and setting, drug absorption, distribution, and elimination.
4. Identify the five classifications or categories of drugs.
5. List the hazards of using narcotic analgesics, and describe the development of tolerance and the symptoms of withdrawal.
6. Describe the major effects of alcoholism.
7. Identify and describe the major effects of central nervous system stimulants.
8. Describe the diseases related to using tobacco.

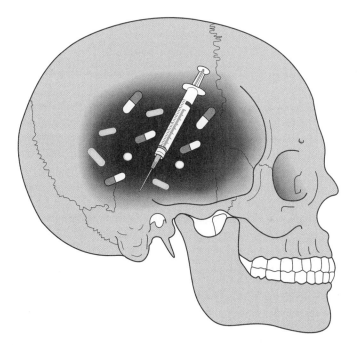

9. Describe the major and adverse effects of hallucinogens.
10. Describe the major and adverse effects of *Cannabis sativa.*
11. Describe the major and adverse effects of inhalants and PCP.
12. Identify the drugs used to increase athletic performance and endurance.

⋇ Scope of the Alcohol/Drug Problem

In 2006, the National Survey on Drug Use and Health (SAMSHA 2007) estimated that 22.6 million Americans (12 or older) were classified with substance dependence or abuse (9.2 percent of the population). Of this group, 3.2 million abused alcohol and illicit drugs, and 15.6 million abused only alcohol.

Between 2002 to 2006 alcohol and drug dependency rates stayed about the same.

C H A R T   3 . 1

Dependence on or Abuse of Illicit Drugs

2002	2003	2004	2005	2006
3.0%	2.9%	3.0%	2.8%	2.9%

Dependence on or Abuse of Alcohol

2002	2003	2004	2005	2006
7.7	7.5	7.8	7.7	7.6

(National Survey on Drug Use & Health, SAMSHA, 2007)

Every neighborhood and community is affected in some way by problems with alcohol/drugs. No house, farm, tenement, high-rise, or alleyway is immune from alcohol/drugs. Many streets of inner cities are infected with crack cocaine, and other streets are contaminated by heroin. Perhaps families on your own block have problems with alcohol, cocaine, hallucinogens, or marijuana. Perhaps families who live down the street are mixing highly explosive chemicals to produce methamphetamine. Even in rural areas, children might be inhaling the fumes of gasoline to get high, growing marijuana in secluded areas, or harvesting hallucinogenic mushrooms. Every family in every community is vulnerable to the problems associated with alcohol and drugs.

⋇ Drugs in Our Society

The 1960s and 1970s were truly the birth of the modern drug revolution. Marijuana, hallucinogens (especially LSD), and other drugs became a major part of the hippie movement of that time. It was a time when young people rebelled against their parents' traditional values by using drugs, dressing differently, growing their hair long, espousing open love, and listening to rock 'n' roll. They also staged protests against civil rights violations, the war in Vietnam, and the traditional values of our political system.

In the 1980s, cocaine became the rage—a drug that was first thought to produce only psychological dependence. However, over the next 10 years this drug would cause us to dramatically change our definition of addiction and our whole outlook on drug abuse. Cocaine was soon being used intravenously and smoked in the form of *freebase cocaine*. Comedian Richard Pryor set himself on fire while smoking freebase cocaine, and John Belushi died when he overdosed by injecting cocaine and heroin ("speedballing"). Both of these unfortunate tragedies brought cocaine to the forefront. A dramatic and tragic victim of cocaine was Len Bias, a talented college basketball player who had been drafted by the Boston Celtics. Boston fans were elated at the prospect of Bias and Larry Bird being on the same team. Unfortunately, on the evening he was drafted by the Celtics, Bias celebrated with freebase cocaine and died.

Soon cocaine was being converted to *crack cocaine*. Crack addicts in the inner cities became a major addict population that quickly challenged our treatment and criminal-justice system. Babies born to mothers who were addicted to crack cocaine were another casualty of this new drug.

It is fair to say that cocaine changed our entire outlook about addiction. Even individuals who thought that drugs were rather benign and produced only psychological dependence could not ignore the high addiction potential of cocaine. This short-acting drug created addicts very quickly, with dramatic and disastrous effects on their lives. It also affected people from all socioeconomic levels.

Another group of drugs that came to our attention in the mid-1980s was synthetically produced drugs. In an attempt to subvert existing controlled substance laws, underground chemists created new drugs that were chemically different (by a molecule or two) from those banned by existing drug laws.

Donald Wesson, an expert in the alcohol/drug field, defined designer drugs as "substances wherein the psychoactive properties of a scheduled drug have been retained, but the molecular structure has been altered in order to avoid prosecution under the Controlled Substance Act." The potency and volume of production of these drugs challenged our perception of illicit drug manufacturing. There was no need for the large production and distribution networks like those used for cocaine and marijuana. There was no harvest of the drug. Instead, one chemist with the basic raw materials could produce enough of the drug to supply the entire United States.

In the early 1990s, another new drug brought to public attention was *ice*. Ice is a transparent, sheetlike crystalline structure that is a purified form of the drug methamphetamine hydrochloride. In the early 1990s, ice was imported to the mainland United States by eastern drug cartels operating out of Oahu, Hawaii. In January 1990, authorities busted the operation of an ice factory in northern California. At that time, the National Institute on Drug Abuse reported the use of ice in cities such as Atlanta, Dallas, Los Angeles, Phoenix, San Diego, and Seattle. Attempts to develop ice on the East Coast did not pan out. Much as crack is to cocaine, ice is to methamphetamine. Ice is a smokable and more powerful form of methamphetamine hydrochloride. Smoking ice allows more rapid absorption into the blood via the lungs. Unlike the extremely short-acting high of freebase and crack cocaine, the ice high can last from 7 to 30 hours. Dr. David Smith, of the Haight-Ashbury Free Clinic, has noted, "Ice did not replace crack, it widened the group of people who use drugs."

⬦ Drug Update—In the New Millennium

Crystal Methamphetamine

The United States is currently experiencing an upward cycle of stimulant abuse, with a dramatic increase in the availability and use of crystal methamphetamine, in a potency, purity, and accessibility unlike that found at any previous time in our history. This is a substance that does not occur in nature and thus must be synthesized in a laboratory.

Street names for this drug include speed, crank, crystal, ice, meth, chalk, chicken powder, peanut butter-crank, go-fast, crystal meth, shabu-shabu, glass, go qip, chris, and christy, depending on the geographical area, the dealer, and the physical form, crystal versus powder.

The name *ice* has been used by dealers to represent methamphetamine as well as other substances, including methamphetamine mixed with heroin, cocaine or other adulterants, quartz, and rock salt.

Part of this alarming trend is ascribed to the takeover of the manufacture and distribution of speed, formerly the province of outlaw fringe individuals, by Mexican nationals, who already had a strong, well-organized distribution network. This has resulted in a much purer, significantly more potent, and lower-priced drug, precipitating a sharp increase in the number of users, including much younger users.

Methamphetamine enters the brain more rapidly than any other CNS stimulant, rapidly producing a "rush" of euphoria when injected or smoked. Many people who try methamphetamine go on to compulsive abuse of the drug. Typically, small doses can have a profound effect, including stimulated movement and increased speech, feelings of excitement and euphoria, and decreased appetite. A significant rise in pulse rate and blood pressure occurs, as well as a sensation often described by users as "my heart pounding out of my chest." This may progress to irregularities in heart rhythm, a dramatic rise in body temperature, convulsions, cardiovascular collapse, and death.

Populations Using Methamphetamine

- Traditionally associated with white, male, blue-collar workers, methamphetamine is now reportedly being used by diverse groups in all regions of the country.
- Use is increasing among men who have sex with men and use other drugs, making this population more vulnerable to contracting and spreading sexually transmitted diseases, especially HIV/AIDS.
- Young adults who attend "raves" or private clubs are increasingly using methamphetamine.
- Notable increases are occurring among homeless and runaway youth.

- Increasing use of methamphetamine is reported among male and female commercial sex workers who also trade sex for drugs and among members of motorcycle gangs. Also, people in occupations that demand long hours, mental alertness, and physical endurance (such as long-haul truckers) have been using this drug at increased rates. (National Institute on Drug Abuse 1998)

Methamphetamine Use by Adolescents

There are mixed reports on methamphetamine use by young people. The U.S. federal government statistics in a nationwide survey of 12th graders indicates a significant downward trend of lifetime methamphetamine use by adolescents from 1999–2005 (4.75 to 2.5 percent). Yet, state and local drug treatment programs report that more than 20 percent of adolescent admissions report methamphetamine abuse and dependence (Rawson 2007).

Methamphetamine use by adolescents can also cause significant problems including:

- Different types of neurological and psychiatric consequences (since the adolescent brain is still developing)
- High levels of depression and suicidal ideation compared to other substance abuse (e.g., marijuana, alcohol)
- Implications in risky sexual behavior
- Problematic among girls (i.e., much higher admissions to treatment programs than boys) (Rawson 2007)

You Can Identify Methamphetamine Users by . . .

- Signs of agitation, excited speech, decreased appetites, and increased physical activity levels. Other common symptoms include dilated pupils, high blood pressure, irregular heartbeat, chest pain, shortness of breath, nausea and vomiting, diarrhea, and elevated body temperature.
- Occasional episodes of sudden and violent behavior, intense paranoia, visual and auditory hallucinations, and bouts of insomnia
- A tendency to compulsively clean and groom and repetitively sort and disassemble objects, such as cars and other mechanical devices. (National Institute on Drug Abuse 1998)

Chronic use leads to a state of paranoia, with individuals displaying behaviors strikingly resembling those of someone experiencing an acute episode of paranoid schizophrenia. Tolerance develops quickly, and chronic users must increase their dose, which, in turn, leads to magnification of the side effects and may lead to permanent brain damage.

In addition to the physical symptoms, the chronic user will experience a profound depression, with low energy levels, anhedonia (the total inability to experience any pleasurable feelings), and such a profound craving for the drug, remembering when the drug "worked" for them, that the cycle is often repeated many times, often with tragic results.

Ice, the smokable form of methamphetamine, is of extremely high purity—greater than 90 percent—and can lead to "runs" of 4 to 5 days without any sleep and often without food or even fluids. Then a "crash" of 4 days or so occurs, before the user begins another "run."

The drug, regardless of form, is often used concurrently with alcohol, either to blunt some of the stimulant effect or to help the user "come down" after a protracted period of use. The use of other depressant psychoactive substances leads to a poly-drug use pattern that can be extremely dangerous.

MDMA (Ecstasy)

MDMA is better known as Ecstasy, XTC, X, Rave, or Adam. Although MDMA was first synthesized and patented in 1914 as an appetite suppressant, it became popular in the 1980s with college students. Prior to July 1985, when it became illegal to sell MDMA, or Ecstasy, the drug was legally sold in bars in Texas catering to college students. A major factor that contributed to MDMA's emergence in the rest of the country was publicity—associated with the drug being blatantly sold in bars and then with its being scheduled as a controlled substance. In 1985, *Newsweek, Time, Life,* and other magazines sensationalized the euphoric, therapeutic, and aphrodisiac qualities of the drug. MDMA is related to both mescaline and amphetamines and could be best described as a "mood-enhancing stimulant." It is often perceived as "mild speed," and users often claim that it increases empathy and communication, which is why it is also called the "hug drug." A subculture has evolved around the drug, with resultant Ecstasy and rave parties, which are often clandestine (although most young adults seem to have no problem knowing where they are), changing location as often as every weekend.

Even though it is often referred to as hallucinogenic, it rarely produces delusions. MDMA is most frequently taken orally, with reports of a variety of psychological effects, including the following:

- Positive mood change
- Dramatic drop in defense mechanisms
- Increased empathy for others
- Increased self-esteem and elevated mood

Combined with the stimulant effect, these also may produce an increase in communication, intimacy, and enhanced pleasure of touching, yet MDMA inhibits orgasm and interferes with erection.

Negative effects include overdose potential, extreme fatigue with too much use, dilated pupils, dry mouth and throat, tension in the lower jaw, grinding of the teeth, and too much stimulation.

Although users tend to perceive MDMA as harmless, there are reports of cases of acute and chronic paranoia associated with usage, and even panic reactions requiring emergency care. As with other central nervous stimulants, a rise in blood pressure accompanies its use; this is of no consequence to most otherwise healthy young adults but can have a potentially deadly effect on someone with an underlying cardiac problem or a congenital abnormality.

There often appears to be a hangover effect, consisting of muscle aches, especially of the jaw and facial muscles (clenching of the teeth is common); generalized fatigue; decreased concentration; and insomnia. Tolerance to the mood- and mind-altering effect does develop, with subsequent increase in the "unwanted" side effects. See Table 3.1 for a summary of the effects of MDMA.

OxyContin Abuse: A Prescription Addiction

OxyContin is a semisynthetic opiod analgesic prescribed for chronic pain. It is often prescribed for cancer patients with chronic, long-lasting pain, or for other related chronic pain. It is effective and beneficial for chronic pain sufferers because it is a long-acting medication that is time-released over 12 hours, so patients need to take it only twice a day.

The active ingredient in OxyContin is oxycodone. OxyContin contains a much larger amount of oxycodone than other prescription opiate pain medications—between 10 and 150 milligrams of oxycodone in each time-release tablet.

OxyContin abusers are seeking a quick, powerful rush. They crush the OxyContin tablets and inject or snort the powder, or mix it in water and drink it. This disarms the timed-release mechanism, resulting in a quick, powerful high.

By prescription, OxyContin costs about $4 for a 40-milligram pill. On the street, the cost escalates to $20–$40 for a 40-milligram pill. As a result, many pharmacies are being robbed for OxyContin, and many prescriptions are being forged to obtain OxyContin (CSAT Advisory 2001).

Rohypnol

Rohypnol is also known as narcozep, rohipnols, and roiphol. It is the brand name for flunotrazepam, a sleeping pill legally manufactured and prescribed for use in Europe, Mexico, South America, and the Asias. It is from the benzodiazepine class (e.g., Valium, Xanax, Restoril) and is not available on the formulary of drugs that may be legally prescribed in the United States. All rohypnols in the United States are therefore illegally purchased. Common street names are rohies, ropies, roofies, wheels, and row-shapys.

Like other benzodiazepines, when taken alone, Rohypnol is unlikely to cause problems. But if combined even with a small amount of alcohol, the intoxication effects may be extreme, leading to severely impaired judgment and motor skills. Individuals given such a combination often "come to" anywhere from 8 to 24 hours later, with no memory of any events that transpired after the time they ingested the drugs (blackouts).

Teens and young adults often follow the abuse pattern of taking the drug in combination with alcohol, as an "alcohol extender." There is a synergistic effect that increases the impairment of memory and judgment. It may also be used by drug addicts to "boost the high" or to "parachute down" from a cocaine binge. Rohypnols have been widely implicated in date rape, in which the female victims are seduced or tricked into ingesting the drug plus alcohol. The disinhibition effect, as

TABLE 3.1

Effects of MDMA

Minor Adverse Effects (relatively common and generally short-lived reactions, which occur shortly after taking a dose)

Mydriasis (dilated pupils)
Photophobia (discomfort when looking at bright lights)
Headache
Anorexia (diminished appetite), nausea, dry mouth, abdominal cramps, diarrhea
Sweating, tachypnea (rapid breathing), tachycardia (rapid heart rate), palpitations, tremor
Bruxism (grinding of teeth)
Trismus (uncomfortable rigidity of the jaw muscles)
Gait disturbance, ataxia (difficulty walking)

Serious Acute Adverse Effects (uncommon reactions)

Hallucinations, severe anxiety, agitation, panic attacks, paranoia
Hypertension (increased blood pressure)
Cardiac arrhythmias (irregular heart rhythms)
Severe central chest pain (probably due to intercostal muscle spasm)
Severe abdominal cramps
Urinary retention (due to alpha-adrenergic stimulation of bladder neck)

Adverse Effects Only in Certain Circumstances

Overexertion, dehydration, collapse
Hyperpyrexia (increased body temperature)
Convulsions (seizures)
Rhabdomyolysis (muscle breakdown)
Disseminated intravascular coagulation (blood clots throughout the body)
Cerebrovascular accident (stroke), intracerebral hemorrhage
Acute renal failure
Polydipsia (excessive drinking), low sodium levels, and stupor
Road traffic accidents
Facial dermatosis (pimples)

Delayed Reactions to Exposure

Jaundice, hepatotoxicity
Tooth wear
Possible congenital anomalies
Poor concentration and attention, memory impairment, depression
Sleep disturbance
Weight loss, exhaustion

SOURCE: Holland 2001.

well as amnesia for the subsequent events, are why these drugs have been given the appellation "leg splitters."

The federal government has begun the process of classifying this drug as a Category I substance, putting it into the same category as narcotics. This would bring with it severe penalties for dealing and possession of the drug.

Heroin

The 1990s saw a significant increase in the use of heroin. The number of hard-core users, estimated by the National Institute of Drug Abuse (NIDA), has remained fairly constant over the past 25 years, at 750,000 to 1 million. However, the past several years have seen a disturbing number of heroin users who are dramatically unlike the stereotypical heroin addict. The profile now contains well-educated, often female individuals, frequently employed in white-collar and even professional capacities. The age of users is also alarming, considering reports of use in high schools and even middle schools.

The reasons for this trend are many. For one, heroin use has assumed the trappings of glamour, often associated with the "arts," fashion, and entertainment world. It is now much purer, and thus more potent, which enables the user to inhale it, either through smoking it, "chasing the dragon," or snorting it in its powder form. The very fact that it does not have to be injected makes it more attractive by alleviating the aversion most people have to needles (i.e., needle phobia, stigma, risk of AIDS virus). There is also the widespread misbelief, and rationalization, that if one smokes or snorts heroin it will be nonaddicting.

To add to its "attractiveness," it is also relatively inexpensive, especially compared with crack cocaine. A bag of heroin containing enough to get the user high for 6 to 8 hours may be purchased for as little as $3 in New York City and will be of significant purity and potency, whereas a $10 bag of heroin purchased on the streets in 1980 was about 4 percent pure. Today it is not uncommon for a sample to be 65 percent pure, or even higher.

Another factor is that the drug is more easily obtained. The neophyte user is no longer forced to venture into dangerous neighborhoods to purchase the drug. It may be as easy as paging the dealer, who then delivers it, or it may be available on certain street corners in middle-class or industrial neighborhoods or even at the workplace.

One of the more insidious aspects of the drug is that, unlike cocaine and even alcohol, heroin use may exist for a significant period of time before its use is suspected. Individuals may be fairly high and functioning for quite a while, and, if they are careful, it may take months before they have to increase their dose and risk getting toxic. By the time it becomes obvious, the problem has progressed to the point where medical treatment and appropriate intervention is most often necessary to treat the addiction.

Heroin-related emergency department visits doubled from 33,900 in 1990 to 70,500 in 1996. In 1993, more than 3,805 deaths nationwide were related to heroin. "Both urban and suburban emergency departments treat patients with heroin overdoses daily and hospitalize 3 to 7 percent of these patients for related complications" (Sporer 2000).

Heroin use can no longer be confined along geographic, economic, or social lines. It is in "Heartland USA," as well as in suburbia and in the urban centers of the nation. It is found among the unemployed and disadvantaged, blue-collar workers, professional workers, the economically advantaged, and even homemakers.

Inhalants

In addition to glue, paint, room deodorizers (e.g., Glade), butane, and even propane, there are commercial products that are often inhaled to get high. This includes ethyl chloride and nitrous oxide, which are known as "whippets," found in whipped cream canisters. It is estimated that at least 10,000 common household products contain ingredients that can be abused.

The most commonly used inhalants by young people are glue, shoe polish, and gasoline. Other inhalants include nitrous oxide, lighter fluid, and aerosol sprays. There are also gender differences in inhalant use, with boys more likely to use gasoline or nitrous oxide, while girls favor glue, shoe polish, spray paints, correction fluid, and aerosol sprays (*Washington FOCUS* 2004).

The earlier children use inhalants, the more likely they will become dependent.

Adolescents who reported first use of inhalants at age 13–14 were six times more likely to be dependent on inhalants than those who started using inhalants at age 15–17. (*Washington FOCUS* 2004)

⋇ Definitions of Terms

Physical Dependence

Physical dependence is the altered state that develops when a person cannot stop taking a certain drug without suffering from withdrawal.

Withdrawal

Withdrawal symptoms are physical symptoms resulting from stopping the use of a drug (see Table 3.2). These vary according to the specific drug, the amount used, and the length of time over which it has been used. Because the body has actually adapted metabolically to the presence of the drug, when it is withdrawn (or even tapered off too rapidly), the reactions may vary from mild, flulike symptoms for a person coming off of opiates to a severe, potentially life-threatening situation when withdrawing from alcohol or other sedative hypnotics.

Psychological Dependence (Formerly, Habituation)

A user with a profound emotional or mental need for the repetitive use of a drug or a class of drugs is **psychologically dependent.** The user becomes so preoccupied with taking the drug to achieve the optimal level of functioning or to maintain a sense of well-being that it becomes extremely difficult to abstain. Psychological dependence is a subjective state that is almost impossible to quantify; therefore, it is of limited usefulness in establishing a diagnosis of chemical dependency.

TABLE 3.2

Diagnostic Criteria for Drug Withdrawal

Opioid	Alcohol	Cocaine	Nicotine
Dysphoric mood	Autonomic	Dysphoric mood	Dysphoric or
Nausea	hyperactivity	Fatigue	depressed mood
or vomitin	Hand tremor	Unpleasant	Insomnia
Muscle aches	Insomnia	dreams	Irritability
Lacrimation	Nausea	Insomnia or	Anxiety
Rhinorrhea	or vomiting	hypersomnia	Difficulty
Pupillary	Hallucinations	Increased appetite	concentrating
dilatio	Illusions	Psychomotor	Restlessness
Piloerection	Psychomotor	retardation	Decreased heart rate
Sweating	agitation	or agitation	Increased appetite
Diarrhea	Anxiety		Weight gain
Yawning	Seizures		
Fever			
Insomnia			

SOURCE: Data are from the *Diagnostic and Statistical Manual of Mental Disorders* 4th ed., American Psychiatric Association, 1994

Tolerance

Tolerance to a drug develops when the individual requires increasingly larger doses to achieve the desired optimal effect. In other words, users require larger doses to achieve the same high produced previously by a smaller dose of the same drug.

Cross-Tolerance

Cross-tolerance is a diminished or reduced response to the effect of a psychoactive drug. This response is due to prior use of other psychoactive drugs, usually in the same drug category.

Synergism

In a synergistic process, one chemical enhances, or adds power to, the effect of another. The combined effect of two or more drugs is therefore greater than the effect of each agent added together (e.g., $1 + 1 = 3$ or more).

Antagonism

The opposite of synergism, antagonism occurs when the combined effect of two drugs is less than the sum of the drugs' effects acting separately (e.g., $1 + 1 = $ less than 2). For example, the depressant effects of alcohol are counteracted by the stimulant effects of cocaine.

Routes of Administration

The route of administration is the method by which the alcohol/drug is ingested. Ingestion may be oral, through the skin, by injection, by smoking, or through other orifices (e.g., suppositories). The most rapid reaction occurs after inhalation while smoking a drug; injection is the next most rapid route. Oral administration and absorption through the skin are the slowest routes. (See Figure 3.1.)

Set and Setting

Set refers to the user's state of mind at the time of use. *Setting* refers to the physical environment or environmental factors surrounding alcohol/drug use. The differences in set and setting can account for different reactions to the drug. The same individual using the same dose and same drug can vary in reaction to the drug based on the set

1. Mouth—Alcohol is drunk.

2. Stomach—Alcohol goes right into the stomach. A little of the alcohol passes through the wall of the stomach and into the bloodstream. Most of the alcohol continues down into the small intestine.

3. Small intestine—Alcohol goes from the stomach into the small intestine. Most of the alcohol is absorbed through the walls of the intestine and into the bloodstream.

4. Bloodstream—The bloodstream then carries the alcohol to all parts of the body, such as the brain, heart, and liver.

5. Liver—As the bloodstream carries the alcohol around the body, it passes through the liver. The liver changes the alcohol to water, carbon dioxide, and energy, The process is called *oxidation*. The liver can oxidize only about one half ounce of alcohol an hour. Thus, until the liver has time to oxidize all of the alcohol, the alcohol continues passing through all parts of the body, including the brain.

6. Brain—Alcohol goes to the brain almost as soon as it is consumed. Alcohol continues passing through the brain untill the liver oxidizes all the alcohol into carbon dioxide, water, and energy.

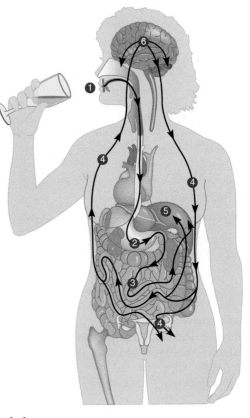

FIGURE 3.1   *How alcohol is absorbed in the body.*
SOURCE: National Institute on Alcohol Abuse and Alcoholism. *Alcohol Health and Research World.* Washington, DC: U.S. Department of Health and Human Services, 1988.

and setting. The hallucinogens are the most dramatic example of the importance of set and setting. A "bad trip" can occur under the influence of hallucinogens if the set and setting are negative. For example, a man takes a hallucinogen and goes to a party with his girlfriend. She breaks up with him at the party, telling him she has been cheating on him for months, and leaves the party with the other guy. He's now at the party, alone, and doesn't know anyone. He is pretty angry and upset and accidentally bumps into a bunch of rowdy, drunk guys. You can imagine the rest.

A woman gets a promotion at work and is affirmed for her diligence, intellect, and good management of a major project. Several co-workers invite her out for a drink on Friday at the close of business. Compare her reaction to that of another woman in the same office who is warned that her performance is poor and placed on probation pending a review by her supervisors. She is not invited to go out with the first group, but instead goes off by herself to a bar with the express intention of getting drunk. You can clearly predict based on set and setting the different reactions that each woman will have to drinking alcohol that Friday evening.

⚔ Definition of Addiction

Historically, there has been a wide range of definitions of addiction—for example:

> A chronic, progressive, and potentially fatal disease. It is characterized by tolerance, psychological and physical dependence, pathogenic organ changes, all of which are the direct or indirect consequence of the alcohol ingested. (National Council on Alcoholism)

> An illness characterized by preoccupation with alcohol and loss of control over its consequences, which usually leads to intoxication if drinking is begun; by chronicity; by progression; and by the tendency to relapse. Typically associated with physical disability and impaired emotional, occupational, and/or social adjustments as a direct consequence. (American Medical Association 1957)

As described throughout this textbook, the current definition of addiction used in the alcohol/drug field is the one developed by Dr. David Smith. An expanded version of that definition of addiction follows:

1. Compulsion and obsession

   a. The compulsive use of the chemical despite its no longer having the desired effect
   b. The fear of being without the substance
   c. The compulsion to substitute other drugs if that particular substance is unavailable
   d. Thoughts about the drug as a dominant theme or integral part of one's life

2. Loss of control or inability to stop

   a. The inability to limit the amount of use
   b. The inability to refuse the substance if available
   c. The inability to stop using the substance for three months or longer
   d. Binge patterns of use

3. Continued use despite known adverse consequences
    a. Medical complications
    b. Psychiatric complications ranging from mood swings and anxiety to depression, panic disorders, and paranoid-schizophrenic reactions or other psychoses
    c. Social consequences, the deterioration of family and other significant relationships, work status, and legal complications

A simple way to remember this behavioral definition is the 3Cs mnemonic:

- **C**ompulsion
- **C**ontrol
- Continued use despite negative **C**onsequences

A more diagnostic definition of substance abuse and dependence can be found in Chapter 4.

Drug Absorption, Distribution, and Elimination

Drug absorption is the process and actions that occur when drugs are taken into the body and absorbed into the bloodstream. Several factors determine the absorption, including the route of administration, the dose of the drug, and the dosage form (e.g., pill/tablet, capsule, liquid, injection, spray, patch, or gum). For the desired effect or effective administration, the drug must be absorbed in adequate concentrations over time and must reach the desired site of action.

There are nine methods of absorption, or routes of administration (see Tables 3.3 and 3.4):

- Oral
- Rectal
- Inhalation
- Mucous membranes
- Skin
- Injection
- Intravenous
- Intramuscular
- Subcutaneous

The drug enters the bloodstream at the site of absorption and is pumped throughout the body. It takes approximately 1 minute for the drug to circulate throughout the body, depending on the size of the individual. Side effects occur because the drug is everywhere in the body, not just at the desired site of action.

Drugs leave the body through the kidneys, the lungs (breath), the bile, and the skin.

⊀ Classification of Drugs

Drug may be most simply defined as a nonfood substance intended to affect the structure and function of the body, most often to diagnose, cure, mitigate, treat, or prevent disease.

TABLE 3.3

Methods of Absorption

Oral
Must be soluble and stable in stomach fluids
Contents of stomach drain into intestine
Pass through lining of intestines into bloodstream
Liquid form faster than tablets
75 percent of drug is absorbed within 2–3 hours
Can lead to vomiting and stomach pain
Amount of absorption varies between individuals

Rectal
Most commonly used when vomiting, unconscious, or can't swallow
Not good absorption; irritates lining

Inhalation
Popular method
Lungs large surface area, fast absorption into bloodstream
Into pulmonary capillaries to heart and out to body
Very fast effects
May even have faster effects than intravenous injection

Mucous Membranes
Mouth or nose

Skin
Patches provide continuous metered release of drug over long time
Absorbed into systemic circulation
Slowly absorbed so level of intake is easily kept constant

Injection
Intravenous
Intramuscular
Subcutaneous
Faster absorption than oral administration
Easy to give accurate dose because it's not absorbed through membranes
Rapid rate of absorption can make it dangerous for overdose or reaction
Can be exposed to bloodborne pathogens

Intravenous
Directly to bloodstream
Precise dosage
Allows for slow administration of drug to watch for symptoms
Most dangerous because enters straight into bloodstream

Intramuscular
Absorbed faster than through stomach
Not as fast as intravenous
Need larger amount than intravenous

Subcutaneous
Fast when injected under the skin

TABLE 3.4

Some Characteristics of Drug Administration by Injection

Route	Absorption Pattern	Special Utility	Limitations and Precautions
Intravenous	Absorption circumvented Potentially immediate effects	Valuable for emergency use Permits titration of dosage Can administer large volumes and irritating substances when diluted	Increased risk of adverse effects Must inject solutions slowly as a rule Not suitable for oily solutions or insoluble substances
Intramuscular	Prompt action from aqueous solution Slow and sustained action from repository preparations	Suitable for moderate volumes, oily vehicles, and some irritating substances	Precluded during anticoagulant medication May interfere with interpretation of certain diagnostic tests (e.g., creatine phosphokinase)
Subcutaneous	Prompt action from aqueous solution Slow and sustained action from repository preparations	Suitable for some insoluble suspensions and for implantation of solid pallets	Not suitable for large volumes Possible pain or necrosis from irritating substances

SOURCE: Modified from Benet, Mitchell, and Sheiner, p. 6, in *A Primer on Drug Action*, 9th edition, by Robert M. Julieu, 2001.

There are many ways to classify drugs, such as by chemical structure or by specific effects on particular organ systems. Most frequently, drugs are classified as nonpsychoactive and psychoactive. **Nonpsychoactive drugs** are substances that in normal doses do not directly affect the brain, such as vitamins, antibiotics, and topical skin preparations. **Psychoactive drugs** affect brain functions, mood, and behavior and are subdivided primarily on the basis of physiological and psychological effects. The psychoactive drug classification includes the following:

1. Narcotic analgesics: painkillers and designer drugs (fentanyl)
2. Central nervous system depressants: sedative hypnotics, alcohol, tranquilizers, and barbiturates
3. Central nervous system stimulants: amphetamines, cocaine, nicotine, and caffeine
4. Hallucinogens
5. *Cannabis sativa:* marijuana and hashish
6. Inhalants: volatile solvents
7. Phencyclidine (PCP)

Narcotic Analgesics
Definition

The term *narcotic* comes from the Greek word *narkosis,* which means "to numb or to be in a stupor." *Analgesia* means "to relieve pain, without producing unconsciousness."

The narcotic analgesics (morphine, codeine, and heroin) come from the poppy plant (*Papaver somniferum*). (See Table 3.5.) The narcotic analgesics category also includes synthetic and semisynthetic drugs that have morphinelike action, such as meperidine (Demerol), methadone, Dilaudid, and Percodan.

The term *narcotic* was often incorrectly applied to a wide variety of drugs, including marijuana, alcohol, and cocaine. This was the result of a legal classification system rather than a medical classification. The emotional overtone of *narcotic* was frequently misapplied to those drugs considered dangerous by legislators and policymakers.

The term *narcotic* has a variety of meanings. Its scientific meaning is drugs related botanically to the opium poppy and pharmacologically to opium, morphine, and heroin. Its medical meaning is synthetic drugs having morphinelike effects on a user. Its legal meaning is anything the legislature of a state wants to classify. Its public meaning is anything the general public wants to label as belonging to a particular drug category. In some states, this includes all drugs having morphinelike action. Elsewhere the term may also be applied to drugs chemically unrelated to narcotics (e.g., cocaine and marijuana).

Additional analgesics are nonnarcotic and satisfy other functions, such as reducing fever (antipyretic) and reducing inflammation (anti-inflammatory). Other nonnarcotic analgesics include aspirin, phenacetin, and Darvon. Nonsteroidal anti-inflammatory drugs (NSAIDs) include Naprosyn and Motrin.

Heroin

There are an estimated 166,000 heroin users in the United States (SAMHSA 2004).

Common street names for heroin include big bag, big H, blanco, bomb, boy, brother, brown, brown rocks, brown sugar, caballo, cat, chich, Chinese red, Chinese white, chiva, crap, dogie, doojee, dope, duji, dust, eighth, flea powder, garbage, good stuff, H, hard stuff, harry, H-caps, henry, him, horse, hombre, jones, joy powder, junk, Mexican mud, mojo, muzzle, pack, poison, powder, pure, red chicken, red rock, rock, scag, schmeck, smack, stuff, tecata, thing, white boy, white junk, and white stuff.

TABLE 3.5			
Narcotic Analgesics Classification			
Natural Opioids	**Synthetic**	**Semisynthetic**	**Antagonists**
Morphine	Demerol	Dilaudid	Narcan
Codeine	Meperidine	Percodan	Naloxone
Opium		Talwin	

Brief History of the Narcotic Analgesics   The opiates have been used for medicinal purposes and pleasure since prehistoric times. Opium eating has been known in Asia for thousands of years. A brief history follows:

1806: Friedrich Wilhelm Adam Serturner, a German chemist, isolated morphine from opium.

1832: Codeine was isolated.

1845: Alexander Wood invented the hypodermic syringe.

1861–65: Approximately 45,000 U.S. Civil War soldiers were addicted to morphine.

1874: Alder Wright, a London chemist, first synthesized heroin from morphine.

1875: A San Francisco ordinance prohibited the smoking of opium in public houses and opium dens.

1906: U.S. Pure Food and Drug Act required all medicines containing opiates and certain other drugs to list them on the labels.

1914: Harrison Narcotics Act required licensure of drug manufacturers, importers, pharmacists, and physicians marketing or prescribing narcotics. Patent medicine manufacturers were exempt from the act, provided that their products did not contain more than two grains of opium, or one-eighth grain of heroin per ounce.

1942–43: During World War II, a German chemist, Aschenbrenner, synthesized methadone and named it Dolophine, after Adolph Hitler.

1970s: Most addicted U.S. soldiers returning from Vietnam withdrew from heroin on the trip back to the United States or shortly thereafter. The anticipated need for heroin treatment was not realized.

1978: Scientists discovered endorphins; these proteins play an important role in the body's pain suppression system.

Chemists first isolated morphine in the early nineteenth century. During the Civil War, doctors widely used morphine in injectable form. Addiction to morphine was very common at that time, resulting in a significant addict population. Fortunately, society attached no stigma to the soldiers' addiction to morphine; it was commonly referred to as "soldiers' disease." Most soldiers withdrew from morphine on their own or under medical supervision, and there was minimal social impact.

Around the 1870s, manufacturers added tincture of opium to many patent medicines sold over the counter for treatment of diarrhea in infants and children. When first introduced at the end of the nineteenth century, heroin was thought to cure opium dependence and morphinism.

Routes of Administration   Users may inject narcotics either intravenously, subcutaneously (under the surface of the skin—known as skin popping), or deep within the muscle. They can also snort narcotics intranasally, smoke it, or absorb it into their bodies via the mucous membranes of the mouth or rectum (using suppositories). The route of administration determines how quickly the drug affects the brain: A drug that is smoked reaches the brain in 5 seconds; one injected intravenously reaches the brain in 14 seconds. A drug taken by mouth takes 30 to 45 minutes to hit the brain.

The intensity of the drug effect and the complications are also influenced by the route of administration. Intravenous use can lead to infection, local abscesses, disseminated infections (HIV, hepatitis B, pulmonary emboli), and local damage to the lungs and lining of the nose.

Major Effects

1. Pain relief (analgesia)
2. Euphoria (sense of well-being)
3. Cough suppressant (antitussive)
4. Respiratory depression
5. Sedation or drowsiness
6. Constriction of the pupils (pinpoint pupils)
7. Nausea and vomiting
8. Itching
9. Decrease in gastrointestinal activity (constipation)

Hazards   Even while using low to moderate doses, users face many hazards related to the circumstances of illicit use, such as drug impurities, infection, and the consequences of the addict lifestyle. By using dirty and shared needles, they contract infections such as HIV/AIDS, hepatitis, tetanus, and all other bloodborne infections (septicemia) leading to endocarditis and to liver, brain, and skin abscesses.

Other hazards include allergic (anaphylactic) reactions to the narcotic or substances used to cut or dilute the narcotic. Overdosing causes cardiac arrest, lung reaction, and the narcotic's direct actions on the brain, leading to coma, shock, respiratory arrest, and death.

Tolerance   Tolerance develops to a rapid degree with the effects of analgesia, respiratory depression, sedation, and feelings of euphoria. In effect, users must take more and more of the narcotic to get the original effect.

The rate of tolerance depends on the pattern of use, route of administration, and physical aspects of each individual. Even though some addicts build to phenomenally high doses, inevitably there is always a final dose that can produce death from respiratory depression.

Tolerance often returns to normal after withdrawal. Many narcotic addicts have fatally overdosed by returning to their normal and customary doses after detoxification.

Cross-tolerance exists even between chemically dissimilar opioids.

Withdrawal   Withdrawal symptoms and their severity depend on the specifics of the drug being used. With low doses of intermittent narcotic use, withdrawal symptoms may be negligible or perhaps resemble mild, flulike symptoms. Anyone who has ever been seasick can identify with these feelings. Withdrawal symptoms include the following:

- Appetite suppression
- Nausea and vomiting
- Dilated pupils

- Gooseflesh, or increased pylomotor activity—the skin resembles a plucked turkey, hence the expression "going cold turkey"
- Restlessness
- Intestinal spasms
- Abdominal pain
- Muscle spasms
- Kicking movements—hence the expression "kicking the habit"
- Occasional diarrhea
- Increased heart rate and blood pressure
- Chills alternating with flushing and sweating
- Irritability
- Insomnia
- Violent yawning
- Severe sneezing and runny nose (rhinorhea)
- Crying and tearing, nasal inflammation
- Depressive mood and tremor

The peak intensity of withdrawal occurs at 48 to 72 hours (2 to 3 days) for heroin, but for methadone the peak withdrawal is from 5 to 7 days.

Despite these symptoms, the management of withdrawal from opiates is far less dangerous than the management of alcohol withdrawal. The effects of the withdrawal are not life threatening but may need medical attention. The medical conditions worthy of attention may be excessive weight loss, dehydration, body chemistry disturbances, and stress on the cardiovascular system. Without treatment, symptoms usually disappear in 7 to 10 days for heroin but may last 2 to 3 weeks for methadone (see Table 3.2).

Opiates and Pregnancy Chronic use of opiates, especially heroin, results in a variety of obstetrical compromises. Because withdrawal in an addicted mother may lead to spontaneous miscarriage, the consensus of the medical community to date is to stabilize the heroin-addicted mother on methadone during the pregnancy. However, these babies tend to be born prematurely, with a lower birth weight. Born addicted, these babies may display withdrawal symptoms and have significant neonatal difficulties, with lifelong negative effects on psychomotor development.

Central Nervous System Depressants

Most central nervous system (CNS) depressants are sedative hypnotics. These include alcohol, barbiturates, and tranquilizers.

Alcohol

Alcohol acts as a depressant on the central nervous system. Once absorbed, it is distributed throughout the body, enters the brain easily, and is uniformly found in all body fluids. In pregnant women, alcohol crosses the placental barrier into the fetus.

A blood alcohol level of 0.05 percent or higher produces some driving impairment. In all U.S. states, anyone driving with a 0.10 percent blood alcohol level is driving under the influence. Alcohol is metabolized at a relatively constant rate, which depends primarily on the body weight of the drinker. A 150-pound man metabolizes approximately three-quarters to one ounce of alcohol in an hour.

Brief History of Alcohol

1500 B.C. : Book of the Dead mentioned "hek," a form of beer made from grain.

2225 B.C. : The Code of Hammurabi, Assyria, involved rules for the keeping of beer and wine shops and taverns.

400 B.C. : Plato wrote rules for the leader of the "symposia" to try to control the excessive drinking that went on. This was probably an ancient version of the "designated driver" (of course, back then it was the chariot driver).

Eighth century: Numerous taverns and beer houses were established in Britain.

Sixteenth century: Through the distillation process, Irish settlers manufactured and distributed "usquebach," or whiskey.

1660: Distilleries were licensed and the popularity of gin became widespread.

1770s: The British brought beer and alcohol to Colonial Americans.

1777: After the American Revolution, there was an increase in rum consumption as a new American freedom, when prior to the revolution there was some success in regulating taverns. Corn whiskey became popular after the Louisiana Purchase added new American corn-growing territories.

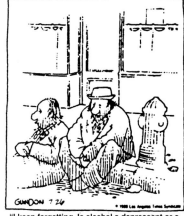

"I keep forgetting. Is alcohol a depressant or a stimulant?"

Alcohol is a CNS depressant.
© 1980 Richard Guindon. Reprinted by permission.

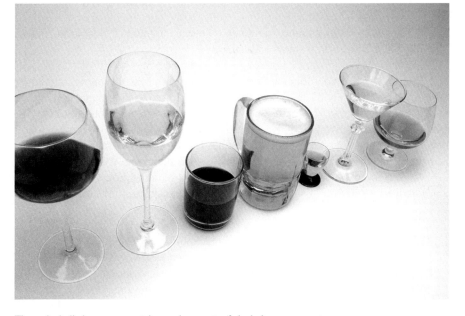

These alcoholic beverages contain equal amounts of alcohol.

> Late 1700s: Dr. Benjamin Rush, champion of the temperance movement and author of *An Inquiry into the Effects of Ardent Spirits,* inspired the nineteenth-century American temperance movement.
>
> 1917: Alcohol Prohibition came about with the Eighteenth Amendment to the Constitution.
>
> 1920s: The Roaring Twenties brought bootlegging, bathtub gin, homemade beer, and speakeasies.
>
> 1932: The Twenty-first Amendment to the Constitution repealed the highly unpopular Eighteenth Amendment.
>
> 1970–present: Numerous alcohol products have been developed and marketed, especially to young people (e.g., malt liquors, wine coolers, a variety of beers).

Estimates of Alcoholism   Other than tobacco products containing nicotine, beverage alcohol (ethanol) is the most widely used psychoactive drug known to humanity. In 2004, about half (50.3%) of Americans aged 12 or older reported being current drinkers of alcohol. This translates to an estimated 121 million people. About 16.9 million Americans (6.9 percent of the population) reported heavy drinking (SAMHSA 2004).

Major Effects   The range of physical reactions to varying doses of alcohol is vast. The effects depend on the amount consumed, the circumstances of consumption (set and setting), the drinker's body size, and the experience of the drinker. Someone unaccustomed to alcohol use is more likely to show signs of impairment than a conditioned drinker who has learned to compensate for impaired behavior. One or two alcoholic drinks may induce talkativeness in one individual, along with slight flushing, and reduce the drinker's inhibitions, so he or she appears more expansive and more animated, perhaps grandiose at times. The same amount of alcohol in another individual may induce drowsiness and lethargy.

Alcohol in even moderate doses generally reduces one's performance in tasks that require physical coordination or mental agility, such as driving a car. Larger doses can alter perception and cause staggering, blurred vision, and the manifestations of drunkenness. However, one person may become emotional or amorous, while another becomes aggressive and hostile. Extremely high doses—typical during binges—can knock out a drinker, even kill the person, if the central nervous system is depressed to the point that body functions, such as breathing, cease altogether.

Alcohol is a toxic drug with irritating as well as sedative properties. It can have a negative effect on every tissue in the human body, as shown in the following:

1. Brain

    a. Amnesia—most commonly called blackouts—causes partial, or sometimes temporary, loss of memory, often following binge patterns of alcohol use. Blackouts can occur even after low-dose alcohol consumption, or first-time alcohol consumption by someone who has a family history of alcoholism. Blackouts may be a significant early indicator of a diagnosis of alcoholism.

    b.   Permanent loss of memory and mental confusion, as in Wernicke-Korsakoff's syndrome

    c.   Damage to the cerebellum, affecting balance and coordination

2.   Peripheral nerves

    a.   Usually in the legs and sometimes other extremities, alcoholics experience pain, loss of sensation, and general weakness.

    b.   Optic nerves are damaged, causing blurred or dimmed vision.

3.   Gastrointestinal tract

    a.   Gastritis and esophagitis, irritation of the lining of the esophagus and stomach, causing mild to severe pain; may aggravate an ulcer

    b   Peptic ulcer at the outlet of the stomach (duodenal)

    c.   Fatty liver, hepatitis, or cirrhosis (a scarring of the liver that destroys the tissue and is a leading cause of death from alcohol)

    d.   Pancreatitis, in which muscle spasms block the duct from the pancreas, causes the acidic juices to back up and start digesting the pancreas. This is often very painful and can also cause death.

4.   Heart and blood vessels

    a.   Heart muscle becomes weaker, and heart expands because it is working harder. Alcohol complicates problems with heart disease.

    b.   Peripheral blood vessels are dilated by alcohol. Initially, this causes a sensation of warmth, followed by serious heat loss in the cold. The old habit of drinking alcohol to fend off the cold actually makes the person more susceptible to the cold.

    c.   High blood pressure is often associated with alcoholism, but the relationship is not clearly established.

5.   Lungs: emphysema occurs most frequently in the alcoholic who also smokes. Alcohol seems to have a direct toxic effect on the cells lining the alveoli, or small air sacs in the lungs, as the alcohol is excreted into the air.

Sobering Up Contrary to much public opinion, steam baths, vigorous exercise, black coffee, and other sobering-up agents have no effect on the rate at which alcohol is metabolized. Time is the only thing that works.

Tolerance Tolerance to most of the immediate effects of alcohol develops with frequent use. Regular heavy drinkers may be able to consume two or three times as much alcohol as novice drinkers. Heavy drinkers have to drink more and more to achieve the desired effect.

Stage 1 Withdrawal Symptoms Withdrawal from alcohol usually begins 6 to 12 hours after the last drink and may even begin in the presence of significant blood alcohol levels. Table 3.6 lists the Stage 1 withdrawal symptoms. These symptoms, in varying degrees, may last anywhere from 3 to 5 days and are relieved by drinking more alcohol.

TABLE 3.6
Stage 1 Alcohol Withdrawal Symptoms
1. Psychomotor agitation
2. Anxiety
3. Insomnia
4. Appetite suppression
5. Gastrointestinal disturbances
6. Elevated heart rate, blood pressure, sweating, and tremors

Stage 2 Withdrawal Symptoms   The onset of Stage 2 withdrawal symptoms is usually within 24 hours after the last drink but may occur as long as 3 days later. Stage 2 consists of the symptoms in Stage 1, plus hallucinations. These may be visual, auditory, tactile, olfactory (smell), or mixed. Although the visual hallucinations usually predominate, olfactory hallucinations are a particularly more ominous sign and may be accompanied by seizures. The delirium tremens—disorientation to person, place, or time—also can be life threatening; this is a true medical emergency, with a 15 percent mortality rate if untreated.

Related Illnesses   Alcoholics have twice the chance of experiencing premature deaths as nonalcoholic persons. Liver disease of varying types is one of the most prominent manifestations of alcoholism. Among young males 20 to 40 years of age, liver cirrhosis is the third fastest growing cause of death, after heart disease and lung cancer. Alcoholics also show higher than normal rates of peptic ulcers, pneumonia, cancer of the upper digestive and respiratory tracts, heart and artery disease, tuberculosis, and suicide.

Many heavy drinkers also suffer vitamin deficiencies, gastritis, sexual impotence, and infections. The more serious alcohol-related neurological disorders include peripheral neuritis (loss of sensation), Korsakoff's psychosis (loss of memory), and Wernicke's encephalopathy (mental confusion).

Fetal Alcohol Syndrome   Alcohol use and abuse by pregnant women is the third leading cause of birth defects, exceeded only by Down syndrome and spina bifida. The four basic abnormalities characteristic of fetal alcohol syndrome (FAS) are as follows:

1. Distorted facial features. A baby born with FAS has short fissures in the eyelids, a small or underdeveloped upper lip with thinned vermilion, and a diminished philtrum, the line running between the upper lip and nose.
2. Prenatal onset growth deficiency. Babies with FAS are usually two standard deviations below normal in weight and height; they exhibit little or no indication of growth spurts to catch up after birth.
3. Reduced central nervous system performance. As a result, babies with FAS have mild to moderate mental retardation; microcephaly, or disproportionately small heads; poor coordination; irritability in infancy; and hyperactivity in childhood.

4. Increased frequency of major abnormalities. Such disorders range from gross cardiovascular abnormalities and congenital heart disease to abnormal and malformed limbs.

Alcohol use during the first trimester is often responsible for stillbirths. Research further supports the position that even small doses of alcohol affect the development of the fetus, especially in the first trimester. The only safe dose of alcohol during pregnancy is no alcohol at all.

Antabuse Some alcoholics have extreme difficulty in abstaining from alcohol. Usually, they choose Antabuse (disulfiram) when other methods to stop drinking have failed. At early stages of recovery, alcoholics may use Antabuse as a deterrent to drinking alcohol, but it must not be viewed as the only modality. (See Chapter 11.)

Alcohol is metabolized by a liver enzyme (aldehyde dehydrogenose) to form acetaldehyde. Normally, acetaldehyde is rapidly metabolized by another enzyme, which breaks it into inert substances, eventually becoming carbon dioxide and water. Antabuse interferes with the enzyme that breaks down acetaldehyde. A person taking Antabuse and drinking alcohol would have a sharp increase in acetaldehyde, resulting in extreme feelings of discomfort, which include nausea and vomiting, flushing, sweating, palpitations, increased heart rate, breathing difficulty, and anxiety. Blood pressure may first rise and then fall, making the person appear to be in shock. Feelings of drowsiness may occur later. People rarely die from an alcohol-Antabuse reaction, but they feel so sick they think they will die. Nevertheless, some people continue to drink alcohol while on Antabuse.

Barbiturates

Barbiturates also belong to the sedative-hypnotic class of drugs and are widely prescribed to decrease central nervous system activity (e.g., induce sleep, relax the nervous system). Barbiturates and barbiturate-like drugs seem to affect the cortex of the brain or those areas related to sleep more than other sedative hypnotics.

Medical Uses In low doses of 25 to 50 milligrams, the short- or intermediate-acting compounds such as amobarbital (Amytal), pentobarbital (Nembutal), secobarbital (Seconal), and butabarbital (Butisol) treat or prevent acute convulsions associated with tetanus; epilepsy; and an overdose of stimulants such as strychnine, nicotine, or cocaine and the withdrawal symptoms associated with alcoholism and other sedative drug dependence. (See Table 3.7.)

For years, doctors prescribed barbiturates in the treatment of asthma, premenstrual tension, motion sickness, nausea and vomiting, peptic ulcer and other gastrointestinal disturbances, hyperthyroidism, high blood pressure, and other cardiovascular diseases. Now doctors can prescribe many newer drugs, which have fewer side effects and less potential for abuse.

Estimates of Use and Addiction After minor tranquilizers, barbiturates are prescribed more than any other psychoactive drug in the United States. Most individuals are introduced to barbiturates by physicians, who prescribe them as mild tranquilizers or sleeping pills.

T A B L E   3 . 7

Classification of Barbiturates and Their Street Names

Short-Acting

Amobarbital (Amytal)—known as blues, blue angels, bluebirds, blue devils, blue bullets

Pentobarbital (Nembutal)—known as yellows, yellow jackets, yellow bullets, nembies Butabarbital (Butisol)

Intermediate-Acting

Phenobarbital (Luminal, Eskabarb)—know as phennies

Secobarbital (Seconal)—known as reds, pinks, red birds, red bullets, red dolls, seccies, F-40s

Long-Acting

Pento-secobarbital (Tuinal)—known as trees, tootsies, double trouble, gorilla pills, rainbows

---

Many individuals find barbiturates make coping with life easier. As tolerance to the tranquilizing and sedating effects set in, individuals increase their doses, often without their physicians' knowledge. Teenagers and young adults take enough barbiturates orally to produce highs the same way as alcohol might be taken. The sources of the supply for these young people are often the black market, the family medicine cabinet, and sometimes manipulation of otherwise legitimate prescriptions.

Illicit use of barbiturates has been on the decline for the past several years in North America. Because they are still prescribed so often for a variety of medical conditions, however, their pharmaceutical use remains widespread, as is their abuse by those who have obtained legitimate prescriptions.

Routes of Administration Usually taken orally, barbiturates are readily absorbed by the stomach and small intestine. Absorption into the bloodstream can be rapid, especially on an empty stomach. Most barbiturates are white powders, odorless but with a slightly bitter taste. Most often packed in capsules and tablets of varying colors, they are also available as liquids, injectable solutions, and suppositories.

Major Effects The short-term effects of barbiturates are very similar to those of alcohol. At low doses, barbiturates tend to induce relaxation, a sense of well-being, and drowsiness. At higher doses, the drug reduces the individual's ability to react quickly and to perform skilled, precise tasks. Often there is a feeling of sedation, and the individual may alternate between feelings of euphoria and hostility and aggressiveness. This is very similar to the high-dose reactions under the influence of alcohol.

At still higher doses, the symptoms may be similar to those of drunkenness, with confusion and difficulty communicating. The person may fall into a stupor or sleep. If the dose is high enough, it may impair the respiratory function so severely that the individual stops breathing and dies.

Barbiturates and Sleep Barbiturates are generally considered by the public as sleep medication. However, long-term barbiturate use can interfere with the rapid eye movement (REM) phase of sleep. REM sleep is associated with an essential feature of healthy sleep—dreaming. Normal functioning is further disturbed with the disruption of REM sleep. When the individual stops taking barbiturates, there is often a rebound effect and more REM sleep occurs. But the dreaming is more intense and frequently turns into a nightmare. The user interprets this as poor sleeping and again takes sleeping pills, often escalating the dose, and a vicious cycle is put into play.

Barbiturates and Pregnancy Barbiturates should never be taken during pregnancy, unless advised by a physician, because they could cause birth defects. Also, the baby may be born addicted to barbiturates and have potentially dangerous withdrawal symptoms.

Tolerance Barbiturates used repeatedly over a long period can induce tolerance and physical and psychological dependence. Tolerance to the euphoric effects of the drug develops quickly in many users, so larger and larger amounts of the drug must be taken to achieve the same high.

The lethal dose is usually only ten to fifteen times the therapeutic dose, so the margin of safety is low. As tolerance develops, the difference between the amount needed to get high may be only one or two pills away from an overdose; such an amount is also potentially lethal in combination with alcohol use.

Withdrawal Table 3.8 lists typical symptoms of barbiturate withdrawal; these and other symptoms may last for days or even months. Anyone greatly addicted to barbiturates also runs a risk of having a grand mal seizure. Grand mal seizures can occur up to two weeks after the barbiturates are withdrawn and can be fatal. This is why it is essential that barbiturate addicts withdraw under a doctor's supervision, preferably in a medical facility.

TABLE 3.8

Barbiturate Withdrawal

The withdrawal symptoms may include
1. Physical weakness
2. Dizziness
3. Anxiety
4. Tremors
5. Sleeplessness
6. Nausea
7. Abdominal cramps and vomiting

From day 3 to day 7 of withdrawal, the user may experience
1. Delirium
2. Delusions
3. Hallucinations

Overdose Signs and Symptoms   The signs and symptoms of an overdose include the following:

1. Mood alteration ranging from depression to euphoria
2. Sedation or drowsiness proceeding to stupor and coma with increasing doses. Paradoxical excitement rather than drowsiness may occur, especially in the young or the old.
3. Confusion and disorientation
4. Slurred speech (dysarthria)
5. Staggering gait (ataxia), indicating that motor coordination is impaired
6. Nystagmus, or involuntary rapid eye movement from side to side
7. Pupils constricting a little at first; later as the level of unconsciousness deepens, they dilate.
8. Respiratory depression, with a decrease in the oxygen supply to the brain; this can cause death.

Barbiturates Used with Other Drugs   Barbiturates are often used in conjunction with stimulants. Amphetamine users often use barbiturates to come down after a prolonged period of amphetamine use. Barbiturates are also used by heroin addicts when their drug of choice is not available.

Barbiturates plus other central nervous system depressants can have a synergistic effect when taken together. People who drink alcohol and use barbiturates run the risk of accidental overdose. Overdoses on barbiturates plus alcohol are more common than on barbiturates alone.

Methaqualone   Methaqualone is one of several nonbarbiturates that have barbiturate-like effects (see Table 3.9). Methaqualone was introduced to the American medical market in the mid-1960s for the treatment of insomnia and anxiety. It was originally believed to have none of the abuse potential of short-acting barbiturates. It was alleged to be a safe, nonaddictive sedative; however, this drug has an extremely high abuse potential.

The popularity of methaqualone grew swiftly, given its enthusiastic medical use and street use. Among its most enthusiastic users were college students in the 1970s.

TABLE 3.9

Nonbarbiturates with Barbiturate-Like Action

- Chloral hydrate (Noctec)—known as Mickey Finn, or knockout drops when used with alcohol
- Methaqualone (Quaalude, Sopor)
- Flurazepam (Dalmane)
- Glutethimide (Doriden)—known as goofers
- Ethchlorvynol (Placidyl)
- Methyprylon (Noludar)
- Paraldehyde

Since then, methaqualone has spread not only to high school and college campuses throughout the United States but also into the adult population. Methaqualone use has also become popular among methadone maintenance patients because of the additive high the drug produces in combination with methadone.

Some street names for methaqualone are sopors, ludes, and love drug.

Principally, younger age groups use this illicit drug, with the heaviest concentration of use between high school age and people in their mid-30s. The cost of illicit methaqualone ranges from $4 to $8 per tablet.

Methaqualone is usually taken orally in pill form. Since 1984, pharmaceutical companies can no longer legally produce methaqualone in the United States. The drug is most often found on the street in bootlegged forms, which look real but may or may not contain actual methaqualone.

Following its ingestion, methaqualone is readily absorbed from the gastrointestinal tract. Once transported into the blood plasma, it is distributed in body fat, the liver, and brain tissue.

Relatively low doses (75 milligrams four times a day) produce sedation; larger doses of 150 to 300 milligrams lead to sleep. Those who use the drug to get high often take far larger doses, sometimes 600 to 900 milligrams and much more if they have been using the drug steadily enough to develop a tolerance.

Users describe the sensation produced by methaqualone as "a peaceful calm, a rush, a drunk." Some describe it as a love drug due to methaqualone's alcohol-like symptoms (e.g., loss of motor and muscle control, loss of inhibitions), although, just as with alcohol, actual sexual performance is reduced.

Basically, intoxication with methaqualone is similar to intoxication with barbiturates or alcohol and subjects the individual to similar risks: death by overdose and accidents due to confusion and impaired motor coordination.

Methaqualone has induced headaches, hangovers, fatigue, dizziness, drowsiness, torpor (extreme sluggishness, apathy, dullness), menstrual disturbances, dry mouth, nosebleeds, diarrhea, skin eruptions, lack of appetite, numbness, and pain in the extremities. Researchers have found that a coma occurs following 2.4 grams of Quaalude. Eight to 20 grams have produced severe toxicity and death.

Methaqualone overdoses are less often associated with cardiac and respiratory depression than are overdoses of the oral barbiturates. However, shock and respiratory arrests may occasionally occur. Methaqualone overdose can also result in delirium, restlessness, hypertonia (excessive tension), and muscle spasms leading to convulsions.

As with barbiturates, tolerance to the intoxicating effects of methaqualone develops more rapidly than does tolerance to the lethal dose. Withdrawal from methaqualone dependence carries approximately the same risks as withdrawal from the short-acting barbiturates and can be quite severe for a large addiction.

Japanese researchers have provided a good deal of the information about methaqualone's addiction potential. In Japan, where this drug was once available over the counter, it was widely abused by young people (Tamura 1989). From 1963 to 1966, a survey of drug addicts, in Japan found that 176 out of 411 (41.8 percent) were addicted to methaqualone. Withdrawal convulsions occurred in 7 percent of the methaqualone addicts, and 9 percent developed delirium tremens symptoms. Subsequent studies in England and in the United States have documented cases of physical

TABLE 3.10

Classification of Minor Tranquilizers (Antianxiety Agents)

Benzodiazepines	Meprobamate	Sedating Antihistamines
Valium (diazepam)	Equanil	Atarax, Vistaril (hydroyzine)
Librium (chlordiazepoxide)	Miltown	Benadryl (diphenhydramine)
Serax (oxazepam)		Sleep-Eze, Sominex, Nytol
Tranxene (chlorazepate)		
Ativan (lorazepam)		
Xanax (alprazolam)		
Halcion (triazolam)		

dependence as manifested by a withdrawal syndrome. The symptoms include insomnia, abdominal cramps, headaches, anorexia, and nightmares.

Research conducted in Philadelphia and at the Haight-Ashbury Free Clinic in San Francisco has also documented the high abuse potential and dependence-producing properties of methaqualone, as well as its cross-tolerance with the short-acting barbiturates.

Tranquilizers

Minor tranquilizers are drugs that act primarily as antianxiety agents (Table 3.10). They reduce anxiety and tension. Major tranquilizers—drugs that are used over the long term in the treatment of mental illnesses, such as schizophrenia—are antipsychotic agents (Table 3.11).

All of the antipsychotic drugs can produce Parkinson-like signs and symptoms with tremor, rigidity, and shuffling gait. To counteract these side effects, one of the following anti-Parkinsonism drugs is often prescribed along with the antipsychotic drug: Artane, Cogentin, Kemadrin, or Benadryl.

Because the major tranquilizers do not produce pleasant psychological effects, they are rarely used nonmedically and have no illicit attraction. The focus of this section is on the minor tranquilizers, which do have an abuse and dependence potential.

Medical Uses Doctors prescribe the minor tranquilizers mainly for treatment of tension, insomnia, behavioral excitement, and anxiety. Some treat convulsive disorders, symptoms of barbiturate-alcohol dependence, and the anxiety and panic that sometimes result from the use of hallucinogenic drugs. Although fairly high doses are necessary, some minor tranquilizers are also effective muscle relaxants (e.g., Valium may be used in injectable form for this purpose).

Estimates of Use Most Americans are introduced to minor tranquilizers by physicians, and most use them according to prescription, but there are large numbers who do not stay within the physician's guidelines. Recent statistics show that the prescribing of tranquilizers is on a downward trend, and some authorities believe this trend may continue.

TABLE 3.11

Classification of Major Tranquilizers (Antipsychotic Agents)

Phenothiazines	Butyrophenones	Thioxanthenes	Other
Thorazine (chlorpromazine)	Haldol (haloperidol)	Navane (thiothixene)	Serpasil (reserpine)
Mellaril (thioridazine		Taractan	Moban (molindone
Stelazine (trifluoperazine)		(chlorprothixene)	hydrochloride)
Compazine (prochlorperazine)			Loxitane
Trilafon (perphenazine)			
Prolixin (fluphenazine)			

Routes of Administration Most minor tranquilizers are usually taken orally as tablets, capsules, or liquids. Occasionally, they are injected for both medical and nonmedical purposes.

Major Effects With normal therapeutic doses, individuals usually feel well, feel relaxed, and may lose some of their inhibitions. They feel a lessening of anxiety, tension, and agitation.

As the dosage is increased, patients usually feel more sedated and may have a sensation of floating. Many individuals at this dosage level experience some depression of nervous and muscular activity, mental confusion, and physical unsteadiness. High doses may produce the following:

- Drowsiness
- Loss of muscle coordination
- Lethargy
- Disorientation and confusion
- Low blood pressure
- Memory impairment
- Rage reactions
- Moodiness and personality alterations
- Symptoms resembling drunkenness

Obviously, the ability to drive a car under high-dose levels is also impaired. Other side effects may include skin rashes, nausea, loss of sex drive, and menstrual and ovulatory irregularities.

The margin of safety of minor tranquilizers is so wide that death rarely results from use of these drugs alone, with the lethal dose being 100 or more times the effective dose. Where death has occurred, it has often been due to an interaction between the tranquilizer and other drugs, such as alcohol.

Tolerance With regular use, tolerance can develop to most of the effects of these sedatives. This means that the user has to take increased doses to get the desired effect.

Dependence and Withdrawal Even though physical dependence and withdrawal can occur with most tranquilizers, these effects are infrequent in relation to the large number of people who take these drugs. On a therapeutic dosage level, addiction may still occur. Escalation of the amount and frequency of the dose without a doctor's orders increases the chance of physical dependence.

Withdrawal from a large habit may involve anxiety states, apprehension, tremors, insomnia, rapid pulse, fever, loss of appetite, nausea, vomiting, stomach cramps, sweating, fainting, and other symptoms. Withdrawal from high-dose tranquilizer dependence is often done gradually as the individual is tapered off of the medication. A quick withdrawal can produce life-threatening withdrawal symptoms.

Addiction Potential with Alcoholics/Addicts   Physicians should not prescribe minor tranquilizers for patients who are addiction-prone. Pharmaceutical manufacturers warn physicians through medical journal ads and the *Physicians' Desk Reference* that tranquilizers are capable of abuse and dependence, especially when prescribed to addiction-prone individuals. Many patients deny or are unaware of their problems with alcohol and/or drugs, however, and fail to report this to their physicians. A thorough assessment for alcohol/drug problems is necessary before prescribing minor tranquilizers. "Non-medical use of benzodiazepines in the general population is rare and of little or no consequence; on the other hand, benzodiazepines are used with some frequency among populations with histories of drug abuse" (Woods et al. 1988).

Central Nervous System Stimulants
Amphetamines

Overview   Amphetamines are central nervous system stimulants (Table 3.12). Until recently they were widely prescribed by physicians for conditions such as obesity, depression, and narcolepsy (uncontrolled fits of sleep). For certain kinds of hyperactive behavior in children, Ritalin is most commonly prescribed.

Doctors also prescribe amphetamines for Parkinson's disease, epilepsy, nausea during pregnancy, bed-wetting, asthma, sedative overdoses, and hypotensive states associated with anesthesia. Because amphetamines relieve sleepiness and fatigue, they are widely used nonmedically by students cramming for exams, long-distance truck drivers, night-shift workers, and individuals seeking general stimulation.

TABLE 3.12

Classification of Stimulants

Amphetamines	Cocaine (Benzoylmethylecognine)	Other Stimulants
Benzedrine (amphetamine)		Ritalin (methylphenidate)
Dexedrine (dextroamphetamine)		Preludin (phenmetrazine)
		Tenuate (diethylpropion)
Methedrine, Desoxyn (methamphetamine)		INH (isoniazid)
		Coffee, colas, tea (caffeine)
		Tobacco (nicotine)

In the mid-1960s, a phenomenon new to North America emerged: intravenous use of massive doses of amphetamines (usually methamphetamines) by chronic abusers, or speed freaks. This abuse pattern had been common in Japan and some parts of Europe following World War II, when stockpiles of amphetamines used by the military were diverted to more general use.

As a result of amphetamines' abuse potential, physicians have sharply restricted their use. Now they prescribe amphetamines primarily for narcolepsy, hyperkinetic syndrome in children, certain mental conditions, and short-term weight control. David Smith and Donald Wesson (1988) note that in 1972, when the U.S. government put federal control over stimulants in the same category as narcotic control, legitimate production of stimulants was reduced by 80 percent.

Street Names for Amphetamines Common street names are A, AMT, bam, beans, bennies, black beauties, black mollies, brain ticklers, brownies, bumblebees, cartwheels, chalk, chicken powder, crank, Christmas trees, crossroads, cross tops, crystal, dexies, diet pills, dolls, double cross, eye openers, fives, footballs, forwards, hearts, jam, jellybeans, leapers, lid poppers, lightning, meth, pep pills, purple hearts, rippers, sparkle plenties, sparklers, speed, splash, sweets, tens, thrusters, truck drivers, turnabouts, uppers, uppie, ups, wake-ups, water, and white crosses.

Estimates of Use The Substance Abuse and Mental Health Services Administration (SAMHSA 2004) reports that the number of recent methamphetamine users was 318,000 in 2004.

Routes of Administration Amphetamines are available in a variety of forms; tablets and capsules are the most common. Amphetamines are usually taken orally or injected intravenously.

Methamphetamine (speed) is usually in powder or crystal form and is made illicitly. The solid form of methamphetamine with the street name ice was first cooked up in Hawaii. Ice is smoked much like freebase or crack cocaine.

Major Effects Typical therapeutic doses of amphetamines stimulate the central nervous system, increase blood pressure, widen the pupils, increase respiration rate, depress the appetite, relieve sleepiness, and decrease fatigue and boredom. Other effects include increased awareness and alertness, slight euphoria, elevation of mood and self-confidence (although the ability to perform complex tasks is usually diminished), increased talkativeness and excitement, reduced nausea and gastrointestinal upset, and dry mouth.

Adverse Effects In some individuals, even a moderate dose of amphetamines can have adverse effects, such as agitation, an inability to concentrate, anxiety, confusion, blurred vision, tremors, and heart palpitations. Higher doses of amphetamines can produce quite severe adverse reactions, which include the following:

- Tremors, palpitations
- Dilated pupils (mydriasis)
- Sweating and flushing, abdominal cramps, nausea
- Tachycardia (rapid heartbeat), heart abnormalities

- Hypertension (later hypotension), circulatory collapse
- Anxiety, agitation, and panic
- Aggression and violent behavior often associated with paranoia
- Rapid breathing, respiratory collapse
- Hallucination (visual and auditory), delirium
- Extremely high fevers
- Convulsions and seizures

Although death reports from amphetamine use are rare, some individuals who are unusually sensitive to these drugs have died as a result of burst blood vessels in the brain, heart failure, or high fever. Amphetamine psychosis, a mental disturbance similar to paranoid schizophrenia, is sometimes associated with high-dose amphetamine use, but many of its symptoms have been observed with moderate dose levels.

Injecting amphetamines causes other complications: unsterile and shared needles cause problems with tetanus, AIDS, abscesses, and hepatitis. The injection of insoluble particles in street speed also causes many problems.

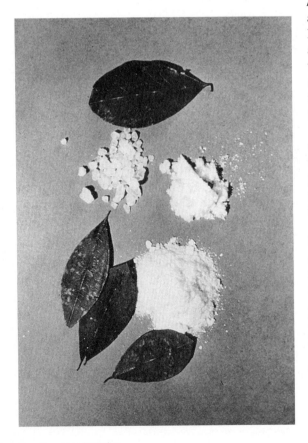

Coca leaves and cocaine.

Dependence and Withdrawal Abruptly stopping amphetamines after chronic heavy use is often followed by symptoms such as fatigue, brain wave abnormalities, prolonged sleep, voracious appetite, stomach cramps, muscle pains, lethargy, and severe emotional depression. Some of these symptoms seem just as dramatic as withdrawal symptoms from depressant drugs.

Withdrawing amphetamines from chronic users does not seem as physically distressing as withdrawal from depressant drugs. There is little evidence of any physical dependence on moderate doses of amphetamines, but researchers frequently report psychological dependence on even low doses.

Prolonged use of amphetamines leads to a broad range of illnesses. Chronic users suffer dehydration, weight loss, and vitamin deficiency. Their reduced resistance to disease allows sores, nonhealing ulcers, and chronic chest infections. Users have a higher than normal rate of liver and cardiovascular disease, hypertensive disorders, and psychiatric problems.

Bootlegged Amphetamines The newer, tighter regulations imposed on the legitimate prescribing of amphetamines have caused the widespread bootlegging of amphetamines and substitution of other substances to mimic the amphetamine high. The most common substitutes include ephedrine—a mild stimulant found in some over-the-counter asthma remedies—and phenylpropanolamine, or PPA, the ingredients in most legal diet capsules. The moderate to large amounts of caffeine in most illicit amphetamines sometimes account for the bulk of the ingredients.

Cocaine

Cocaine is a central nervous system stimulant that has gained great popularity in a variety of drug forms. At first, cocaine was expensive; only the wealthy could afford it. Today, crack cocaine is used by every socioeconomic class, making it the scourge of humanity.

Brief History of Cocaine

2500 B.C : Coca leaves were found in burial sites in Peru.

500 B.C : In Columbia, South America, large stone monolithic idols possessed puffed-out cheeks, representative of a coca chewer.

Tenth century: Incas started to use the plant referred to as "Mama Coca," and the coca tree was pictured as a beautiful woman.

Eighteenth century: The Spanish took coca leaves back to Europe. However, there was general disinterest in coca by Europeans. One can speculate that the sample of coca leaves taken from South America lost its potency during the trip.

1786: Lamarck named the species of the coca plant *Erythroxylum coca.*

1844: Conflicting reports stated that either Albert Nieman or Gaedecke isolated cocaine.

1878: W. H. Bentley espoused cocaine as a cure for morphine addiction.

1883: Aschenbrandt prescribed the use of cocaine to counteract the battle fatigue of the Bavarian troops.

1883: Sigmund Freud wrote *Über Coca* praising the medicinal effects of cocaine.

1887: Sigmund Freud recognized cocaine addiction and wrote a book titled *Fear of and Craving for Cocaine.*

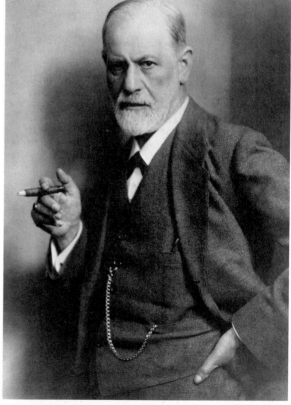

Sigmund Freud.

Cocaine is obtained from the leaves of *Erythroxylum coca,* a bush grown in parts of South America. Mountain Indians of Peru and Bolivia have chewed coca leaves as a social ritual for more than a thousand years.

The coca leaf was taken to Europe in the nineteenth century and became quite popular in certain circles. Sigmund Freud, the father of psychoanalysis, used cocaine extensively. In 1883, he recommended cocaine for treatment of morphine addiction, alcohol dependence, asthma, digestive disorders, and depression and fatigue. Freud frequently recommended the drug for what was then called neurasthenia (i.e., nervous anxiety). Freud soon realized cocaine was addictive; in 1887, he wrote *Fear of and Craving for Cocaine,* describing dependence on cocaine.

One of the most popular soft drinks of all time, Coca-Cola, originally contained extracts of the coca leaf. Coca was also present in wines such as Vin Mariani, a wine that was extremely popular with the pope and the royal families in Italy and other countries. Today, a little more than 100 years after the cocaine problems of the 1880s, we have another cocaine problem caused by coca products that are far more addicting than those of the past. Cocaine was also used as a topical anesthetic (e.g., in eye surgery) and as a local vasoconstrictor.

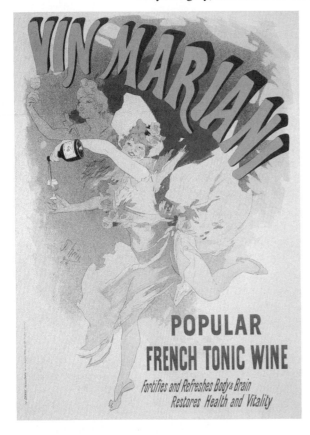

This late-nineteenth-century ad for Mariani wine, which contained cocaine, portrays the beverage as a panacea for all ills.

Street Names for Cocaine There are several street names for cocaine: Bernice, bernieds, big C, blow, bombita, bouncing powder, burese, C, charles, charlie, coke, cola, corrine, dream, dust, flake, fly, girl, gold dust, heaven, heaven dust, her, ice (not to be confused with the form of methamphetamine), incentive, jay, joy powder, lady, lady snow, nose candy, nose powder, paradise, poison, powder, rock, schoolboy, snow, star dust, sugar, white, white lady, white powder, and white stuff.

Estimates of Use An estimated 2 million Americans are current cocaine users, 467,000 of whom use crack (SAMHSA 2004).

Routes of Administration Cocaine can be inhaled, injected, or smoked. Cocaine hydrochloride is snorted or injected, while crack cocaine is smoked.

Freebase cocaine is another smokable form of cocaine. Heating up cocaine hydrochloride with a volatile solvent (usually ether) and a base (baby laxative) results in cocaine free of its hydrochloride base, with by-products of water and salt.

$$\text{Cocaine HCl} + \text{ether} + \text{base} + \text{heat} = \text{pure cocaine} + \text{NaCl (salt)} + \text{H}_2\text{O (water)}$$

Because this cocaine is extremely pure, the volatile point, or the temperature at which cocaine burns, is raised. This allows freebase cocaine to be smoked without burning it. Simply burning cocaine does not produce a high. Freebase cocaine smoke goes from the lungs to the brain in 6 seconds, resulting in an immediate and intense high. This high lasts only 40 to 50 seconds and requires repeated doses, making it extremely expensive to maintain a habit. Crack cocaine is formed by combining cocaine with baking soda; this overrides the hydrochloride acid and allows the crack to be smoked. Crack is sold in small rocks at lower prices to lower economic populations.

Major Effects The cocaine user experiences 15 to 30 minutes of excitation and euphoria, tends to talk a lot, and feels energetic and self-confident. The effect of cocaine often gives the individual a supreme feeling of well-being, control, and enjoyment of activities that may previously have been mundane. At early stages of use, men report feeling a stimulation of sexuality. Cocaine is very short-acting because it has an extremely short half-life; after the euphoria, psychological depression, nervousness, fatigue, and irritability set in. (See Table 3.13.)

Adverse Effects With heavy regular use, depression and anxiety can be so severe that the user continues to snort, smoke, or inject cocaine every 20 minutes or so for several hours to avoid the onset of depression. This pattern may develop into binges—or 24 to 48 hours of cocaine use.

Another method to take the edge off cocaine is to inject heroin with cocaine (speedballing). This form of cocaine use was implicated in the death of comedian and actor John Belushi. Addicts frequently turn to the sedative hypnotics (alcohol, tranquilizers, and barbiturates) to counteract the downside after using cocaine. This pattern of sedative hypnotic use may also cause a dependence on drugs in this classification. Acute toxicity can occur from any method of cocaine use. In the past, cocaine was thought of as a rather benign drug. Today, we know that cocaine-related deaths are more common than once thought. Cases of sudden death from cocaine use are increasing. Large doses of cocaine may cause shallow breathing, fever, restlessness, anxiety, and confusion. Even small doses of cocaine can cause a slowing of the heart rate. Cocaine use can also result in arrythmia and heart attack. High doses also have an impact on the motor systems in the brain and spinal cord, resulting in

TABLE 3.13

Cocaine Clinical Syndromes

Cocaine Euphoria	Cocaine Dysphoria	Cocaine Schizophreniform Psychosis
Euphoria	Sadness	Anhedonia (inability to feel pleasure from what would have normally given pleasure)
Affective lability	Melancholia	
Increased intellectual function	Apathy	Disorientation
Hyperalertness	Inability to concentrate	Hallucinations
Hyperactivity	Painful delusions	Concern with minutia
Anorexia	Anorexia	Stereotyped behavior
Insomnia	Insomnia	Paranoid delusions (parasitosis)
Hypersexuality		Insomnia
Proneness to violence		Proneness to violence

tremors and convulsive movements. Long-term chronic snorting of large amounts of cocaine can destroy tissue in the nose. Nausea, vomiting, and abdominal pains can occur. Death from cocaine overdose is usually due to convulsions, respiratory arrest, and/or the Casey Jones reaction, a condition during which the body acts like a runaway train exceeding its own metabolic limits. People have done and seen some bizarre things under the influence of cocaine. Case studies in Chapter 5 describe these in more detail.

Tolerance and Withdrawal According to our behavioral definition of addiction, cocaine is the most addicting drug known today, especially freebase cocaine. However, a physical tolerance to cocaine does not develop. When cocaine is used, the dopamine neurotransmitters are blocked from reuptake, stranding them in the synaptic clefts. This causes a cessation of stimulant response. However, this is not a classical tolerance reaction. This was one of the factors that led to the tragic miscalculation that cocaine was not an addicting drug. Its intense high and the user's need to avoid the crash or depression makes cocaine highly addicting and contributes to the binge patterns of cocaine use. Cocaine is one of the few chemicals (other than amphetamines and other stimulants) that exist outside of the body and stimulate catecholamine. Catecholamines are responsible for extraordinarily intense reactions to stressful situations (e.g., a father lifts a car to release his child pinned beneath it). The Casey Jones reaction mentioned above is directly related to this catecholamine-enhancing property of cocaine. Once this reaction is set in motion, it usually results in death. Some people die from nontoxic doses of cocaine due to a phenomenon known as the kindling effect. The brain is primed for, sensitized to, the effect of cocaine, so that one additional dose may trigger firing or discharge, leading to sudden death.

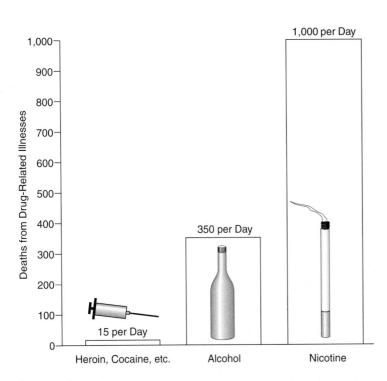

This graph shows the number of deaths from drug-related illnesses for illicit drugs (heroin, cocaine, etc.) and licit drugs (alcohol and nicotine).

Cocaine Additives Cocaine purchased on the illicit market is very seldom, if ever, pure by the time it reaches the consumer. As it makes its way from the original source down to the illicit market, the drug's purity is cut with various substances. These additives include mannitol (a mild baby laxative), lactose (milk sugar), or the psychoactive drugs procaine (Novocain), Lidocaine (Xylocaine), benzocaine, tetracaine, and amphetamine. Some individuals have allergic reactions to these substances.

Tobacco

Tobacco is the most widely abused drug. Despite warnings regarding the health hazards, approximately 70.3 million Americans (29.2% of the population aged 12 or older) were current users of tobacco products in 2004: 59.9 million smoked cigarettes, 13.7 million smoked cigars, 7.2 million used smokeless tobacco, and 1.8 million smoked tobacco in pipes (SAMHSA 2004). Tobacco use remains the single leading cause of preventable death in this country. The numbers of tobacco-related deaths are far higher than those related to alcohol or other drugs.

Diseases Related to Smoking Tobacco

1. Heart disease (coronary heart disease, increased artherosclerotic disease). Smoking elevates low-density lipoproteins (LDL, or bad cholesterol) while reducing high-density lipoproteins (HDL, or good cholesterol).
2. Peripheral vascular disease
3. Cerebrovascular disease
4. Cancer (lung cancer; cancer of the larynx, mouth, esophagus; contributing factor in urinary cancer, kidney cancer, and pancreatic cancer)
5. Chronic obstructive lung disease and colds (chronic bronchitis and emphysema)

Health Consequences

- More women die from lung cancer than breast cancer each year.
- Twenty to 25 percent of female smokers don't stop during pregnancy.
- Over three-fourths of smokers start during the developmental teenage years.
- One out of every five high school seniors smokes cigarettes on a daily basis.
- Chewing tobacco (smokeless tobacco) is the leading cause of oral cancer.
- Approximately 75 to 80 percent of recovering alcoholics smoke cigarettes.

In recent years, there has been a decrease in use of tobacco products by the general public, yet the use of tobacco, especially by young people, makes them a significant population at risk for the development of smoking-related diseases.

Hallucinogens
Definition

The term *hallucinogen* is derived from the Latin word *hallucinari,* which means "to dream or to wander in the mind." Other terms describing hallucinogens are *psychedelic* ("alters consciousness"), *psychotomimetic* ("mimics psychosis"), and *psychotogenic* ("produces psychosis").

Hallucinogens are capable of altering time and space perception; of changing feelings of self-awareness and emotion; of changing one's sense of body image; and of increasing sensitivity to textures and shapes, sounds, and taste. In addition, these drugs bring visions of luminescence, flashes of light, kaleidoscopic patterns, and landscapes. They can also induce hallucinations and feelings of enlightenment and spiritual or religious awakening.

In the past, any substance whose function is to change the habitual way of perceiving and orienting oneself toward one's physical, psychological, and social environment was considered a hallucinogen. As a result, many drugs such as marijuana, PCP, and even cocaine are inappropriately classified as hallucinogens because that is the category they seem to fit best.

In the 1960s, Timothy Leary advocated LSD as a means of "turning on, tuning in, and dropping out" of mainstream lifestyles and thinking. Of the many natural and synthetic hallucinogens, LSD is the most potent by weight and the most thoroughly researched.

Other hallucinogens include mescaline, which is derived from the dried buttons or heads of the peyote cactus; peyote buttons, which can be eaten or made into a tea; and psilocybin, which is found in a wide range of American and Mexican mushrooms. Some street names for peyote are bad seed, big chief, buttons, cactus, P, peyotl, and topi. Common street names for mescaline include beans, big chief, buttons, cactus, cactus buttons, mesc, mescal, and moon topi. (See Table 3.14.)

LSD

Common street names for LSD are acid, barrels, beast, Big D, blotter, blue acid, blue cheer, blue heaven, blue mist, brown dots, California sunshine, cap, chocolate chips, contact lens, cubes, cupcakes, D, deeda, domes, dots, electric Kool-Aid, flash, ghost, hawk, haze, L, lysergic, mellow yellows, microdots, orange cubes, paper acid, peace,

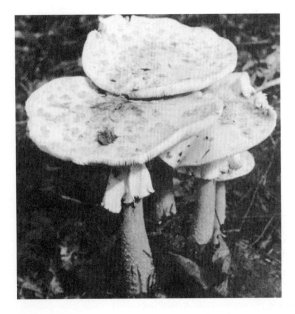

Panther mushroom.

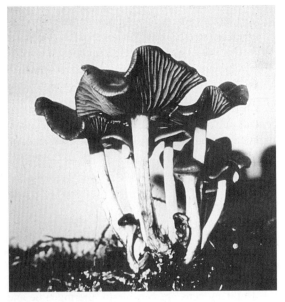

Psilocybe mushroom.

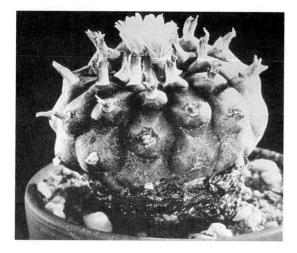

Peyote cactus.

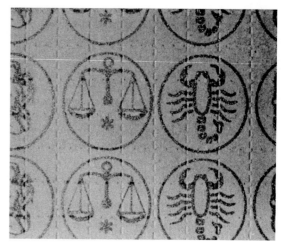

LSD blotter paper

pearly gates, pellets, pink owsley, purple haze, sacrament, strawberries, strawberry fields, sugar, sugar cubes, sunshine, tabs, ticket twenty-five, wedges, white lightning, window pane, and yellow.

Brief History of LSD and Other Hallucinogens

1000 B.C. or earlier: Hallucinogenic mushrooms were used in religious and tribal use.

700 B.C. : Hallucinogenic mandrake root was referred to by the Assyrians and mentioned in the Bible as a fertility substance.

T A B L E   3 . 1 4
Classification of Hallucinogens
LSD-25 (lysergic acid diethylamide)
Dimethyltryptamine (DMT)
Psilocybin (mushrooms)
Psilocin
Bufotenine
Harmine
Mescaline (active part of peyote cactus)
Diethytryptamine (DET)
Dipropryltryptamine (DPT)
Dimethoxymethamphetamine (DOM/STP)
Methylenedioxyamphetamine (MDA)
Belladonna alkaloids (atropine, scopoliamine, and stramonium are found in many medicines for asthma and stomach cramps)
Nutmeg (myristicin)

38: Datura was used by the early Incas and other Indians of South America. Peyote cactus (mescaline) was used by Incas and later by Native Americans.

1899: Oklahoma was the first state to outlaw the use of peyote.

April 16, 1943: Albert Hoffman, a chemist who discovered aspirin, working at Sandoz Laboratories in Basel, Switzerland, discovered LSD-25 and experienced the first LSD-25 trip.

Until mid-1960s: LSD was used in experiments in mental hospitals and laboratories to explore the treatment of mental disorders and as a means of studying psychotic behavior.

1960: Timothy Leary, Ph.D., a research professor in the Department of Social and Human Relations at Harvard University, reported a "full-blown conversion experience" after eating psilocybin mushrooms. He and Richard Alpert, Ph.D. (today known as lecturer Ram Dass), distributed psilocybin.

1961: Leary and Alpert distributed LSD.

1963: Leary and Alpert were dismissed from Harvard, giving them tremendous publicity. They coined the famous phrase "Turn on, tune in, and drop out."

1965: At an LSD conference, Sidney Cohen summarized the research on LSD use with psychiatric patients and other experiments.

1969: The Woodstock Festival took place in Woodstock, New York.

1960s and 1970s: LSD was extremely popular on the streets, especially among young people and college students.

1992–93: An increase in the trend of LSD use by young people became evident.

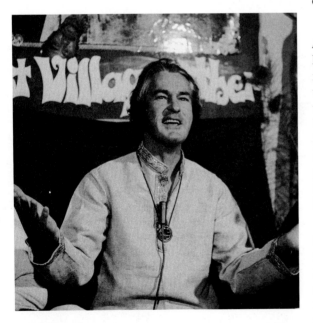

Timothy Leary was influential in the popularization of LSD in the early 1960s.

Estimates of Use In comparison with the use of hallucinogens in the late 1960s, today's use rate is smaller. But, contrary to media reports, that use has not all but died out. These drugs continue to be taken by almost a million people in the United States each year (929,000 per SAMHSA 2004). LSD is the most commonly used hallucinogen. LSD is manufactured, and hallucinogenic mushrooms grow wild in some states, as do many plants with hallucinogenic or toxic-hallucinogenic properties.

Routes of Administration Hallucinogens are usually ingested orally, but they may be smoked, snorted, or injected. Because such small amounts are required at any one time (25 to 150 millionths of a gram), LSD is often impregnated in sugar pills, blotter paper, or small gelatin squares. The nasty taste of some hallucinogens requires mixing them with other substances to counteract their taste. Teas and broths are a common method of ingesting hallucinogens.

Major Effects The effects of hallucinogens are influenced by the personality of the user, the expectations of use, the user's general experience with drugs, the mind-set of the individual, and, most important, the setting. The right group of trusting friends, a comfortable, soothing environment (e.g., dim lights and soft music), and someone experienced with hallucinogens are described as integral in developing a good hallucinogenic trip.

As a result of all these variables, users of hallucinogens report a wide range of reactions. Some individuals feel an insight and expanded consciousness, while others report a discomfort and fear of losing control that is quite disturbing. Generally, low to moderate doses of hallucinogens produce mood and perceptual alterations. LSD and other hallucinogens can produce profound effects on the user's thinking, self-awareness, and emotions. Hallucinogens distort time and space perception and induce hallucinations.

Adverse Effects Hallucinogenic experiences can sometimes add to existing neuroses, or character disorders, and can produce transient waves of mild anxiety, paranoia, or severe panic. Flashbacks (recurrences of negative hallucinogenic experiences) usually occur within a year or less from the previous use of hallucinogens. However, the incidence of flashbacks is relatively small. Flashbacks can occur in individuals who have used hallucinogens excessively and in the occasional or first-time user.

Accidents are very common under the influence of hallucinogens. The high degree of suggestibility and perceptual distortions and hallucinations often lead to accidents. Such accidents include walking through a plate glass window; jumping from a roof due to the coaxing of a friend (high degree of suggestibility); and suffering accidental falls, drownings, and car accidents.

Tolerance and Dependence Researchers have observed psychological dependence in long-term LSD users but have rarely reported dependence as a consequence of other hallucinogenic use. Hallucinogenic trips can be of long duration, compared with other drug use. Users tend to trip for from 4 to 6 hours to 12 to 24 hours. Following these trips, users are usually quite tired. This often necessitates periods of getting back to normal functioning before again using hallucinogens. Because of this pattern of occasional or intermittent use of hallucinogens, physical dependence is unlikely under most conditions. Tolerance has been shown to develop to some of the psychological and physiological effects of LSD. Quite frequently, there is cross-tolerance to other hallucinogens. For example, an individual who has recently been taking LSD generally shows a reduced response to mescaline and psilocybin.

Cannabis Sativa

Cannabis refers to any product of the plant *Cannabis sativa,* which grows in most parts of the world. In North America, the most commonly used products derived from this plant are marijuana and hashish. Marijuana is the unprocessed, dried leaves, flowers, seeds, and stems of the plant. Hashish is a more potent product processed from the resin of this herb. Researchers have obtained more than 300 cannabis

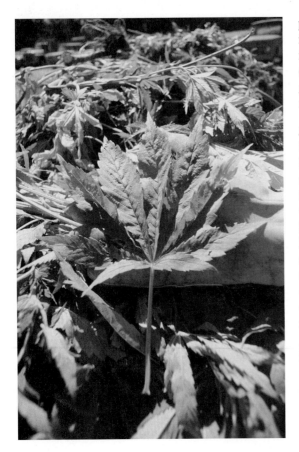

Gloved hand holding marijuana leaves.

products (cannabinoids) from cannabis. They have isolated and synthesized the most active ingredient in marijuana. This product, tetrahydrocannabinol (THC), is the psychoactive compound found in the greatest amount in the plant; it is thought to produce most of the high.

Street Names Common street names for marijuana include Acapulco gold, ace, African black, aunt mary, baby, bale, bomb, boo, brick, broccoli, bush, Canadian black, charge, Colombian, doobie, dry high, fatty, fingers, flowers, gage, ganga, gauge, giggleweed, grass, green, grefa, greta, grifa, grillo, grunt, hay, hemp, herb, homegrown, Indian hay, Indian hemp, J, jane, jay smoke, joint, joy stick, juanita, kick sticks, kif, killer, killer weed, kilter, loco, mary, maryann, maryjane, mary warner, mary weaver, meserole (messerole), Mexican brown, Mexican green, Mexican locoweed, MJ, mooca, moota, mooters, mootie, mota, mother, mu, muggles, muta, number, Panama gold, Panama red, panatella, pin, pode, pot, ragweed, rainy day woman, red dirt, reefer, roach, root, sassafras, sinsemilla, smoke, snop, stick, sweet lucy, tea, Texas tea, twist, weed, wheat, yerba, and Zacatecas purple. Street names for hashish include black hash, black Russian, blond hash, canned sativa, hash, Lebanese, and mahjuema.

Brief History of Marijuana

2737 B.C. : The earliest reference to marijuana by a Chinese treatise on pharmacology was attributed to Emperor Shen Nung.

Second century B.C. : The Scythians, a warlike and mobile Middle Eastern tribe, spread cannabis into Egypt and then northward to Russia and Europe. They had a ritual of throwing hemp seeds on heated stones and inhaling the vapors (funeral rite).

650 B.C. : The use of cannabis was mentioned in Persia and Assyria.

400 B.C. : The use of cannabis was mentioned in Rome.

1545: The first record of a marijuana plant in the New World occurred when Spanish traders introduced marijuana to Chile.

1611: Sir Walter Raleigh was ordered by the British to grow hemp in his Virginia colony. Hemp was much needed for the strong shipbuilding industry of the time.

1765: George Washington grew marijuana hemp and is said to have experimented with the medicinal or intoxicating potency of the plants.

1804–44: Jacques-Joseph Moreau of France used marijuana in the treatment of melancolia, hypomania, and other forms of mental disorder.

1839: W. B. O'Shaughnessy, a young chemistry professor, used marijuana for
   medicinal use as an anticonvulsant and an appetite stimulant.

1846: A group of French writers formed the "Club des Hachichias," meeting in
   Paris once a month, where they often smoked marijuana. The meetings were
   attended by Victor Hugo, Baudelaire, Dumas, Gautier, and De Nerval.

Early 1900s: It is believed that the drug and use of the word *marijuana* were
   introduced to the United States by migrant Mexican laborers.

1937: Henry Anslinger, commissioner of the Bureau of Narcotics, campaigned
   on the dangers of marijuana.

1937: The federal government developed the Marijuana Tax Act and used
   taxes to outlaw the drug.

October 1969: A Gallup Poll estimated that 10 million Americans, half of them
   under 21 years of age, have smoked marijuana.

1970: The Controlled Substance Act, supported by the American Medical
   Association, reported that marijuana had no potential medicinal use,
   ignoring years of medical evidence to the contrary.

Estimates of Use   Marijuana is the most widely used of all illicit drugs. Past-month
users number 14.6 million (61.1 percent of U.S. population) (SAMHSA 2004).

Medical Uses   Cannabis, primarily in the form of synthetic THC, has been under
scientific investigation in recent years to ascertain its potential therapeutic uses. One
approved therapeutic use is as an antiemetic (antivomiting) agent for the nausea
and vomiting associated with chemotherapy treatment for cancer patients. It is also
medically used to relieve the intraocular pressure accompanying glaucoma. Both
of these medical uses are the most well researched. Other potential medical uses of
marijuana researched thus far include spasm relief, asthma relief, anxiety reduction,
and relief of alcohol withdrawal symptoms. Studies in these areas have not been as
prolific, or as conclusive, as those regarding chemotherapy and glaucoma (Solomons
and Neppve 1989).

   As of 2001, thirty-four states had statutes on the books allowing marijuana,
typically in the form of THC, to be used in medical research and/or medical treatment as a part of a clinical investigation. The number of states that have actually
implemented these procedures is much smaller. The political and moral/ethical emotionality of our times may further hinder these investigations into the effectiveness
of marijuana in medical research. For this reason, other synthetically produced cannabis derivatives are also under investigation.

Routes of Administration   Marijuana can be smoked in hand-rolled cigarettes, or
joints. Today's higher-potency marijuana is usually smoked in a pipe—most frequently, a water pipe. This allows the most intense high with the least waste of the
marijuana.

   Generally, hashish has a much higher THC content, though it varies widely in
potency. Hashish can be crumbled and rolled into a cigarette for smoking; often, it is
mixed with a lower-grade marijuana or tobacco. In this country, hashish is normally
smoked in a water pipe.

Marijuana and hashish can also be eaten in cookies, brownies, and other food or made into a tea. In this form, the high lasts longer, since it is slowed down by the digestive processes.

Cannabis resin is not water soluble, so the drug cannot be injected. The few who have tried using it this way usually experienced violent convulsions.

Major Effects   The effects of cannabis depend on the potency of the drug, the method of use, and the experience and expectations of the user regarding what will happen. For low-dose periodic use, the common effects of marijuana use are these:

- Intensification of thoughts and feelings
- Feelings of exhilaration, relaxation, giddiness
- Minor increase in heart rate
- Drowsiness, dry mouth and throat, bloodshot eyes
- Impaired short-term memory
- Altered states of time and space
- Dilated pupils

For a list of experiences that adult users tend to describe as positively affected by marijuana use, see Table 3.15.

Increased Potency of Marijuana   You might remember hearing about types of marijuana such as Acapulco gold, Maui Wowi, or Panama red. Most of the potent

---

TABLE 3.15

Aspects of Life Experience Adult Daily Users Most Frequently Described as Positively Affected by Marijuana

- Ability to relax and enjoy life
- Enjoyment of food
- Ability to overcome worry and anxiety
- Ability to sleep well
- Ability to avoid feeling bored
- Enjoyment of sex
- Understanding of others
- Creativity
- Ability to avoid feeling angry
- Ability to enjoy varied activities
- Self-understanding
- Overall happiness
- Ability to avoid feeling depressed
- Ability to be tolerant and considerate of others

SOURCE: Herbert Hendin et al., *Living High: Daily Marijuana Use by Adults,* Copyright © 1987 Human Sciences Press. Reprinted by permission of Insight Books, New York, NY.

marijuana in the 1960s was imported from these places. Today, homegrown marijuana is the staple of American pot smokers. The more than 14 million pot smokers in the United States prefer the high-potency sinsemilla grown in hidden caches throughout the United States. Humboldt County in California is a well-known locale of this homegrown cultivation. The California gold rush continues there in the form of marijuana crops, despite increased eradication efforts.

In the 1960s, the THC content of marijuana was 1 to 2 percent in potency. Most users would smoke half a joint to get high. Two or three joints passed among friends could get everyone high. Today, the THC content of marijuana averages 6 percent. One hit is enough to keep an individual loaded. Today, hashish is 10 percent THC, and hash oil is 20 percent THC. This increase in the potency of marijuana means we are looking at a new drug with new problems. The research of the past with marijuana in the 1 to 2 percent THC level does not apply to marijuana now in use.

Subjective effects of cannabis intoxication have been reported in hundreds of different ways. Common reports include happiness, warmth, conviviality, camaraderie, and the ability to enjoy music and art better than when sober. Reactions to marijuana depend a great deal on the attitude of the user and the compatibility of the surroundings (set and setting). Cannabis is sometimes classified as a mild hallucinogen. With the increase in potency of marijuana, this classification may be warranted.

Adverse Effects The long-term effects of chronic cannabis use are at the heart of the current medical debate on this drug. Strong psychological dependence does develop in many regular users of marijuana, as evidenced by a need for cannabis use every day to perform certain tasks, to relax and unwind, or to sleep. The individual's life begins to revolve around the use of marijuana as a primary activity. The user tends to use marijuana more frequently throughout the day and evening.

Withdrawal symptoms after steady use may include irritability, decreased appetite, restlessness, sleep disturbances, sweating, nausea, or diarrhea. Hangovers are not uncommon. However, unlike the alcohol hangover, which causes headaches and sensitive optic nerves, the cannabis hangover is more likely to be light-headedness characterized by the inability to gather thoughts. When the drug is ingested, the effect can linger on for an entire day, along with nausea, body aches, and other symptoms.

Despite the lack of classic withdrawal symptoms, some patterns of marijuana use fit the behavioral definition of addiction. Researchers have well established the fact that chronic marijuana use can cause physical dependence by identifying full-blown withdrawal symptoms in the newborn babies of marijuana-dependent mothers. Treatment for the addiction to marijuana requires the support of an outpatient treatment counselor knowledgeable about alcohol/drug recovery and marijuana dependence. Marijuana Anonymous groups have also developed to meet the rising incidence of dependence on marijuana.

Anxiety and panic reactions are common with chronic marijuana use. Many individuals who have used marijuana to self-medicate affective disorders, such as depression and bipolar disorder, can experience severe anxiety and panic reactions. Individuals experiencing psychologically negative reactions may require temporary hospitalization so they don't lose control and hurt themselves or others.

Damage to the Respiratory System The tars in cannabis smoke are 50 percent greater by weight than tobacco tars and 70 percent higher in cancer-producing substances. Considering that marijuana is deeply inhaled and the smoke is held in the lungs, instead of passively inhaled, as in cigarette smoking, the cancer-causing risk is increased by marijuana smoking.

Long-term, heavy smoking of cannabis is associated with bronchial problems, sore throat, and chronic coughing. These conditions may be more severe in chronic hashish users. In addition, those who smoke tobacco as well as cannabis products have an added risk of bronchial problems and cancer.

Immune System Effects Research suggests that cannabis, particularly when used regularly, tends to suppress the body's immune response and ability to combat infections (Cohen 1986). Marijuana temporarily arrests the maturation of developing T cells, which protect the body from colds and other bacterial infections. This increases the chances of illness due to either bacteria or viruses. The most prominent indication of this effect is the higher incidence of bronchial infections, coughing, bronchitis, and pneumonia noted among chronic, heavy marijuana users.

Reproductive System Effects Chronic use of cannabis decreases sperm motility and serum testosterone in men and interferes with the menstrual cycle in women, thus affecting fertility. Most of these effects are reversed after marijuana use is discontinued. Marijuana is suspected to be harmful to the fetuses in pregnant women; research with rhesus monkeys has shown pregnancy problems such as stillbirth and spontaneous abortion. Reduced birth weight is also a characteristic of surviving fetuses.

Brain System Effects Considerable debate continues over the effects of cannabis on the brain. A certain percentage of users develop lethargy, apathy, and disorientation, which persist long after chronic use has been discontinued. Fortunately, these effects appear to wear off gradually. Some researchers claim that long-term changes occur in some brain wave patterns; these claims are being investigated further.

Impairment of Maturation Process Most researchers agree that cannabis use, during the primary developmental years of 11 to 15, in particular, interferes with physical and mental maturation processes and impedes emotional development. Research describes an amotivational syndrome with symptoms of apathy, lethargy, and a general lack of involvement and motivation in growth and developmental activities.

Marijuana and Driving Cannabis intoxication and chronic marijuana use impair short-term memory, alter the user's sense of time and space, and impair overall coordination and motor functioning. The ability to track other vehicles is also impaired and is a major problem in driving a car. Tracking involves judging time, distance, and the speed of other cars. Skills such as merging into traffic, making U-turns, and performing other driving tasks require tracking skills. Adding another drug, such as alcohol, only makes the situation worse. Many persons insist that their driving performance is improved under the influence of marijuana. This is due to their increased sensitivity to enjoying driving, not to a realistic evaluation of driving ability.

Smoking marijuana also makes it very dangerous to operate machinery and other equipment, since perception and timing are off, and the drug may also produce fatigue and drowsiness.

A study of airplane pilots reported that, after smoking marijuana, performance was impaired up to 2 to 3 days later, despite the pilots' thinking that they did extremely well on simulated tests (Rohr 1989). Other problems include (1) true allergic reactions to cannabis for a small minority of users, (2) gastrointestinal disturbances and weight loss among a small percentage of heavy users, and (3) difficulty in medical control of some diabetic users.

Inhalants

From time to time, the phenomenon of inhalant use is brought to public attention. In the 1960s, there was an epidemic of glue sniffing. Nowadays, there is still a consistent use of various solvents, aerosols, and other gases that people inhale to get high. Inhalant use is more prevalent in young people, people of color, and minorities who do not have the money to buy drugs. And, in certain locations, the problem is much more serious because of the number of young people who use inhalants to get high, yet this is hardly a modern-day phenomenon. Table 3.16 lists some common inhalants.

Brief History   Some inhalants and anesthetics, such as nitrous oxide, ether, and chloroform, were used recreationally in the nineteenth century, especially during times of liquor scarcity. This occurred in Europe, Great Britain, and North America, where ether inhalation parties were common among students and physicians.

In the 1960s, the inhalation of volatile substances such as plastic model glue, nail polish removers, and aerosol sprays occurred frequently among adolescents. A wave of anti-glue-sniffing publicity at the time resulted in many local and state laws prohibiting minors from buying such substances. In spite of these laws, inhalant vapors and sprays continue to be used today, partially because of the widespread application of such products in household use and partially because of ineffective legislation and enforcement.

In the 1970s and 1980s, paint became the primary inhalant of abuse. Users sprayed cans of paint, preferably gold and silver, into rags that they stuffed under their noses to inhale the fumes. These huffers (paint inhalers) were often inner-city

---

TABLE 3.16

Classification of Inhalants

A wide variety of names apply to inhaled substances. Many liquids also contain alcohol and petroleum distillates.

Naphtha	Fluorocarbon propellants
Benzene	Nitrous oxide
Acetone	Amyl nitrite, butyl nitrite
Toluene	Anesthetic gases (e.g., ether, chloroform)
Carbon tetrachloride	Gasoline

Latinos and other young people of color. Native American youth have an extremely high incidence of gasoline inhalant use. In 2004, an estimated 856,000 persons had used inhalants for the first time in the past 12 months (SAMHSA 2004). Inhalants—particularly volatile solvents, gases, and aerosois—are often among the first drugs that young children use. One national survey indicates that about 6 percent of U.S. children have tried inhalants by fourth grade (NIDA 2004).

Route of Administration   Inhalation accomplished is in any number of ways, depending on the ingenuity of the user. Inhaling fumes can be accomplished by placing the substance on a rag; placing or spraying the substance in a plastic bag; or, in the case of some pressurized gases, filling up a balloon, then waiting for the frozen vapor to warm up (if necessary) before inhaling. Users also sometimes go into a food market, smash the bottom of whipped cream cans, and squirt the gas from the broken containers into the backs of their throats. This aerosol freon gives them a cheap high.

Absorption of gases and volatile liquids is efficient and rapid. Absorption into tissues begins with the nasal mucous membranes. The major absorption site is the lungs, where substances enter the bloodstream. From the lungs, substances are distributed directly to the brain and other organ systems. They also enter fatty tissue.

Available Forms of Inhalants   Glue, model cement, fingernail polish removers, various cosmetics, various cleaning solvents, gasoline, paint, paint thinners, lighter fluids, antifreeze, aerosol cans, and white correction fluids can all be inhaled.

Major Effects   Users report a feeling of well-being, a reduction of inhibitions, and an elevated mood. In many respects, the effects are similar to those produced by alcohol and other sedatives. Higher doses often produce laughing and giddiness, feelings of floating, dizziness, time and space distortions, and illusions. (See Table 3.17.) Some substances induce psychedelic effects. An inhalant's effects may last anywhere from 5 minutes to an hour, depending on the substance and the dose.

Many people do not understand why anyone would actively seek a high from inhalants. They forget how young children often twirl to feel the effect of dizziness and how children, adolescents, and even adults are exhilarated by the rides

---

TABLE 3.17

Signs and Symptoms of Inhalant Use

1. Slurred speech
2. Odor of the substance being used
3. Mental disorientation or confusion
4. Headaches, dizziness, and weakness
5. Muscle spasms in the neck, chest, or lower extremities
6. Euphoria, exaggerated feeling of well-being
7. Loss of balance and ataxia (uncoordinated walk)
8. Nystagmus (eye movement from side to side)

at amusement parks, especially the rides that give them feelings of vertigo. These effects are altered states of consciousness that are reinforcing to many individuals. Such is the case with inhalant abusers. Other reasons for using inhalants include (1) recreation (fun, mood elevation, the high); (2) peer group influence ("it was what everyone was doing"); (3) cost effectiveness (a quick and cheap high); and (4) easy availability.

Tolerance and Dependence When use of volatile substances continues for a long time and becomes heavy, tolerance may develop. Physical dependence with withdrawal symptoms has also occurred among some chronic users. These withdrawal symptoms include hallucinations, headaches, chills, delirium tremens, and stomach cramps. Hangovers lasting several days have also occurred.

There is cross-tolerance between some solvents and central nervous system depressants. For example, skid row alcoholics inhale hydrocarbon vapors from kerosene or spray paint when they run out of liquor. These solvents forestall withdrawal symptoms from the alcohol, especially delirium tremens.

Alcohol and barbiturates potentiate some of the adverse effects of certain solvents. Consequently, users risk unconsciousness or even heart failure if they add the effects of alcohol to the effects of volatile solvents.

Acute Adverse Effects Acute use of solvents often brings on confusion, drunkenness, slurred speech, numbness, runny nose, tears, headache, and muscular incoordination. Frequently, there is nausea and vomiting. Due to impaired judgment from solvent use, users often feel confusion, panic, irritation, tension, and hyperactivity and become physically aggressive.

In cases of high dosage, the general sedative-anesthetic effects take over, resulting in drowsiness, stupor, respiratory depression, and unconsciousness. Extremely heavy use can inhibit breathing and bring on death.

Many of these substances are capable of sensitizing the heart to adrenaline. Since the early 1960s, heart failure due to this effect has been suspected in hundreds of users. This has been referred to as sudden sniffing death syndrome (SSD).

Some deaths have been directly attributed to solvent use. Most of them are due to suffocation when the users faint from inhalation and their noses and mouths remain covered by the plastic bags or when they suffocate in their own vomit. Additional acute adverse effects depend on the specific products and their chemical makeup.

Long-Term Effects Some temporary abnormalities take place in liver and kidney function and bone marrow activity; gastritis, hepatitis, jaundice, blood abnormalities, and peptic ulcers also occur.

Chronic users have exhibited slow-healing ulcers around their mouths and noses. Other effects are loss of appetite, weight loss, and nutritional disorders. Brain damage also results from regular solvent use; most of the time, this has been reversible (without permanent effect) once the use was stopped.

With so many different kinds of solvents and hydrocarbons with chemically different structures, it is impossible to predict the long-term effects of the inhalation of all possible substances. Recent information suggests that some substances, such as toluene, may actually be less harmful than previously believed. On the other hand, long-term use of other substances, such as n-hexane, which is commonly found in some plastic cements, gasoline, various adhesives, and rubber cements, may cause permanent damage to the muscles. Because spray paint, aerosols, glues, and other such substances often contain a half-dozen or more ingredients in combination, researchers have had a great deal of difficulty ascertaining the exact damage potential for humans (Ashton 1990).

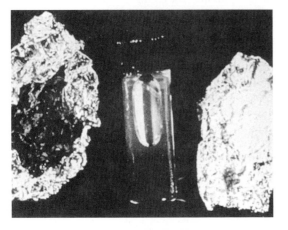

Phencyclidine (PCP).

Phencyclidine

Phencyclidine (PCP) is a drug that cannot be classified properly as a hallucinogen, a stimulant, or a depressant, causing it to be listed in a separate drug category. Originally, PCP was developed in the 1950s as a sedative, general anesthetic, and analgesic. In clinical testing, it worked fine as a painkiller, although subjects often developed visual disturbances, severe agitation, and other unpleasant side effects. These side effects caused its discontinued use with humans. Until 1978, phencyclidine was sold as a veterinary medication for immobilizing primates and other large animals. Its use as an illicit drug began in the mid-1960s.

Street Names for PCP Common street names for PCP are angel dust, animal trank, aurora borealis, DOA, dust, elephant, hog, peace, peace pill, rocket fuel, supergrass, and tic tac.

Estimates of Use The geographic patterns of PCP use are haphazard. It has long been popular on the West Coast and in certain large cities; recently, the geographical pattern of use has become more widespread.

The majority of users are young, approximately 12 to 18 years of age, though there is use by young children and adults. (PCP users inadvertently exposed infants to PCP when they stored their drugs in empty milk bottles.) Few users have been involved for as long as 10 years, probably due to negative effects, resulting in discontinuance or a switch to another intoxicant (Thombs 1989).

Routes of Administration PCP is a white, crystalline powder, soluble in water. Most commonly smoked or ingested, it may occasionally be injected. As tablets or capsules, PCP commonly comes in various sizes and colors. When PCP is smoked, users sprinkle the drug over mint leaves, marijuana, tobacco, or other substances, or they spray PCP liquid onto the substance to be smoked. One popular method is to dip cigarettes into liquid PCP. Given all these possibilities, this drug may appear as a drug or be disguised to look like any number of other substances.

Major Effects With a moderate or low dose, PCP produces a state of euphoria lasting 3 to 5 hours when smoked or 5 to 8 hours when eaten. Reactions to the drug vary greatly; much depends on the personality of the user and the circumstances surrounding the use (set and setting). Users who have bought this drug thinking it was THC have sworn that the high was like a heavy marijuana intoxication. When PCP is misrepresented as a hallucinogen, users report LSD experiences. Users who believe they are getting PCP, however, seldom have these convictions.

The most common reactions from moderate to low doses are auditory, visual, time, and other sensory disturbances. The most consistent effect is deadening of the extremities. Due to the drug's anesthetic properties, users lose control of their muscles. Depending on the individual, the overall reaction may vary anywhere from hyperactivity to complete immobility. The drug, though not a true hallucinogen, may mimic hallucinogenic drugs in some ways. It has been described by one authority as a *delusionogen,* a term that may more accurately describe its effect on the user.

Intoxication by PCP produces an experience of tranquilization, euphoria, inebriation, dissociation, and usually tactile and auditory hallucinations. The most common effects are changes in body imagery, perceptual distortions, and feelings of apathy and estrangement. The experience often includes drowsiness, inability to verbalize, and feelings of nothingness or emptiness. Reports of difficulty in thinking, poor concentration, and preoccupation with death are frequent.

Adverse Effects As with most other drugs, for some users occasional recreational or social use of small amounts of PCP does not cause undesirable side effects. However, this situation is likely to change when users take or smoke larger doses or smaller amounts consistently day after day. Users often smoke or ingest other drugs in addition to PCP, causing many unusual reactions.

Accidents With high doses of PCP, accidents are common. Because PCP produces a loss of feeling, users frequently report cuts, bruises, and torn muscles and ligaments. The dissociative effects of PCP may make users believe these injuries are happening to someone else at the time.

In the heyday of PCP use in southern California in the 1960s, high doses resulted in many drownings. In those drownings, the individuals unde the influence of PCP became disoriented; once underwater, they did not know which way was up. Drownings also result when users are so anesthetized that they forget to breathe; friends who are also stoned may not realize what is taking place (Thombs 1989).

Violence Higher or consistent doses of PCP have also led to incidents of violence. These vary widely, but many are characterized by the user's inability to feel pain. The result is a situation where the user feels extraordinary strength and immunity to pain. Police have reported high-dose PCP users breaking out of steel handcuffs, failing to stop an attack even though shot several times, coming forward and attacking police, or bleeding to death because of an inability to feel the injury inflicted during an attack. Despite several hundred reports of incidents like these, in relation to the millions who use this drug, they are considered rare.

More common adverse reactions include the following:

- Paranoia
- Severe agitation

- A severe withdrawn or isolated feeling
- Bizarre delusions
- Increases in heart rate, blood pressure
- Sweating, salivation, and flushing of the skin (these increase according to the dose)
- Nystagmus (jerky eye movements) and other reactions

PCP is unsafe to use during pregnancy, though the exact potential for damage to the fetus is unknown. PCP may also interfere with the hormones governing normal growth and development in the adolescent user. The principal proven negative effects on youthful users, however, relate to a decreased learning capacity, difficulty in concentration, poor grades, and poor social adjustment.

Unpredictable episodes of panic may occur. Latent psychopathology may be unmasked or triggered either by acute doses or by patterns of chronic use, as evidenced by episodes of violence, paranoia, and so forth. With prolonged regular PCP use, the effects can linger after the intoxication has worn off, necessitating therapy or rehabilitation. Flashbacks are also reported from prolonged PCP use. With very large doses, convulsions or coma may occur.

Several PCP deaths have been due to the direct effects of the drug. Other deaths have been attributed to PCP combined with other drugs, particularly central nervous system depressants. As mentioned earlier, deaths are more frequently due to accidental causes while under the influence.

Tolerance and Dependence PCP does not appear to be physically addictive, even though some tolerance does develop in regular users. When used orally, PCP is most often used only occasionally. When smoked, it is very often used more frequently and can create a very strong psychological dependence. Few data substantiate a withdrawal syndrome with PCP, though the drug often produces aftereffects lasting many months after use is discontinued. One of these aftereffects is depression, which can last up to a year; if untreated, it can lead to relapse and suicide.

⚹ Athletes and Drugs

Athletes have been using drugs to enhance their performance since ancient times. The use of drugs by athletes is almost as old as the Olympic Games themselves.

In the marathon event of the 1904 Olympic Games in St. Louis, Missouri, the winning runner was American Thomas Hicks, who was aided by a heady cocktail of brandy and strychnine (a stimulant at low doses, a poison at high doses). Today, more than fifty psychomotor stimulant drugs are banned from use during an Olympic competition.

The use of performance-enhancing drugs continues to be a current problem. Professional baseball players Roger Clemens, Barry Bonds, and many others were implicated in the use of these drugs. Olympic gold-medal winner Marion Jones has admitted to doping. The Tour de France has had drug-related scandals as well. Practically every professional and amateur sport has had concerns about athletes using these drugs to improve their performance.

Steroids

All of the previously described drugs used in sports and athletics can be labeled *ergogenic* because they are performance-enhancing substances. By far, the most controversial ergogenic drug used by many athletes—especially young, developing boys and girls—is steroids.

Brief History

Steroids were developed in the 1930s for the treatment of anemia and a variety of diseases that wasted away muscles. Physicians have also used steroids to treat cancer, burns, intestinal problems, asthma, and emaciation. After World War II, steroid use restored body tissue to victims of starvation. The increased aggressiveness caused by steroid use was one of the benefits sought by German soldiers in World War II.

In 1988, Canadian sprinter Ben Johnson lost his Olympic gold medals because he tested positive for steroids. Today, steroid use is a problem not only with world-class Olympic athletes but also with teenagers. Steroid use became the adolescent rage of the 1990s. Studies indicate that 6 to 10 percent of high school boys will use steroids by graduation, as will 1 percent of girls. Unfortunately, two-thirds of these young people will start to use steroids before the age of 16. Most young people who use steroids do so to enhance their performance in sports, yet a surprisingly large percentage (25 percent) use steroids for appearance. The skinny boy on the beach who gets sand kicked in his face no longer chooses the old Charles Atlas weight-training program to bulk up. Instead, steroid use with weight training and diet create the hulking bodies that young men desire. Beefing up and strengthening their bodies give these young people added self-confidence because they feel attractive (Hough 1988).

Steroids are illegal without a prescription. Federal officials estimate the illicit steroid market at $400 million.

Terminology

Androgenic steroids, which include testosterone, primarily develop and maintain male sex characteristics. So-called **anabolic** steroids are synthetic derivatives of testosterone developed in an attempt to minimize testosterone's androgenic or masculinizing effects on the individual while promoting protein synthesis and muscular growth.

Because none of these compounds is purely anabolic or purely androgenic in its effects, and since athletes usually stack, or use the steroids in combination, technically the more correct designation is "anabolic-androgenic steroids (A-AS)" rather than just anabolic steroids (AS).

Major Effects

Many of the early studies regarding the effectiveness of steroids produced conflicting results. More recent studies have clearly indicated significant increases in strength as a result of steroid use. The American College of Sports Medicine in its position statement on steroids in 1989 concluded that "gains in strength can occur through a variety of mechanisms in the highly trained athlete who takes steroids."

Increases in lean body mass do occur in A-AS steroid use. In the past, this was thought to be the result of water retention. It is now clear that there is an actual increase in muscle tissue and enhancement of muscle contractility. In addition, some reports cite an increase in actual bone density. However, most of these changes do not increase strength unless their use is combined with high-intensity weight training and a properly balanced diet.

Anabolic-androgenic steroids also increase the ability to perform high-intensity training sessions. In part, this is due to increased protein metabolism as well as the inhibition of the metabolic (breaking down) effects of corticosteroids, which are released in increased amounts whenever the body is stressed. The result is that the body requires less recuperation time between intensive workouts to repair itself. However, most studies have also shown that aerobic capacity is not affected or improved at all with steroid use.

Adverse Effects

The problem with steroids is that they do not act exclusively on one muscle or tissue group. Therefore, they stimulate all muscles and tissues, making the individual at risk for other adverse effects. The body's homeostasis is disrupted with the use of steroids, causing a variety of physical problems. "Heart disease will probably be the most widely noted side effect with anabolic steroid abuse. Blood pressure elevates significantly when an individual takes anabolic steroids due to the retained fluid and increased blood volume. . . . High Density Lipoproteins (HDL-C) that aid the body in removing cholesterol, and are important to cardiac longevity, are drastically reduced with the use of androgens" (American Osteopathic Academy of Sports Medicine 1989).

For adolescents, the drug can cause stunted growth and the premature closing of growth plates. Other problems resulting from steroid abuse by men include the following:

- Liver and kidney damage
- Breast development
- Acne, baldness
- Cysts
- Shrinking of the testicles and sterility
- Reduced sex drive
- Headaches, nausea, and dizziness

For women the drug can cause the following:

- Infertility
- Clitoral enlargement
- Breast atrophy
- Menstrual irregularities
- Male pattern baldness and voice change

More and more evidence is accruing that the most significant effect of A-AS use may be psychiatric. Psychological reactions such as extreme aggressiveness, mood swings, depression, and delusions are reported in some individuals. Signs and symptoms similar to drug and alcohol dependence (e.g., loss of control; continued use despite known adverse consequences, tolerance, and withdrawal) suggest that both physical and psychological dependence can occur with A-AS use.

Amphetamines

The first widespread abuse of drugs in professional sports occurred in the late 1960s and early 1970s, when professional football players used amphetamines. Mandell (1979) reported this as a so-called Sunday syndrome of amphetamine use to enhance performance. However, athletes in many other sports—notably, those involved in endurance events—also have used amphetamines.

Amphetamines have an appetite-suppression effect attractive to a variety of athletes for whom making and keeping a required weight is essential (e.g., jockeys, gymnasts, wrestlers, and boxers). Numerous studies have attempted to document the effects of amphetamines on performance. Some have looked at psychomotor tasks, others have examined certain variables related to overall performance, and still others have studied athletic performance (Derlet and Heischober 1990).

Smith and Beecher (1959) reported that approximately 75 percent of trained swimmers, weight lifters, and runners showed improvements in performance after administration of amphetamines. However, Karpovich (1969) found improvement in only three of twenty athletes, and one athlete actually performed more poorly. A review in 1981, using criteria based on knee-extension strength and running to exhaustion, showed that performance usually improved by only a small percentage. However, in highly competitive sports, even a 1 percent improvement can mean the difference between victory and defeat.

Most people also would probably agree that the alertness of the fatigued person, whether an athlete, a truck driver, a student, or a subject of an experiment, increases with the use of amphetamines. However, Chandler and Blair concluded in 1980 that "amphetamines do not prevent fatigue but rather mask the effects of fatigue and interfere with the body's fatigue-alarm system which could lead to disastrous results, especially under extreme environmental conditions."

Deaths caused by amphetamine use have involved cerebral vascular accidents (strokes) secondary to hemorrhages in the brain, acute heart failure with arrhythmias, and hyperthermia. The elevation of body temperature, if not fatal, can combine with heat exhaustion and circulatory collapse to cause heat stroke, because amphetamines obscure the athlete's normally protective physiologic fatigue level.

By diminishing pain thresholds, amphetamines allow athletes to continue to compete despite injury, thus potentially causing more tissue damage to the injured areas. Finally, there is an added potential for injury to others in contact sports because of the increase in aggressiveness caused by amphetamine use.

Chewing Tobacco

Epidemiologically, the percentage of smokers among athletes in the United States has declined, along with the decreasing trend in the general population. The use of chewing

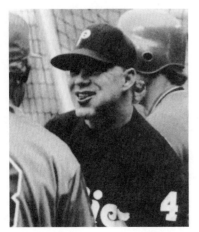

America's favorite pastime: baseball. Players still chew tobacco. Bettmann Archive.

tobacco, however, remains inordinately high among athletes. Part of this can certainly be ascribed to new marketing and promotion campaigns by the tobacco companies, as well as the almost mythic, traditional relationship of "chawing tobacco to the great American pastime of baseball. Ironically, the original baseball cards advertised tobacco. Long ago, politicians recognized the health hazards and declared chewing and spitting tobacco illegal in most places—except the baseball park.

From 1978 to 1985, celebrity athletes promoted chewing tobacco. Free supply programs and heavy advertising at sporting events stimulated the sale of chewing tobacco. As a result, chewing tobacco saw a 55 percent rise in sales at a time when cigarette sales dropped off. In 1970, men 55 and older were the heaviest users of chewing tobacco. By 1985, males under the age of 20 displaced them. Smokeless tobacco, a marketing label for chewing tobacco, is used by kindergarten children in Arkansas and Alaska; in Texas, reportedly, up to one-third of varsity football and baseball players use smokeless tobacco (Lombardo 1985).

Many people have been misled into thinking that smokeless tobacco is a safe alternative to smoking. The surgeon general's *Report on the Health Consequences of Smokeless Tobacco Use* concluded that smokeless tobacco is causally related to oral cancer and gum recession, that it can lead to dependence on nicotine, and that it is not a safe alternative to cigarettes (U.S. Surgeon General 1988). In 2004, 7.2 million Americans used smokeless tobacco (SAMHSA 2004).

Nonetheless, some athletes use nicotine products for their perceived stimulating effect before their events, while others paradoxically use the tobacco for its calming effect. Still others state they use nicotine for its effect on the satiety center ("I'll gain weight if I stop smoking"). Some just use tobacco products for personal rather than performance reasons.

Regarding the widely held misconception that smokeless tobacco enhances performance, it is critical to make known that nicotine does not heighten energy or strength. In reality, the user who smokes, chews, or snorts nicotine is simply experiencing elevation in heart rate and blood pressure. The perceived relaxation is actually relief from the craving associated with nicotine withdrawal.

Clearly, young people will continue chewing smokeless tobacco unless professional athletes, coaches, and managers act as role models and point out the negative effects of all tobacco products.

Other Drugs/Alcohol in Sports

The pressures of professional athletic competition and the accompanying lifestyle can create a situation in which athletes seek both relief and the enhancement of performance by using alcohol or other drugs. Many high school, college, and even professional athletes are ill prepared for these pressures.

The widespread use of cocaine, marijuana, alcohol, amphetamines, and other drugs in professional sports came to the attention of the general public in the drug scandals of the past three decades. This was an indicator of the high level of denial and enabling behavior by players, coaches, and management. Today, teams are making more concerted efforts at education, assessment, and treatment. They have programs that help athletes develop the skills to deal with the pressures. However, alcohol/drug problems are still enabled and/or denied at many levels of athletic competition. Additional efforts are needed to resolve the issue of alcohol/drug abuse and addiction at all levels of athletic endeavor.

⋇ In Review

- Alcohol and other drugs are found in each neighborhood and community in our society, and every family is vulnerable to the problems associated with alcohol/drugs.
- You can identify methamphetamine users by
  - Signs of agitation, excited speech, decreased appetites, and increased physical activity levels. Other common symptoms include dilated pupils, high blood pressure, irregular heartbeat, chest pain, shortness of breath, nausea and vomiting, diarrhea, and elevated body temperature.
  - Occasional episodes of sudden and violent behavior, intense paranoia, visual and auditory hallucinations, and bouts of insomnia
  - A tendency to compulsively clean and groom and repetitively sort and disassemble objects, such as cars and other mechanical devices.
- The most commonly used inhalants by young people are glue, shoe polish, and gasoline. Other inhalants include nitrous oxide, lighter fluid, and aerosol sprays.
- A simple way to remember the behavioral definition of addiction is the 3*C*s mnemonic:
  - **C**ompulsion
  - **C**ontrol
  - Continued use despite negative **C**onsequences
- Nine methods of absorption:
  - Oral
  - Rectal
  - Inhalation
  - Mucous membranes
  - Skin
  - Injection
  - Intravenous
  - Intramuscular
  - Subcutaneous
- *Set* refers to user's frame of mind at time of use. *Setting* refers to the physical environment or environmental factors surrounding alcohol/drug use.
- Drugs are classified as nonpsychoactive and psychoactive. *Nonpsychoactive drugs* are substances that in normal doses do not directly affect the brain, such as vitamins, antibiotics, and topical skin preparations. *Psychoactive drugs* affect brain functions, mood, and behavior and are subdivided primarily on the basis of physiological and psychological effects.

- The psychoactive drug classification includes the following:
  - Narcotic analgesics: painkillers and designer drugs (fentanyl)
  - Central nervous system depressants: sedative hypnotics, alcohol, tranquilizers, and barbiturates
  - Central nervous system stimulants: amphetamines, cocaine, nicotine, and caffeine
  - Hallucinogens
  - *Cannabis sativa:* marijuana and hashish
  - Inhalants: volatile solvents
  - Phencyclidine (PCP)
- Definition and sources of narcotic analgesics: The term *narcotic* comes from the Greek word *narkosis,* which means "to numb or to be in a stupor. *Analgesia* means "to relieve pain, without producing unconsciousness.

    The narcotic analgesics (morphine, codeine, and heroin) come from the poppy plant (*Papaver somniferum*). The narcotic analgesics category also includes synthetic and semisynthetic drugs that have morphinelike action, such as meperidine (Demerol), methadone, Dilaudid, and Percodan.
- Narcotic analgesics have the following major effects:
  - Pain relief (analgesia)
  - Euphoria (sense of well-being)
  - Cough suppressant (antitussive)
  - Respiratory depression
  - Sedation or drowsiness
  - Constriction of the pupils (pinpoint pupils)
  - Nausea and vomiting
  - Itching
  - Decrease in gastrointestinal activity (constipation)
- Most central nervous system (CNS) depressants are sedative hypnotics. These include alcohol, barbiturates, and tranquilizers.
- Amphetamines are central nervous system stimulants. Until recently they were widely prescribed by physicians for conditions such as obesity, depression, and narcolepsy (uncontrolled fits of sleep). For certain kinds of hyperactive behavior in children, Ritalin is most commonly prescribed.

    In some individuals, even a moderate dose of amphetamines can have adverse effects, such as agitation, an inability to concentrate, anxiety, confusion, blurred vision, tremors, and heart palpitations. Higher doses of amphetamines can produce quite severe adverse reactions, which include the following:
  - Tremors, palpitations
  - Dilated pupils (mydriasis)
  - Sweating and flushing, abdominal cramps, nausea
  - Tachycardia (rapid heartbeat), heart abnormalities
  - Hypertension (later hypotension), circulatory collapse
  - Anxiety, agitation, and panic
  - Aggression and violent behavior often associated with paranoia
  - Rapid breathing, respiratory collapse

- Hallucination (visual and auditory), delirium
- Extremely high fevers
- Convulsions and seizures
- Cocaine is obtained from the leaves of *Erythroxylum coca,* a bush grown in parts of South America. Mountain Indians of Peru and Bolivia have chewed coca leaves as a social ritual for more than a thousand years.
- Diseases related to smoking tobacco include the following:
  - Heart disease (coronary heart disease, increased artherosclerotic disease). Smoking elevates low-density lipoproteins (LDL, or bad cholesterol), while reducing high-density lipoproteins (HDL, or good cholesterol).
  - Peripheral vascular disease
  - Cerebrovascular disease
  - Cancer (lung cancer; cancer of the larynx, mouth, esophagus; contributing factor in urinary cancer, kidney cancer, and pancreatic cancer)
  - Chronic obstructive lung disease and colds (chronic bronchitis and emphysema)
- The health consequences of tobacco use include these:
  - More women die from lung cancer than breast cancer each year.
  - Twenty to 25 percent of female smokers don't stop during pregnancy.
  - Over three-fourths of smokers start during the developmental teenage years.
  - One out of every five high school seniors smokes cigarettes on a daily basis.
  - Chewing tobacco (smokeless tobacco) is the leading cause of oral cancer.
  - Approximately 75 to 80 percent of recovering alcoholics smoke cigarettes.
- *Cannabis* refers to any product of the plant *Cannabis sativa,* which grows in most parts of the world. In North America, the most commonly used products derived from this plant are marijuana and hashish. Marijuana is the unprocessed, dried leaves, flowers, seeds, and stems of the plant. Hashish is a more potent product processed from the resin of this herb. Researchers have obtained more than 300 cannabis products (cannabinoids) from cannabis. They have isolated and synthesized the most active ingredient in marijuana. This product, tetrahydrocannabinol (THC), is the psychoactive compound found in the greatest amount in the plant; it is thought to produce most of the high.
- Glue, model cement, fingernail polish removers, various cosmetics, various cleaning solvents, gasoline, paint, paint thinners, lighter fluids, antifreeze, aerosol cans, and white correction fluids can all be inhaled.
- Signs and symptoms of inhalant use are the following:
  - Slurred speech
  - Odor of the substance being used
  - Mental disorientation or confusion
  - Headaches, dizziness, and weakness
  - Muscle spasms in the neck, chest, or lower extremities
  - Euphoria, exaggerated feeling of well-being
  - Loss of balance and ataxia (uncoordinated walk)
  - Nystagmus (eye movement from side to side)
- The substances that athletes use to enhance athletic performance include caffeine, chewing tobacco, amphetamines, and steroids. Steroid use by athletes, especially young people, can be a major tragedy.

⚗ Discussion Questions

1. Applying the term *dangerous* to a drug is sometimes done from an emotional rather than a factual standpoint. Which drugs do you think are labeled "dangerous" when the adverse effects are in fact not that great?
2. Which drugs do you think pose the "most hazardous" adverse effects? Explain why.
3. Rank the following drugs in terms of most harmful (1) to least harmful (10), and defend your rationale.

    alcohol
    methamphetamine
    marijuana
    glue sniffing
    freebase cocaine
    snorting heroin
    OxyContin
    Xanax
    LSD
    cocaine

4. To what extent do you think steroids and other performance-enhancing drugs are used in professional sports? Explain your reasoning.
5. Do you think marijuana is less harmful than alcohol? Explain your yes or no answer.

⚗ Discussion Exercise

Please rate the following drugs in order: Most hazardous–11; Least hazardous–1. Include your rationale for each drug

Example:	**DRUG**	**RATIONALE**
10	Alcohol	• Most widely abused drug
		• Binge drinking by young people/college students
		• Family problems—impact on children
		• Lost costs to business—sick days, injury, illness
9	Methamphetamine	• Physical and health problems
		• High addiction potential with young people

Rate these 11 drugs or drug categories:

    Alcohol
    Amphetamines
    Cocaine
    Ecstacy
    Heroin
    Hallucinogens (e.g., LSD)
    Inhalants (e.g., sniffing glue, paint)
    Marijuana

Methamphetamine
Painkillers
Tranquilizers

Drug   **Rationale**

11 —

10 —

9 —

8 —

7 —

6 —

5 —

4 —

3 —

2 —

1 —

❊ References

American Osteopathic Academy of Sports Medicine. 1989.

American Psychiatric Association. 1994. *Diagnostic and statistical manual of mental disorders.* 4th ed. Washington, D.C.: Author.

Ashton, C. H. 1990. Solvent abuse: Little progress after 20 years. *British Medical Journal* 300: 135–38.

Chandler, J. V., and S. N. Blair. 1980. The effect of amphetamines on selected physiological components related to athletic success. *Medicine and Science in Sports and Exercise* 12: 65–69.

Cohen, S. 1986. Marijuana research: Selected recent findings. *Drug and Alcohol Newsletter, Vista Hill Foundation* 15(1).

CSAT advisory: Breaking news for the treatment field: Oxycontin. 2001. *Prescription Drug Abuse* 1(1).

Derlet, R., and B. Heischober. 1990. Methamphetamine: Stimulant of the 1990s. *Western Journal of Medicine* 153(6) (December): 625–28.

Holland, Julie, ed. 2001. *Ecstasy: The complete guide: A comprehensive look at the risks and benefits of MDMA.* Rochester, Vt.: Park Street Press.

Hough, D. 1988. Anabolic steroids and ergogenic aids. *Academy of Family Practice* 41: 1157–64.

Goldberg, Raymond. 2003. *Drugs across the spectrum,* 4th edition. Belmont, Calif.: Wadsworth/Thomson Learning.

Goldstein, Avram. 2001. *Addiction: From biology to drug policy,* 2nd edition. New York: Oxford University Press.

Hanson, Glen, et al. 2002. *Drugs and society,* 7th edition. Boston: Jones & Bartlett.

Julien, Robert M. 2001. *A primer of drug action: A concise nontechnical guide to the actions, uses, and side effects of psychoactive drugs,* 9th edition. New York: Henry Holt.

Karpovich, P. V. 1959. Effect of amphetamine sulfate on athletic performance. *Journal of American Medical Association* 170: 558–561.

Lombardo, J. 1990. Stimulants and athletic performance. Amphetamine and caffeine. *Physician and Sports Medicine* 4: 1157–64.

Mandell, A. J. 1979. The Sunday syndrome: A unique pattern of amphetamine abuse indigenous to American professional football. *Clinical Toxicology* 15(2): 225–32.

National Institute on Drug Abuse [NIDA]. 1989. *Drug use among American high school students, college students, and other young adults. National trends through 1988.* Rockville, Md.: Author.

National Institute on Drug Abuse [NIDA]. 1995. *1994 National Household Survey on Drug Abuse.* Advance Report No. 10. Washington, D.C.: Author.

National Institute on Drug Abuse [NIDA]. 1998. *Community drug alert bulletin.* Rockville, Md.: Author.

National Institute on Drug Abuse [NIDA]. 2001. *The National Household Survey on Drug Abuse: Cigar use.* Washington, D.C.: Author.

National Institute on Drug Abuse [NIDA]. March 2004. Inhalant abuse. NIDA Research Report Series. Publication Number 04-3818.

National Survey on Drug Use and Health (NSDUH). 2007. SAMSHA.

Rawson, R., et al. 2007. Use of methamphetamine by young people: Is there reason for concern? *Addiction* 102(7)(July).

Rohr, V. 1989. Withdrawal sequelae to cannabis use. *International Journal of the Addictions* 24: 627–31.

Smith, David, and Donald Wesson. 1988. *Treating cocaine dependence.* Center City, Minn.: Hazeldon Foundation.

Smith, G. M., and H. G. Beecher. 1959. Amphetamine sulfate and athletic performance. *Journal of American Medical Association* 170(5): 542–57.

Solomons, K., and V. M. Neppe. 1989. Review article: Cannabis: Its clinical effects. *South American Medical Journal* 78: 476–81.

Sporer, Karl A. 2000. Acute heroin overdose. In *Heroin overdose: Research and interventions.* San Francisco: Linden Center.

Substance Abuse and Mental Health Services Administration [SAMHSA]. 2004. Overview of findings from the 2004 National Survey on Drug Use and Health. NSDUH Series H-27.

Tamura, M. 1989. Japan: Stimulant epidemics, past and present. *Bulletin on Narcotics* 1: 83–93.

Thombs, D. 1989. A review of PCP abuse, trends, and perceptions. *Public Health Reports* 104(4): 325–28.

U.S. Surgeon General. 1988. *The health consequences of smoking: Nicotine addiction.* Rockville, Md.: U.S. Dept. Health and Human Services.

Washington FOCUS. 2004. Risk factors identified in inhalant abuse. *Washington FOCUS,* 14(3).

Woods, James H., et al. 1988. Use and abuse of benzodiazepines. *Journal of the American Medical Association* 260(23): 3476–3480.

Definitions of Substance Abuse, Dependence, and Addiction

Objectives

1. Identify diagnostic criteria for substance abuse and substance dependence.
2. Explain and give examples of the three *C*s in our behavioral definition of addiction—compulsion, control, and consequences.
3. Identify and describe the stages of drug use from nonuse to addiction.
4. Describe some of the problems in identifying "periodic excessive" substance abuse.
5. Describe the differences between early and late stages of alcohol/drug use.
6. Describe the differences between Jellinek's classifications of the different kinds of alcoholism.
7. Define and describe denial by the addict/alcoholic and his or her family members.
8. Identify important alcohol/drug assessment questions.
9. Identify the varied consequences of alcohol/drug abuse and dependence.
10. Identify the various issues that make adolescents more at risk for substance abuse.
11. Explain the relationship between alcohol/drugs and suicide.
12. Identify the differences between a screening tool and an assessment tool.

⚹ Introduction

The most difficult challenge in the assessment process is in differentiating those individuals who fall in the gray area between occasional, or nonproblematic, use of alcohol/drugs from those who use excessively and/or have an alcohol/drug problem. Assessment is also complicated by the fact that people strongly deny problems with alcohol and drugs. Individual, family, and societal perceptions of alcohol/drugs are distorted by this denial system.

The major goal of this chapter is to help the reader define substance abuse, substance dependence, and addiction, and to identify the various stages of use. The chapter also focuses both on screening and assessment tools and on clinical questions and assessment strategies.

⚹ Diagnostic Categories

The *Diagnostic and Statistical Manual of Mental Disorders,* 4th edition, text revision (*DSM-IV-TR*) (American Psychiatric Association [APA] 2000) is a primary reference used by mental health practitioners to diagnose both mental disorders and substance-related disorders.

Substance-related disorders are divided into two major categories:

1. *Substance-use disorders.* These include substance dependence and substance abuse.
2. *Substance-induced disorders.* These include substance intoxication and substance withdrawal.

The *DSM-IV-TR* also describes substance-induced mental disorders (see Chapter 10 of this textbook).

Substance Abuse

Substance abuse is described by the following diagnostic criteria in the *DSM-IV-TR* (APA 2000):

A. A maladaptive pattern of substance use, leading to clinically significant impairment or distress, as manifested by one (or more) of the following, occurring within a 12-month period:
  1. Recurrent substance use, resulting in a failure to fulfill major role obligations at work, school, or home (e.g., repeated absences or poor work performance related to substance use; substance-related absences, suspensions, or expulsions from school; neglect of children or household)
  2. Recurrent substance use in situations in which it is physically hazardous (e.g., driving an automobile or operating a machine when impaired by substance use)
  3. Recurrent substance-related legal problems (e.g., arrests for substance-related disorderly conduct)
  4. Continued substance use despite having persistent or recurrent social or interpersonal problems caused or exacerbated by the effects of the substance (e.g., arguments with spouse about consequences of intoxication, physical fights)
B. The symptoms have never met the criteria for substance dependence for this class of substances.

Substance Dependence

Substance dependence is described by the following diagnostic criteria in the *DSM-IV-TR* (APA 2000):

A. A maladaptive pattern of substance use, leading to clinically significant impairment or distress, as manifested by three (or more) of the following, occurring at any time in the same 12-month period:
  1. Tolerance, as defined by either of the following:
    a. A need for markedly increased amounts of the substance to achieve intoxication or desired effect

b.   Markedly diminished effect with continued use of the same amount of the substance
2.   Withdrawal, as manifested by either of the following:
a.   The characteristic withdrawal syndrome for the substance
b.   The same (or a closely related) substance is taken to relieve or avoid withdrawal symptoms
3.   The substance is often taken in larger amounts or over a longer period than was intended.
4.   There is a persistent desire or unsuccessful efforts to cut down or control substance use.
5.   A great deal of time is spent in activities necessary to obtain the substance (e.g., visiting multiple doctors or driving long distances), use the substance (e.g., chain-smoking), or recover from its effects.
6.   Important social, occupational, or recreational activities are given up or reduced because of substance use.
7.   The substance use is continued despite knowledge of having a persistent or recurrent physical or psychological problem that is likely to have been caused or exacerbated by the substance (e.g., current cocaine use despite recognition of cocaine-induced depression, or continued drinking despite recognition that an ulcer was made worse by alcohol consumption).

Substance Withdrawal

Substance withdrawal is described by the following diagnostic criteria (APA 2000):

A.   The development of substance-specific syndrome due to the cessation of (or reduction in) substance use that has been heavy and prolonged.
B.   The substance-specific syndrome causes clinically significant distress or impairment in social, occupational, or other important areas of functioning.
C.   The symptoms are not due to general medical condition and are not better accounted for by another mental disorder.

Substance Intoxication

Substance intoxication is described by the following diagnostic criteria (APA 2000):

A.   The development of a reversible substance-specific syndrome due to recent ingestion of (or exposure to) a substance. Note: Different substances may produce similar or identical syndromes.
B.   Clinically significant maladaptive behavioral or psychological changes that are due to the effect of the substance on the central nervous system (e.g., belligerence, mood lability, cognitive impairment, impaired judgment, impaired social or occupational functioning) and develop during or shortly after use of the substance.
C.   The symptoms are not due to a general medical condition and are not better accounted for by another mental disorder.

Definition of Addiction

In the early 1980s, the rise in cocaine use challenged the basic framework of our definition of alcohol/drug addiction. Cocaine was previously thought to be a drug that incurred psychological dependence with no physical dependence. At that time, we defined addiction as a physical dependence measured by a significant and noticeable medical withdrawal symptom. Although cocaine had no significant, medically noticeable withdrawal symptoms, users reported a severe addiction to it. David Smith (Smith and Wesson 1988) was aware of this discrepancy and proposed a more behavioral definition of addiction. Because Smith's definition is more functional, counselors in the fields of chemical dependency treatment and addictionology use it. In fact, counselors can apply this behavioral definition of addiction to a wide variety of types of disorders, including eating, gambling, sex, workaholism, television, smoking, video games, spending/consumerism, and other activities.

Alcoholism and drug addiction are best described metaphorically as "the dragon in the corner, eating its own tail."

The three basic components of the behavioral definition of addiction are the three Cs—*compulsion, control,* and *consequences.*

1. **Obsessive-*compulsive* behavior** with alcohol/drugs. Users think about alcohol and drugs in a vicious negative cycle; their obsessive concern and preoccupation follow an incessant use of alcohol/drugs in a continuous pattern and compulsive lifestyle.
2. ***Control*—Inability to stop** using the substances. Users cannot stop using alcohol/drugs for at least 3 months and/or make feeble attempts to cut back in a stop-then-start pattern. They are unable to refuse readily available drugs.
3. **Continued use despite adverse *consequences.*** Users are caught up in their addictions, illustrating the pervasive defense mechanisms of denial (rationalization and minimization). Eventually, the alcoholic/addict suffers family, social and interpersonal, economic, and spiritual bankruptcy.

Stages of Alcohol and Drug Use

Defining addiction is a challenge; however, defining the stages and patterns of alcohol/drug use that precede addiction is even more challenging. Figure 4.1 outlines the various stages of drug use, which are described in this section of the chapter.

Nonuse of Alcohol/Drugs by Children

The most successful preventive approach is not to use drugs and alcohol, especially at early ages. Not smoking cigarettes at early ages highly correlates with not developing addictions later in life. Children are less likely to develop chemical dependencies later in life, if parents

1. Do not model alcohol/drug use and encourage a healthy approach to life.
2. Encourage children to participate in activities that enhance the development of a strong sense of self.

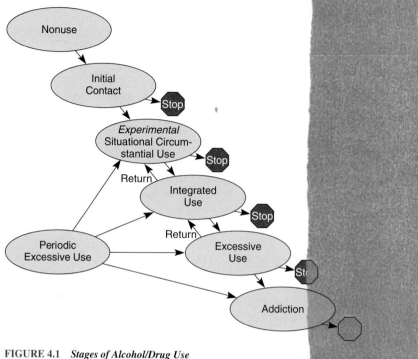

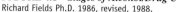

FIGURE 4.1   *Stages of Alcohol/Drug Use*
Richard Fields Ph.D. 1986, revised, 1988.

3. Promote positive alternative activities to alcohol/drug use (see Chapter 8).
4. Are sensitive to what children feel while parents are setting appropriate boundaries.
5. Provide structure, discipline, and consistency.
6. Develop a climate of discussion, which facilitates an effective exploration of values and the development of coping skills in goal setting, decision making, and conflict resolution.

Parents can establish nonuse of drugs and alcohol by teaching children to make positive lifestyle choices that they can maintain throughout adult life. Although the drive or desire to alter one's consciousness is innate, learning to alter one's consciousness with alternatives other than chemicals is a developmental task of childhood. Children can be encouraged to be more active in choosing things to do that change their mood and develop their sense of self, instead of choosing a passive solution, the use of alcohol/drugs.

Nonuse of Alcohol/Drugs by Adolescents

Some young people are able to use alcohol and drugs and not suffer any significant problems. For others, especially those who have family histories of alcoholism and drug addiction, such a trial could be the beginning of a lifelong pattern of addiction.

To help their at-risk adolescents, parents should

1. Establish clear, consistent guidelines and rules regarding alcohol/drugs.
2. Model nonuse of alcohol/drugs.
3. Establish clear, consistent communication of the hazards and potential harm of alcohol/drugs, especially at early ages of adolescence.
4. Encourage the development of alternative activities to alleviate feelings of boredom, depression, and isolation and to promote the development of a strong sense of self.
5. Promote active involvement in school, athletics, social situations, church, and other activities.
6. Encourage active development of skills and talents.
7. Promote trust and establish healthy boundaries in relationships.
8. Support adolescents in their perseverance through their developmental tasks of identity and individuation.

Initial Contact with Alcohol/Drugs

The initial contact stage is defined as the first time one tries alcohol/drugs. Usually, this stage is thought to be relatively harmless, yet there are potential hazards from initial contact, such as the following:

- Anaphylactic (allergic) reactions, which can cause death
- Toxic and lethal doses
- Loss of control and emotional overreactions
- Physical and psychological problems
- Accidents and/or dangerous situations

The three major components of alcohol and drug use are the individual, the drug, and the set and setting in which the drug is taken. Set and setting often determine the individual's reaction to alcohol/drugs.

As mentioned in an earlier chapter, **set** refers to the psychological and emotional frame of mind of a person when using alcohol/drugs. Those who are relaxed, comfortable, and secure in the knowledge that they can handle possibly losing control usually have less trouble with the initial use of alcohol/drugs. Individuals who have a set that can be described as anxious, extremely nervous, or overly concerned with maintaining control are more prone to a negative drug reaction. If a person is not emotionally stable and/or has psychiatric problems, alcohol/drug use can exacerbate those problems. (See Chapter 10.) This is especially true for hallucinogens and marijuana. Set can also be influenced by the person's mood or emotional state at the time of alcohol/drug use. The individual who has just received some bad news or has had a negative experience might be feeling down or depressed; this may result in a negative set and a negative experience with alcohol/drugs. Significant trauma, shame, and embarrassment can also contribute to a negative experience with alcohol/drugs.

Setting involves not only the physical environment but also the social and interpersonal environment. Negative drug reactions may be the result of being in an uncomfortable setting, with unknown people who are not trusted.

Alcohol/Drug Use—A Progressive Disease

Certainly, the beginning of alcohol/drug use starts with initial contact. Because alcohol/drug use is a progressive disease, individuals get more involved as they progress through the stages. A positive initial contact usually leads to the next stage of drug use—experimentation. Experimentation may lead to the subsequent stages, which end in addiction. Richard Rawson (1989) has written about his outpatient treatment of cocaine addicts. He describes the progressive themes at various stages of cocaine addiction, as shown in Table 4.1. These descriptions can easily be adapted to alcohol and other drugs and illustrate the progressive nature of addiction.

As stated earlier, a positive initial contact may be the beginning of a progressive cycle to addiction. This is especially true for those who grew up in alcoholic/addict and/or dysfunctional family systems.

Experimentation

Experimentation is the stage of using alcohol/drugs in different situations and circumstances. People explore and experiment with a drug, testing their own capacity to use alcohol/drugs in different situations and circumstances. Users learn about alcohol/drugs by experimenting with various doses, frequencies of use, methods of ingestion, and sometimes combinations (polydrug use). Each individual's reaction to a drug is also affected by physiological, psychological, and emotional factors. Some factors include not eating prior to use, fatigue, and levels of physical and emotional well-being. During experimentation, individuals change and adjust the drug, the set, and the setting and then determine their reaction.

Experimenters use drugs during this stage in different settings, with different people, and in different frames of mind, or set. A triangular relationship exists among the individual (set), the drug, and the environment (setting). During the experimentation stage, the user adjusts the three elements of this equation to determine the drug's effect.

Many systems that classify the stages of alcohol/drug use often call the experimental stage a *recreational* or *social use* stage. These terms tend to put alcohol/drugs in a more positive, emotion-laden frame of reference. The implication of the term *recreational* is that alcohol/drug use is no more than harmless recreational/ social fun. This view overlooks the potential hazards and problems that may occur.

TABLE 4.1	
Phases of Cocaine Addiction	
Initial contact	"Isn't this a great drug?"
Experimentation	"It's sure expensive, but it's worth it."
Excessive use	"I really should cut down."
Addiction	"I know I have to stop, but I can't."

SOURCE: Rawson 1989.

Parental guidelines during the experimental stage should include the following:

1. Talking with other parents and exchanging information about their children's behavior in the neighborhood, at neighboring homes, at school, or in the general community
2. Knowing where children are and who their friends are, as well as meeting the parents of their friends
3. Developing initiative, responsibility, and appropriate consequences for behavior
4. Evaluating the dynamics of the family and seeking professional help for early alcohol/drug educational advice and assessment
5. Being aware that a child is at risk and seeking family counseling for alcohol/drug education, prevention, and treatment if there is a history of alcohol/drug problems in the family

Integrated Use

At the integrated stage of alcohol/drug use, the person spends more time, thought, and energy in the use of alcohol/drugs. It has become an integrated part of the individual's life. Whether adolescent or adult, the person begins to associate with others who use the same drug. At parties, the marijuana smokers congregate, the alcohol users belly up to the bar, and the polydrug users are the life of the party, drinking at the bar and smoking dope in the backyard.

The individual at the integrated stage buys the drug to make sure that the drug is available. For example, at this stage a person must have the alcohol/drug available when away from home for a vacation or a business trip. Obviously, alcohol/drugs are well integrated into the user's style of life.

Excessive Use

Even for experts, the excessive use stage is difficult to describe because there are different kinds of excessive use. Some people call this stage drug abuse; however, the term *drug abuse* is very arbitrary, emotion-laden, and difficult to define. The second National Commission on Marijuana and Drug Abuse (1973) found that the term had "no functional utility" and "had become no more than an arbitrary code word for that drug use which is presently considered wrong." The commission concluded that the facts of actual drug use are often not distinguished from feelings and opinions. The commission recommended that the term drug abuse be discontinued because of the emotion-laden, subjective interpretation of the term.

Excessive use is an increase in alcohol/drug use that results in significant problems or negative consequences. Users are putting increased time, thought, and energy into buying—perhaps selling—and using alcohol/drugs.

Some people use alcohol/drugs excessively in a periodic pattern, sometimes in the form of binges, which are excessive drug use within a period of 24 to 72 hours. Periodic excessive alcohol/drug use can occur just on weekends, every other week, once in a month, or even as infrequently as once every 3 months. When all the criteria for addiction are met, periodic excessive use is also defined as addiction.

As Figure 4.1 shows, "periodic excessive use" can occur at four stages—experimental, integrated, excessive, and addiction. The key in determining which stage more accurately describes an individual's level of substance use would be to identify the negative consequences of use and the family (genetic) history of addiction.

Addiction

Addiction is the last stage. Based on our definition of addiction and the disease model, an addict cannot return to any of the previous stages of alcohol/drug use. The best recovery strategy is to abstain from alcohol/drug use and to participate in a 12-step recovery program. This usually involves an inpatient program; strong development in self-help support groups, such as Alcoholics Anonymous, Narcotics Anonymous, and Cocaine Anonymous; a relationship with a sponsor; and an aftercare treatment program on completion of the inpatient program. (See Chapter 11.)

Chronic alcoholics and drug addicts spend major portions of their lives addicted to alcohol/drugs. In this late stage of chronic addiction, they are extremely difficult to treat. (See Table 4.2.) Some new approaches are required for this population. Such programs provide basic needs for shelter, food, other health-related services, and educational and counseling services. These programs for chronic alcoholics emphasize maintaining the individual's dignity while providing access to recovery services.

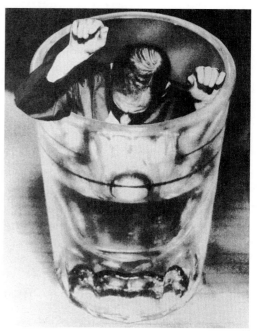

The alcoholic's life is limited, with significant negative consequences, as if he or she "is trapped in a shot glass."

✳ Jellinek's Types of Alcoholics

E. M. Jellinek (1960) believed that persons with certain types of alcoholism suffer through declining stages of functioning. He described five distinct types of alcoholism:

1. Alpha alcoholism: psychological dependence, in which alcoholics increasingly use drinking to help with their problems
2. Beta alcoholism
    a. Physical problems, such as cirrhosis of the liver or stomach problems, resulting from the consumption of alcohol
    b. No physical or psychological dependence
3. Gamma alcoholism
    a. Physical addiction, with withdrawal symptoms occurring whenever drinking is stopped
    b. Loss of control to regulate alcohol use
    c. Severe damage to health, financial, social, and interpersonal functioning
    d. Periods of abstinence (going on the wagon)

TABLE 4.2	
Early and Late Stages of Alcohol/Drug Use	
Early Stage	**Late Stage**
More freedom	Lack of freedom
Fewer risks and less damage	More damage
Possible abuse	Present abuse
No illness	State of illness
Linear operating factors	Vicious cycles

4. Delta alcoholism

   a. Similar to gamma; however, the individual can control intake in given situations
   b. High degree of physical and psychological dependence, making abstinence, even for brief periods, impossible

5. Epsilon alcoholism: periodic, unpredictable drinking binges

⚹ Vulnerability to Relapse

At each of the stages of recovery, individuals are vulnerable to relapse, or a return to alcohol/drug abuse or addiction. Therefore, all chemical dependency treatment programs must address relapse issues. Many experts agree that a longer-term inpatient or residential program is much needed (although financially difficult, due to limitations in insurance reimbursement and managed care). Experts agree that a 6- to 9-month inpatient program would be most effective, considering the high relapse rates. In addition, a 1-year outpatient aftercare program would further enhance the probability of recovery without relapse. It is not surprising that the relapse statistics are high following the traditional 28-day inpatient stay, making it even more important to counsel patients in relapse prevention. (See Chapter 11.)

Many people find it extremely difficult to stop using alcohol/drugs. Danaher and Lichtenstein (1978) describe the natural cycle of smoking, which is similar to the cycle of alcohol/drug use (see Table 4.3).

For more information on relapse, relapse prevention, recovery-prone behaviors, and relapse-prone behaviors, see Chapter 11.

Denial—A Problem in Accurate Assessment

An old joke in the drug/alcohol field is that "denial" is a river in Egypt (de-Nile). A more current description is that D-E-N-I-A-L stands for I **D**on't **E**ven k**N**ow **I** **A**m **L**ying.

The denial of alcohol/drug problems is a major factor in the difficulty of assessment. There is widespread denial, not only by individuals who have drug problems but also by family and friends, as well as society at large. It is often difficult to break through denial and have the courage to admit a problem with alcohol/drugs. Family

TABLE 4.3		
Natural Cycle of Cigarette Smoking		
Reasons for Starting		
Availability	Social confidence	
Curiosity	Modeling of peers, siblings, parents	
Rebelliousness	Other reasons in the psychosocial domain	
Anticipation of adulthood		
Reasons for Continuing		
Nicotine addiction	Avoidance of negative effects (withdrawal)	
Immediate positive consequences	Other reasons in the physiological and	
Signals (cues) in the environment	psychosocial domains	
Reasons for Stopping		
Health	Aesthetics (feeling that it is bad, ugly,	
Expense	and/or unbecoming)	
Social pressure	Example to others	
Self-mastery	Other reasons in the psychosocial domain	
Reasons for Resuming		
Stress	Alcohol consumption	
Social pressure	Other reasons in the psychosocial domain	
Abstinence violation effect		

SOURCE: Brian G. Danaher and Edward Lichtenstein. *Becoming an Ex-Smoker,* copyright © 1978 Brian G. Danaher and Edward Lichtenstein. Reprinted by permission.

members often experience a sense of shame or embarrassment or feelings of responsibility for the alcohol/drug problem of a family member.

The two major defense mechanisms used to deny problems with alcohol and drugs are minimization and rationalization. The following are common examples of minimizations and rationalizations of alcohol/drug problems:

"Now, if I drank and drugged like Shawn, then I would really have a problem."
"I use alcohol and drugs only on weekends; a person with a problem uses everyday."
"I never miss work, no matter how much [alcohol/drugs] I've used."
"The media are just trying to get you scared."
"I don't have a problem. Now, Tiffany has a problem. Why don't you get her into treatment?"

Additional consequences of minimization and rationalization include the following:

- Neglect; emotional, physical, or sexual abuse
- Loss—death, trauma, divorce, separation

- Numerous relocations and unstable home environment
- Parental dysfunction, creating feelings of parental unavailability and/or feelings of abandonment, rejection, or shame

Another reality is that substance abusers often are deceptive, tell half-truths, and outright lie about their use and the behaviors around their use. Of course, the larger the lie, the more unbelievable it is, yet abusers might defend themselves by saying, "Would I make up such an outrageous story?" The answer is often Yes!

⚔ Identification of Adolescent Alcohol/Drug Problems

Adolescent alcohol/drug problems are often harder to assess than adult substance abuse. Trying to clarify and sort out what is "normal" adolescent behavior versus what is an alcohol/drug problem is very difficult.

The following eleven questions can help in identifying an adolescent alcohol/drug problem:

1. *Mood.* Has the child been extremely moody or more upset than usual? Adolescence is a time of fluctuations in mood. A child might be as happy as a lark one minute and quite despondent the next. Therefore, it is difficult to isolate change in mood as being related to alcohol/drug use. However, if a child's mood seems more intense than usual, it could be related to the irritability associated with withdrawal from marijuana, alcohol, or other drugs.

2. *Changes.* Are there some significant changes in the child's choice in friends, grades, dress, general hygiene, and responsibilities? Adolescence is a time of change, a time to explore different aspects of one's identity and personality. However, when these changes are self-damaging and seem more than just the trying on of a different role, it could be a sign for concern.

3. *Responsibility.* Is the child more irresponsible about his or her commitments (e.g., chores, schoolwork, friends)? Is he or she not coming home on time or disregarding rules? It is common for young people to push limits and boundaries. However, doing this on a consistent basis or pushing boundaries beyond reasonable expectations may be a sign of alcohol/drug abuse.

4. *Motivation.* Is there a noticeable decrease in motivation, interest, or activity? Has the child shown disinterest in things he or she is normally interested in (e.g., friends, school, sports, extracurricular activities)? Loss of motivation is indicative of regular marijuana use. Alcohol and other drugs can also impair interest and/or performance in activities normally seen as pleasurable.

5. *School.* Are there signs of problems at school and difficulty in studying, completing assignments, and so on? Has the teacher complained that the youngster is sleeping or inattentive in class? Some common signs of problems are ditching school, having problems with teachers, acting out behavior, getting failing or lowered grades, and having fights and arguments with friends. School problems are usually the first sign of negative consequences that may be related to an alcohol/drug problem.

6. *Negative activities.* Is the child engaging in activities that are not healthy or productive and potentially damaging? Such activities include those that

might provoke physical violence; emotional abuse of others; disregard for others' property; dangerous use of motor vehicles; weekend-long parties or excessive isolation and secrecy about activities; and no accountability or supervision of time. A youngster having problems with alcohol or other drugs will abandon old friends and seek out those with similar attitudes and behaviors.

7. *Lying, stealing, and cheating.* Is money, household objects, or personal property missing? Is alcohol, prescription medication, or perhaps a parent's own stash of drugs missing? Does the child make up stories and lie compulsively? The expense of alcohol/drugs can be overcome by taking things that can be used for cash or bartered for alchohol/drugs. It is probably not forgetfulness or memory loss that has caused things to be either "misplaced" or "missing."

8. *Community.* Has the child been in trouble with neighbors, storekeepers, or other community members? Have concerned friends, neighbors, relatives, or others talked about this child's behavior? Have former friends, teachers, or parents of the child's friends expressed concern or given information that indicates this child may have a problem with alcohol/drugs? You can't go on ignoring the problem when others in the community have seen the child's misbehavior or actual alcohol/drug abuse.

9. *Criminal justice problems.* Has the child been involved in an activity that has caused investigation or charges being made by the police? Examples of these behaviors include disorderly conduct, drunkenness, driving under the influence, stealing, bouncing checks, shoplifting, vandalism, fighting, and breaking and entering. As outlined earlier, alcohol/drug use and antisocial behavior are highly correlated.

10. *Physical signs.* Are there physical signs of alcohol or drug use? Have some of the following been noticed?

    - The smell of alcohol or marijuana on the breath or body
    - Dilated pupils
    - Increase in activity
    - Grandiosity
    - Talkativeness
    - Extreme quietness
    - Slurred or incoherent speech
    - Bizarre behavior
    - Moodiness
    - Aggressiveness and show of temper
    - Fatigue, lethargy

    Has drug paraphernalia been found in the child's room (e.g., rolling paper, syringes, pipes [water pipes], mirrors, razors, baggies)?

11. *Parents.* Do you find yourself justifying your child's behavior? Are you saying things like the following?

    - "He or she will grow out of it."
    - "This is just a stage."

- "Kids will be kids."
- "I went through the same kind of behavior when I was a kid."

If so, you may be denying signs of alcohol/drug abuse. Remember: *Believe the behavior,* not necessarily what the person says.

Case Study 4.1 illustrates that it is not necessary to catch children red-handed using alcohol/drugs. If there is enough evidence of possible alcohol/drug abuse, seek professional help early—don't wait until the problem gets out of hand.

⚹ Alcohol/Drug History

Recovery from alcohol/drugs also involves the family of the alcoholic/addict. The family system is an integral part of the development of the disease. The most difficult work in recovery is dealing with family issues and relationships to help family members recover from dysfunctional patterns in the family system. (See Chapter 5.)

This section is not intended as a clinical skill training, but it lists things you need to be aware of when taking an alcohol/drug history.

The most important task in assessing the potential for problems with alcohol/drugs is determining if there is a family history of alcohol or drug abuse and addiction. Family members may deny the extent of alcohol/drug use in their family. It might take additional questioning to clarify the true dimensions of family use of alcohol/drugs.

Some education for family members and the individual who may have a drug problem might also be necessary to establish a clear perception of the dimensions of substance abuse and addiction. To assess an individual's alcohol/drug problem, counselors need the following information:

- Age of initial drug and alcohol use
- Frequency of use, amounts used, set and setting of use
- Patterns of use, binges, periods of nonuse
- Stage of current use—experimentation, integrated use, excessive use, addiction
- History of negative consequences—physical, psychological, financial, familial, and spiritual
- Medical history—conditions that might be affected by use of drugs/alcohol
- Use of coffee, cigarettes, and medication

Individual Vulnerability to Alcohol/Drugs

Counselors should determine the individual's vulnerability and at-risk factors to alcohol/drug use:

What evidence is there of individual vulnerability?

- Primary alcoholism/drug addiction in the family system of origin
- Inherited or acquired mood disorder
- Psychosis
- Rejection or insensitivity to norms of behavior

Case Study 4.1
The Marijuana Search

Despite Mr. and Mrs. Green being aware of signs of drug use by their 13-year-old son, John, he kept denying he was using. John seemed to have an answer for everything. He would make them feel guilty for doubting his word and not trusting him. As time went on, the deceptions and lies got more and more complicated. John, despite being caught in these lies, insisted that he was not smoking marijuana. The parents were frustrated and felt the only way they could have their son acknowledge his problem was for them either to catch him using marijuana or to find his marijuana.

One day, while their son was out of the house, they searched his room. Despite looking everywhere in the room, they couldn't find any tangible evidence of marijuana use. Curiously, the room seemed cleaner and neater than usual—almost as if their son suspected a search was imminent. Perhaps he heard them talking on the phone to the neighbors when they suggested a search. By chance, the father decided to expand the search to other rooms in the house—bathrooms, family room, bedrooms. They found what they were looking for in the hall closet. They unscrewed the rubberized handle of the vacuum cleaner and found a small stash of marijuana.

When John came home, his parents calmly held a family meeting. They asked him if he had any marijuana in the house. Again, he said he didn't. When they produced the marijuana and told him where they found it, John didn't blink an eye while saying, "Oh, that stuff. I forgot all about it. I've been holding that for the kid down the block for months now—you know, the one who went into drug treatment. I forgot all about it."

Discussion Questions

Explain and describe "parental denial" in acknowledging their child's drug use.
Do you think parents have the right to search their kids' room, etc.?
What do you think about drug testing of children,
> By parents?
> By schools? As a requirement for extracurricular activities? . . .
Are drug tests reliable? Explain "false positives."
Class Project: Visit a drug-testing lab and report on the procedure, tests available, and
> reliability of tests.

What is the individual's attitude toward alcohol/drug use?

- Favorable, unfavorable, nonexistent

What are the environmental factors?

- Family, other

Are drugs available?

- Legally available, readily available illegally
- Individual has the necessary finances for drugs (Rankin 1978)

Counselors should also identify any other significant problems, especially other compulsive behaviors in the family—a family history of

- Alcohol/drug problems, gambling, workaholism
- Eating disorders—anorexia, bulimia, obesity
- Employment and financial problems
- Marital problems
- Psychiatric disorders—depression, anxiety, affective (feeling) disorders, and others

⋊ Consequences of Alcohol/Drug Use

An extremely important area of assessment is the consequences of alcohol/drug use. Remember, the third criteria of addiction is "continued use despite adverse consequences."

A client, who was referred for outpatient counseling after 120 days in a residential and extended care program, was now dealing with significant criminal, civil, and other legal problems, as well as financial, marital, business, and relationship problems. He said, "You can do all the drinking and drugging you want as long as you are willing to pay the consequences."

Perhaps this is a straightforward way of looking at addiction, but it does point out the significant consequences that come with substance abuse and addiction. Pointing out the consequences may be a valuable tool in breaking through denial. A very common exercise used in most drunk driving programs is to have clients figure out how much their conviction has cost them. For some, the amount is staggering when they stop to consider the cost of legal fees, the diversion program, loss of work, and so on.

Arnold Washton (1995) asks several questions in the assessment stage about consequence, covering the physical, psychological, sexual, relationship, job, financial, and legal consequences of alcohol/drug use (Table 4.4).

⋊ Alcohol/Drugs and Suicide

Another key assessment issue with alcohol/drugs is the potential for suicide. Stanton and Landau-Stanton (1985) state that the "recognition of substance abuse as a suicidal endeavor stems from as far back as 1938 when Menninger likened addiction to chronic suicide." Table 4.5 highlights key facts about suicide.

Some common assessment questions for suicide are these:

1. Is there a family history of alcohol/drug problems, suicide, or depression?
2. Do you use alcohol/drugs to

    a. overcome bad/shameful feelings?
    b. deal with sleeping problems, depression, or stress?
    c. quiet suicidal or self-destructive thoughts?

TABLE 4.4

Consequences Related to Alcohol or Drug Use

Check below any PHYSICAL problems caused by or worsened by your use of alcohol or drugs:

- Convulsions with loss of consciousness
- Nasal sores, bleeding
- Chest congestion, wheezing
- Hepatitis or other liver problems
- Severe or frequent headaches
- Drug overdose requiring treatment in an emergency room or hospital
- Coughing up black phlegm
- Severe weight loss (without dieting)
- Sinus problems
- Ulcers or other stomach problems
- Heart palpitations
- Other (specify)

Check below any PSYCHOLOGICAL problems caused by or worsened by your use of alcohol or drugs:

- Irritability, short temper
- Panic attacks
- Violent thoughts
- Severe depression
- Memory problems
- Paranoia, suspiciousness
- Suicidal thoughts
- Other (specify)

Check below any SEXUAL problems caused by or worsened by your use of alcohol or drugs:

- Loss of sex drive
- Sex with strangers
- Sexuality out of control
- Sexual obsession or preoccupation
- Risking of AIDS through sexual behavior
- Other (specify)

Check below any RELATIONSHIP or SOCIAL problems caused by or worsened by your use of alcohol or drugs:

- Arguments with spouse or mate
- Thrown out of household
- Loss of friends
- Arguments with parents, brothers, or sisters
- Spouse or mate has threatened to leave or has already left
- Social isolation
- Other (specify)

Check below any JOB or FINANCIAL problems caused by or worsened by your use of alcohol or drugs:

- In jeopardy of losing my job
- Late to work
- Less productive at work
- In debt
- Already lost at least one job
- Missed days of work
- Missed opportunity for promotion or raise
- Behind in paying bills
- Other (specify)

Check below any LEGAL problems caused by or worsened by your use of alcohol or drugs:

- Arrested for possession of illicit substances
- Arrested for forging prescriptions
- Auto accident while driving under the influence
- Arrested for assaulting someone
- Arrested for embezzlement or check forgery
- Arrested for sale of illicit substances
- Arrested for DWI or DUI
- Arrested for violent or disorderly conduct
- Arrested for theft or robbery
- Other (specify)

SOURCE: Washton 1995.

TABLE 4.5

The Facts about Suicide

1. Suicide is preventable. Most suicide victims do not want to die.
2. Suicide is the eighth leading cause of death and ranks ahead of homicide.
3. Talking about suicide does not cause someone to be suicidal.
4. Suicidal behavior is not inherited, but the risk is higher for family members who have lost a close relative to suicide.
5. The suicide rate is higher for the elderly than any other age group.
6. Suicide is the second leading cause of death among young people. Accidents are number one, but even some of these accidents could be suicides.
7. Suicide claims the lives of at least 30,000 people annually in the United States.
8. Five states have passed legislation providing for school suicide prevention programs.
9. The incidence of suicide among young people has nearly tripled during the past three decades.
10. Three times as many men as women kill themselves, yet three times as many women as men attempt suicide.
11. More than 80 percent of people communicate their intent to kill themselves before they attempt to do so. They leave clues as to their distress and/or plans.

SOURCE: American Association of Suicidology, 4201 Connecticut Ave. NW, Suite 310, Washington DC 20008, (202) 237–2280.

3. Do you have suicidal thoughts?
4. How will you do it? Do you have a plan? (Assess the availability or means to commit suicide and the lethality of the means.)
5. Have you previously had suicidal thoughts and have you attempted suicide before? How frequently do these thoughts occur?
6. What role does alcohol/drug use have in relation to suicide? Does it make you more likely or less likely to follow through?
7. On a scale of 1 to 10, how likely are you to kill yourself?
8. How much do you want to die? to live?
9. What would prevent you from committing suicide?
10. What might occur to make life worth living?

These questions can help you to assess potential suicide:

- Have you been thinking about suicide?
- Do you have a plan to take your life?
- Do you feel hopeless about the future?
- Do you think you are a burden to your loved ones?
- Are you feeling so bad you are considering ending your life?
- Do you ever wish you could go to sleep and never wake up?
- Have you ever wanted to stop living?

If a client is suicidal, an extremely important question to ask is, "What would prevent you from committing suicide?" This will often lead to a dialogue and plan of action that will prevent suicide. Fortunately, the vast majority of suicidal people do not want to die so much as they want to find a way to live. A common practice involves a written contract with a client who may be suicidal. The client agrees to not take action or to call the therapist or a suicide hot line before making an attempt. (See Case Study 4.2.)

(Alcoholics Anonymous)—Silence is the enemy of recovery.

⋇ In Review

- The *Diagnostic and Statistical Manual of Mental Disorders* (APA 2000) establishes standards for assessing mental disorders and substance-related disorders. The major substance-related disorders are substance dependence, substance abuse, substance-induced withdrawal, and substance-induced intoxication. All four of these disorders are described by their diagnostic criteria.
- The behavioral definition of addiction is expressed by the 3Cs mnemonic:

  Compulsion
  Control (inability)
  Continued use despite negative **C**onsequences

- The stages of drug use are nonuse, initial contact, experimentation, integrated use, excessive (continuous and periodic) use, and addiction.
- Denial is the major defense, due to users' minimization and rationalization of their level of involvement with alcohol/drugs, which makes accurate assessment more difficult.
- Assessment of adolescent alcohol/drug problems is very difficult. Trying to clarify the truth and sort out what is "normal" adolescent behavior versus what is an alcohol/drug problem is often difficult. Assessing these eleven topics can help identify an adolescent alcohol/drug problem:

  Mood
  Changes
  Responsibility
  Motivation
  School
  Negative activities
  Lying, stealing, and cheating
  Community
  Criminal justice problems
  Physical signs
  Parents

- Assessment involves not only taking a good alcohol/drug history but also assessing the individual's vulnerability to alcohol/drugs, the consequences of the alcohol/drug use, and the person's suicide potential.

Case Study 4.2
Alcohol, Depression, and Suicide

The names and details of this case study have been changed to maintain anonymity.

Cheryl, a 43-year-old manager of a telecommunications company, struggled with bouts of alcoholism and depression. She originally called, seeking help for marital problems. During the assessment session, Cheryl reported her struggles with alcohol and drugs. She admitted that she was probably addicted to cocaine. She was convinced that she could no longer use cocaine. She still struggled to control her drinking. Cheryl had been through one inpatient treatment program and sporadically attended AA but was able to sustain only short periods of abstinence. Her job was extremely stressful, demanding more of her time and energy. She frequently lost her temper with people she worked with. The counselor listened to her "gripes" about her husband and their marital problems but astutely brought the conversation back to Cheryl's alcohol abuse.

In the third session, Cheryl acknowledged the need to strengthen her efforts to seek recovery from alcohol. She began attending AA and was encouraged to obtain an AA sponsor and attend counseling sessions once a week, yet, as time went on, she got distracted from committing to AA and chose a sponsor whom she rarely interacted with. Despite the counselor's efforts to get her to develop a stronger recovery program, she resisted. In future sessions, Cheryl began to talk about overwhelming feelings of depression and suicidal thoughts. She was referred to a psychiatrist for evaluation and was put on antidepressant medication. At the same time, the counselor and Cheryl wrote a contract that she would not attempt suicide and, if she felt suicidal, she would call the counselor or the suicide helpline.

Several months into treatment, Cheryl's depression was stabilizing and she was attending AA meetings more regularly, but she still had not established an active relationship with a sponsor or others in the program. The counselor suggested a woman's recovery therapy group. Cheryl agreed and attended the therapy group each week. At this time, her marriage was headed for a divorce, and her job was getting worse. She eventually moved out of her house and rented an apartment. During this time, she lapsed back to using alcohol and was more depressed. The counselor and group encouraged her to get more active in AA and to continue with her medication. Unfortunately, Cheryl did the opposite. She stopped taking her medication, rarely went to AA, and immersed herself in her work. She spent excessive hours working overtime and eventually dropped out of group counseling, stating that her schedule and finances made it impossible to attend. Despite efforts by her counselor to have her continue in group at a reduced fee, Cheryl decided against it. She continued, only briefly, with her individual counseling. Despite the counselor's best efforts to point out the need for counseling and renewed recovery efforts, Cheryl did not follow through. She began to miss counseling appointments. The counselor pointed out her pattern of "isolating" and continued to try to reengage her into counseling and recovery. Despite the counselor's best efforts, Cheryl went to counseling less frequently and eventually stopped going.

Nine months later the counselor received news that Cheryl had killed herself. The combination of alcoholism, depression, marital problems, stress at work, and Cheryl's inability to seek connection with others had led to her suicide.

Discussion Questions

Describe the role "pride" and "shame" can play in not seeking help.

As a counselor, what boundaries would you set to deal with a client with suicidal ideation? Would you set up a contingency contract?

List some questions you might ask a client whom you suspect may be suicidal.

What does "Silence is the enemy of recovery" mean?

What signs might make you aware of the potential for suicide?

Have you ever considered suicide? What is your view on suicide?

What conditions increase a person's vulnerability to suicide?

- The most important task in assessing the potential for problems with alcohol/drugs is to determine whether there is a family history of alcohol or drug abuse and addiction. It might take additional questioning to clarify the true dimensions of family use of alcohol/drugs.
- Alcohol and suicide are strongly interrelated. Use these questions to assess potential suicide:

    Have you been thinking about suicide?
    Do you have a plan to take your life?
    Do you feel hopeless about the future?
    Do you think you are a burden to your loved ones?
    Are you feeling so bad you are considering ending your life?
    Do you ever wish you could go to sleep and never wake up?
    Have you ever wanted to stop living?

- Some important questions to ask clients at risk for suicide:

    On a scale of 1 to 10, how likely are you to kill yourself?
    How much do you want to die? to live?
    What would prevent you from committing suicide?
    What might occur to make life worth living?

- A variety of alcohol/drug screening inventories are available for review in Appendix A.

✴ Case Studies

1. Read each case illustration and determine

    - Stage of substance use
    - Significant or important history
    - Other questions you would want to ask
    - What you would address in counseling and how

Stages of Drug Use—Case I: Jake, 13 years old

Jake   13-year-old, male caucasian, seventh grader in a middle surburban junior high school, reports trying marijuana and enjoying it; drinks occasionally at parties, couple of beers, but doesn't really like the taste; likes to get buzzed on alcohol, but prefers marijuana.

Presenting Problem—Found smoking marijuana with ninth graders, after school, behind the stands at the baseball field.

- Makes good grades at school, has gotten into minor trouble for joking around and "goofing" on teachers whom he considers "lame"; otherwise a very responsible student, assignments are in on time, etc.
- Wants to attend a good college, not sure about career
- Likes athletics and all sports, especially baseball
- Reports being withdrawn and introverted until the third grade, no friends, played by himself (e.g., fantasy baseball), then family moved to new

neighborhood (present neighborhood) and he has made friends through playing sports and school

- Family history—father has a temper, clerk at an insurance firm; mother not working; two younger siblings . . . no history of alcohol/drug use in family, describes his father as either angry or sullen (*therapist note:* suspect father is clinically depressed)

Additional Questions

From this limited information, what do you suspect Jake's stage of alcohol/drug use is?

What future areas would you explore for a better evaluation?

Do you think Jake is at risk for marijuana dependence? Cite your reasons why or why not.

Would you continue to see Jake in counseling, and if yes, what would you focus on and for how long?

Stages of Drug Use—Case II: Larry, 46-Year-Old Fireman

- Presenting problem was a marital conflict: In an escalated argument, Larry shoved his wife, and she took the kids and went to her mother's house.
- Larry has a temper, rageful at times; he was adopted at a young age.
- No contact with his birth parents.
- Adopting parents have no history of alcohol/drug use.
- History of drinking regularly as a young man, "getting into his fair share of trouble."
- Currently reports drinking each evening to calm down from the stress of the job; his alcohol use has escalated over the last 5 years. He blames it on the increased marital conflict and disagreements over parenting the children.
- Further evaluation reveals periods of excessive mania, followed by states of depression and despair and increased alcohol consumption.
- Also has a history of PTSD from several incidents on the job, although Larry considers it "normal" stress on the job.

Stages of Drug Use—Case III: Sarah, 34-Year-Old Bookkeeper

- Presenting problem—disabling depression
- Extremely shy and quite introverted
- A virgin at 34, she describes herself as "flawed" and fears being an old maid.
- She drinks alone, 3–4 glasses of wine most evenings, more on Friday and Saturday nights.
- Her father was an alcoholic and died from alcohol-related problems when she was 5 years old.
- Sarah never misses work as a result of drinking and has recently cut back, drinking only three times a week instead of every night.

Stages of Drug Use—Case IV: Barry, 39-Year-Old OBGYN

- Presenting problem—depression related to divorce
- After talking about the divorce, he reveals that he uses OxyContin and cocaine "on occasion."
- He further reports being investigated by the medical licensing board for alleged sexual advances toward one of his patients.
- He believes he is being set up by his former nurse, with whom he had an ongoing affair. She used cocaine with him as well.
- Reports drinking regularly but not excessively

2. Give some examples of denial by the addict/alcoholic and the family members of the substance abuser. Explain what function denial plays in the family system.
3. List and explain some adolescent at-risk factors for substance abuse for these issues: mood, changes, peer group, negative actions, deception and lying, physical signs.
4. What is the most important question to ask when doing an assessment for drug abuse? Why?

⌘ References

American Psychiatric Association. 2000. *Diagnostic and statistical manual of mental disorders.* 4th ed., text rev. Washington, D.C.: Author.

Danaher, B. G., and E. Lichtenstein. 1978. *Becoming an ex-smoker.* Englewood Cliffs, N.J.: Prentice-Hall.

Jellinek, E. M. 1960. *The disease concept of alcoholism.* New Haven, Conn.: Hillhouse Press.

National Commission on Marijuana and Drug Abuse. 1973. *Drug use in America: Problem in perspective.* Second report of the National Commission on Marijuana and Drug Abuse. Washington, D.C.: U.S. Government Printing Office.

National Institute on Alcohol and Alcoholism [NIAA]. 1990. Factors enhancing the reliability and validity of self-reports among substance abusers.

Nowlis, Helen. 1975. *Drugs demystified.* Paris: UNESCO Press.

Rankin, James G. 1978. *Core knowledge of the drug field: A basic manual for trainers.* Toronto: Addiction Research Foundation.

Rawson, Richard. 1989. *Cocaine recovery issues: The neurobehavioral model.* Beverly Hills, Calif.: Matrix Institute on Addictions.

Shedler, Jonathan, and Jack Block. 1990. Adolescent drug use and psychological health: A longitudinal inquiry. *American Psychologist* 45(5):612.

Smith, David, and Donald Wesson. 1988. *Treating cocaine dependence.* Center City, Minn.: Hazeldon Foundation.

Stanton, M. D., and Judith Landau-Stanton. 1985. Treating suicidal adolescents and their families. In *Handbook of adolescent and family therapy,* edited by M. P. Mirkin and S. L. Koman. New York: Gardner Press.

Washton, Arnold M. 1995. *Psychotherapy and substance abuse: A practitioner's handbook.* New York: Guilford Press.

Family

Substance Abuse and Family Systems

Objectives

1. Identify families as systems with key elements of rules, values, verbal and nonverbal methods of communicating, boundaries, roles, and patterns of interaction.
2. Identify the characteristics of family metaphorically as a mobile (Satir) trying to maintain balance.
3. Explain the three rules that children of alcoholics learn, as identified by Claudia Black: "Don't talk. Don't trust. Don't feel."
4. Identify the reasons for using the term *imbalanced* instead of *dysfunctional* family system.
5. Identify the rules, values, and communication styles of the rigid, ambiguous, overextended, and distorted family systems.
6. Identify the ways in which placaters, blamers, intellectualizers, and distracters discount themselves and/or others, as described by Virginia Satir.
7. Identify the characteristics of the roles described by Sharon Wegscheider-Cruse:
   - Family hero
   - Family scapegoat
   - Lost child
   - Family mascot
8. Define and classify enabling behavior as
   - avoiding and shielding
   - attempting to control
   - taking over responsibility
   - rationalizing and accepting
   - cooperating and collaborating (Nelson 1988)
9. Identify and describe the five stages of grieving—denial, anger, bargaining, depression (feeling stage), and acceptance—as they relate to family recovery from an alcohol/drug problem.

⋇ Introduction

A major focus of this book is perceiving alcoholism/drug addiction and substance-abuse problems as having a major impact on the family and its members—the family system. Drug/alcohol abuse does not happen in isolation. This chapter explores the imbalances created in the alcoholic/addict family systems, with specific imbalances in communication, roles, and actions. The chapter lays the foundation for understanding the personal impact on children who grow up in the alcoholic system, which is further explored in Chapter 7 as these children become adults, or adult-children of alcoholics.

⚹ Families as Systems

Initially, one must look at the family as a system. Some key elements of family systems are that they all have rules, values, verbal and nonverbal methods of communicating, boundaries, roles, and patterns of interaction. Systems always seek some level of homeostasis, or balance. Alcoholism and drug dependency are dysfunctional elements in family life. The result is a disequilibrium, or imbalance, forcing family members to compensate and give up aspects of their own sense of self in an attempt to keep the family in balance. The alcoholic/addict family system could be compared with an unbalanced toy top, one so top-heavy that when it tries to spin in a functional pattern, it instead swerves to one side and skids in a diagonal direction until it stops. The individuals in this system are all compensating in different yet similar ways. It's as if they are walking around with a heavy weight on one shoulder; they have to either lean to one side to walk properly or use all their energy to try to compensate and look as if they are walking upright. Both positions require a great deal of energy. Family therapist Carl Whitaker (Whitaker and Napier 1978) has described the family as the source of all kinds of electrical energy, with positive and negative voltages.

Virginia Satir (1967), a famous family therapist, was the first to describe the family using the metaphor of a mobile: if the wires on one of the pieces of the mobile are twisted, the mobile spins improperly. Instead of a delicately balanced mobile, each piece gets entangled and out of balance at the slightest breeze. A well-balanced mobile, or family system, sways and flexes with the strong gusts and heavy winds of life. The family with alcohol/drug problems is described as an imbalanced, or dysfunctional, family system. In a healthy family, the system is flexible and fluid, open (not rigid), predictable (not inconsistent), and balanced in meeting both the individual's and the family's needs.

Looking at the family as a system is imperative in addressing the problem of alcohol/drug dependence and addiction. If the family system does not change and the family members do not do their recovery work, the same dysfunctional styles of communication and interaction make the alcoholic/addict at risk for alcohol/drug relapse or the development of another dysfunctional behavior.

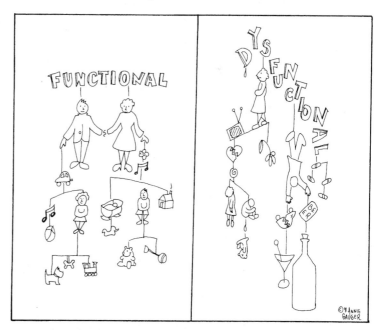

Functional and dysfunctional systems.
Annie Bauger.

To effectively treat the alcoholic/addict, the rest of the family system also needs treatment. The dysfunctional aspect of the disease has affected all family members. The high alcohol/drug relapse rate is often attributable to the lack of recovery by the family members. Too frequently, the alcoholic/addict is the focus of help, and the family members deny their own enabling and codependent behavior. The messages from the family are "Just fix the alcoholic/addict" and "Just get him or her to stop using alcohol/drugs and then everything will be O.K."

Family members avoid being active in treatment because they resist looking at their own behavior; they fear getting in touch with painful feelings, which may be overwhelming.

Another fear is whether the family system can survive reexperiencing these feelings. They wonder, "Has the family been hurt beyond repair?" and "Will the family be able to work through the violations of the past?" These questions and others need to be addressed for the effective recovery of the alcoholic/addict and the family members.

The expression *dry drunk* refers to the alcoholic/addict who is abstaining from alcohol/drug use but either is unaware of other behavioral, personality, and relationship problems or is choosing not to address these maladaptive behaviors. The overall behavior and personality styles of dry drunks are very similar to when they were using alcohol/drugs. Essentially, they have chosen not to deal with the underlying issues that contributed to the negative aspects of their personalities. For some, it is certainly enough that they are sober. Others who are still experiencing feelings of depression, fear, rage, and anxiety may decide to get help and address the problem.

After 1 to 5 years of being sober, many recovering alcoholics/addicts realize that they are still having problems, especially in interpersonal relationships. This is often described as the addicts' "second bottom." The first bottom is the realization that they can no longer continue to use alcohol/drugs. The second bottom is the realization that they are still not having fun, due to unresolved personality issues. They ask themselves the question, "Now that I am years sober, am I having fun yet?" The answer frequently is, "No, my life is more manageable but I'm still not feeling better."

The family of the alcoholic/addict also goes through a kind of dry drunk. The family may glow in the joy of the alcoholic/addict's initial sobriety and may now feel validated that he or she is, indeed, okay. From the viewpoint of friends, neighbors, and community, he or she "did the right thing." There is no discounting that the family members were courageous in struggling to get the alcoholic/addict into treatment. However, they must continue the struggle to develop a healthier family system. In many cases, the family returns to old dysfunctional patterns. It is fair to say that recovery from the diseases of alcoholism and drug addiction is an ongoing process for the individual and the family.

⚹ Family Rules

Each family makes decisions and choices based on the rules, boundaries, and alliances of family members. Family rules often involve rules of communication—who is allowed to express feelings, how and when they are expressed, and how they are received.

Rules in the alcoholic/addict family system often focus on ways to communicate and believe in order to deal with the substance-abusing person. This often involves secret keeping, or what Claudia Black (1982) referred to as the three rules that children of alcoholics often learn to live by: Don't talk. Don't trust. Don't feel."

> Talking, especially about the substance abuse, might cause even more problems. Trusting usually leads to disappointment when parents do not come through with their promises. Feeling is too painful, and expression of feelings is not allowed because it might cause more trouble. (Lawson and Lawson 1998)

⚹ *Imbalanced* versus *Dysfunctional*

Nathan Ackerman first coined the term *dysfunctional family* in 1958, when referring to alcoholic family systems. Throughout the literature of the alcohol/drug and mental health fields—and even in this textbook—we frequently use the term dysfunctional in describing families, systems, relationships, parenting, behavior, and individuals. The term dysfunctional is often a shame-based, negative label, with a negative emotional tone. Labeling them as dysfunctional discourages families and individuals who are struggling with the problems of alcohol/drug dependence. Many people have been annoyed and discouraged at being told they are dysfunctional. It sounds hopeless. For example, what good does it do to tell a patient, relative, or friend, "You come from a shame-based, dysfunctional family system" or "You have a codependent, enabling, dysfunctional relationship with your spouse and children"? This doesn't really help people and it shames them, making them feel helpless and hopeless. Most people feel a sense of betrayal in even thinking about their families in such a derogatory manner.

Instead of using *dysfunctional,* replace it with the term *imbalanced,* for this is truly what we are looking at—an imbalance in the individual and in the family members' lives. Remember Satir's image of an out-of-balance mobile. It is so much more hopeful to seek treatment if one has the expectation of becoming balanced. It is also a far more positive approach.

There is truly an emotional imbalance in the alcoholic/addict family system. The term *imbalance* gives hope that there is a way to get help and better manage the system. The goal is to establish balance and order by addressing the problems in the family.

There are different kinds of imbalance in family systems. Alcohol/drugs serve a different function in each of these imbalanced systems. Next, we examine rigid, ambiguous, overextended, and distorted family systems to better understand imbalanced family systems. In each family system, the drug of choice and its function are for illustration, not an empirically proven fact.

Rigid Family Systems

Rules—Strict interpretation of the rules with no exceptions; inflexibility with no extenuating circumstances. The rules keeper (usually a critical/judgmental father or mother) is exempt from the rules.

Values—"There is only one way to do things and that is the right way—my way." Things are always black or white, right or wrong.

Motto—"Do it right, or else."

Communication—Linear, hierarchical. The father is usually dominant, powerful, and unapproachable. The mother softens the impact of the father's harshness. Or the mother is critical-judgmental, often moralistic and controlling, and the father goes along with the mother, deceptively avoiding conflict and the rage of the mother.

Drugs of choice—Alcohol and/or heroin, other sedative hypnotics, and narcotic analgesics.

Functions of drug—Suppress feelings, especially anger, and stay numb to the trauma in this family system.

Ambiguous Family Systems

Rules—We have rules but we don't enforce them, and we change them if someone is annoyed or inconvenienced.

Values—Forever changing, based on the situation.

Motto—"Keep peace at all costs; avoid conflict."

Communication—Mixed messages that are confusing. "Do what you know we want, without us letting you know what it is we want."

Drugs of choice—Alcohol and/or heroin, marijuana, and hallucinogens.

Functions of drug—Suppress feelings of discomfort, kill pain, shut out reality, and/or distort reality.

Overextended Family Systems

Rules—Be productive, get busy, stay on the move.

Values—Look good, achieve, do it with willpower, feelings are for wimps.

Motto—"We can achieve anything we set our minds to." "The right stuff."

Communication—Feelings are not expressed or integrated; decisions are based on results and what will please the parents.

Drugs of choice—Cocaine, methamphetamine, and other stimulants, alcohol.

Functions of drug—Keep on working/doing, even though feelings are not congruent with work or intimate relationships.

Distorted Family Systems

Rules—Don't let outsiders know we are crazy. Act as if we were a normal family, just a bit eccentric.

Values—Maintain an illusion of normalcy, despite significant physical, emotional, and interpersonal problems of the family. Keep outsiders guessing about us.

Motto—"Aren't most families like ours?"

Communication—Mixed messages; parents and children are unavailable and have limited common perceptions of situations.

Drugs of choice—Alcohol, hallucinogens, marijuana, and inhalants.

Functions of drug—Distort reality, which is already distorted, to try and make sense, or no sense, of it.

Entitled Family Systems

Rules—Rules don't necessarily apply to us because we are special.
Values—Money, status, and who you know.
Motto—We are entitled.
Communication—We are better than others, so we see others as less entitled.
Drugs of choice—Fine wines, champagne, cocaine, Ecstasy, marijuana, and anything we want.
Functions of drug—Pleasure, party, embue life.

⚝ Satir's Family Patterns of Communication

Virginia Satir, author of *Conjoint Family Therapy* (1967) and *Peoplemaking* (1972) and co-author of *Helping Families to Change* (1983), emphasizes the feeling component of family patterns of communication. She describes a dysfunctional family as one that maintains rules that do not fit the reality of what is felt and believed.

Satir's work is monumental and popular. According to Satir, individuals with poor self-concepts see pots that are half-empty. Individuals with the ability to differentiate (i.e., those with good self-concepts) see their pots as half-full. The former group feels hopeless and negative; the latter group is positive and hopeful.

Satir identified the following dysfunctional styles as well as a functional style of communicating:

1. Placaters discount themselves. Their goal is frequently to avoid conflict and to avoid others' anger. Their communication patterns feature the following:

    a. Words that agree and avoid conflict: "Whatever you want is O.K." The placaters' worth is based on others accepting, not rejecting, what they say.
    b. Bodies that placate: "I am helpless." The placaters' worth is based on being physically available, even when that may not be consistent with what they feel.
    c. Feelings: "I am worthless." Placaters believe they have no choices but to be dependent in dysfunctional relationships because there is no way out, and they are not strong enough or worth the struggle.

2. Blamers elevate themselves by discounting others. Their goal is to avoid looking at themselves, their own issues, and their own responsibility. Others' feelings are often discounted. If others would only do it the right way—which is their way—then things would work out. Their communication patterns feature the following:

    a. Words that are critical, judgmental, shaming put-downs: "You never do anything right." "It's all your fault."
    b. Bodies that blame: "I am more powerful, more dominant."
    c. Feelings: "It is your fault that I am unhappy."

3. Intellectualizers discount their own feelings. Their goal is to place rigid emphasis on the cognitive to figure out problems, to deny the role feelings

play in relationships and decisions, and to avoid the emotional impact of feelings. Intellectualizers are the brains, the computers, the cognitive persons who think, "If I can only understand this, I'll be O.K." They often feel that, if they can only find that missing piece of the puzzle, they will find the cause of their problems. They fail to integrate the key elements of the puzzle—their feelings—and fail to realize that the puzzle may not be solvable, especially with their linear approach. Their communication patterns feature the following:

   a.   Words that are extremely logical: "That makes sense and is reasonable."
   b.   Bodies in control or shut down
   c.   Feelings: "I am vulnerable and feel threatened when I get in touch with my feelings, especially feelings of vulnerability."

4.   Distracters discount context. Their goal is to keep others and themselves away from painful feelings, to distract and avoid conflict. Distracters are the elusive, sometimes charming, magicians. They are difficult to hold accountable or responsible because they keep the focus elsewhere, not on themselves. Many alcoholics and addicts are masters of this style of communication and avoid or deny their problems with alcohol and drugs. Their communication patterns feature the following:

   a.   Words that are confusing and irrelevant. They are unable to establish clarity or to set specific goals.
   b.   Bodies that act as if they are somewhere else when the content gets too specific and focused. They want to frustrate, discount, and escape from others.
   c.   Feelings: "Nobody cares. I am not happy."

According to Satir, **leveling** is the healthy state of communication. Words, body, and feelings are consistent with the message. The individual is congruent and acts in a congruent fashion.

⚹ Family System Roles

Wegscheider-Cruse's Alcoholic/Addict Family System Survival Roles

Sharon Wegscheider-Cruse was trained by and has worked closely with Virginia Satir. Wegscheider-Cruse is best known for her books *The Family Trap* (1976) and *Family Reconstruction Therapy: The Living Model* (1994). She is a leader in the field of adult children of alcoholics and family reconstruction and has popularized the concept of survival roles in the alcoholic/addict family system. These roles are labeled in terms of the coping mechanisms members use to survive in a dysfunctional alcoholic/addict family. They include the chief enabler, family hero, family scapegoat, lost child, and family mascot.

The *chief enabler* assumes primary responsibility for the chemically dependent family member. The chief enabler shelters and protects, even denies, the dysfunctional aspects of a family member's alcohol/drug use. The major enabling approaches are the following:

1. Avoiding and shielding
2. Attempting to control
3. Taking over responsibilities
4. Rationalizing and accepting
5. Cooperating and collaborating (Nelson 1988)

The *family hero* is the achiever, the responsible child, the good child, the model child. The family hero is often the firstborn, who escapes the dysfunctional aspects of the alcohol/drug family through personal achievement. The family's sense of self-worth is often the conscious or unconscious responsibility of this family member. Unfortunately, the family hero achieves for the family and ignores personal feelings, values, and goals. The family hero in adulthood often experiences a depression or sense of loss due to the incongruency of internal feelings with external behaviors. The hero may be outwardly successful but feel like a charlatan, or empty inside. When this conflict is not dealt with, the family hero is vulnerable to alcohol/drug problems and/or problems in interpersonal relationships.

The primary function of the *family scapegoat* is to divert the family members away from the real issues in the family (e.g., marital discord, marital infidelity, or parental alcohol/drug problems) and the painful emotionality of these family issues. The family members can then blame the scapegoat for all of the family problems. The family scapegoat often exhibits acting-out behavior in school and at home, antisocial behavior, and substance abuse due to underlying feelings of anger and resentment.

The *lost child*'s role (see Case Study 5.1) is often the most tragic. This is the child whose primary function is to allow the dysfunctional family—especially the parents—to expend less energy. This child often identifies with the pain of his or her parents and other siblings and wants to decrease the family members' level of pain by not contributing to the problem, perhaps even taking on the family's pain. The family inadvertently reinforces this child for not having needs. The child denies feelings and needs, frequently disconnecting emotionally and even physically from the family. At some point, the child can no longer deny personal feelings and pain. Thus, lost children frequently get overwhelmed with emotions and are at risk for suicide.

The primary function of the *family mascot* is to divert attention away from the family issues and family pain. The mascot uses humor, silliness, and even self-disparaging ineptness (making fun of oneself) as a way of diverting the family from its pain. Frequently, the mascot discounts a sense of self as the price to pay for calm in the family. As a result, the mascot may feel unworthy of love, unless able to alleviate someone's pain.

These are just a few family roles. The roles are stereotypic classifications for purposes of identifying some common role features in dysfunctional, or imbalanced, family systems. Please note that the roles are illustrations of dysfunctional patterns of family interaction and should not be used to pigeonhole someone into a static classification. Usually, people maintain a variety of traits from each of the roles. Family roles may also change based on different family situations and adjustments in the family process.

Case Study 5.1
The Lost Child
Michelle

Michelle was beginning her senior year in high school when her family began therapy. At that time, her stepbrother, Jack, was heavily into drugs (marijuana, hallucinogens, speed, and cocaine) and alcohol. Her other sisters were extremely angry with Jack's attitude and behavior. Michelle was an A student and the student body president. She was on the cross-country team and very popular. She had a quiet, affable presence and acted older than her 17 years. She was the only one in the family to whom Jack related. During the course of treatment, it was very difficult for Michelle to express any feelings. Even in individual sessions, she would deny feeling any pain or negative emotions.

Later that year, Michelle was accepted to a college a few hours' drive from home. During her first semester away at school, despite good study habits, she ended up dropping a course and receiving C grades. Also, she didn't make any friends at school. Michelle was running on the college track team but was unmotivated and not running to her true potential. This was quite traumatic for Michelle because she had been so popular and such a good student and athlete in high school. Michelle set up an individual counseling appointment during her college break. For the first time, she was in touch with her pain and grief. If she had not reached out for help, Michelle would have been another college student unable to cope with the pressures or to deal effectively with backlogged feelings, which eventually might have caused her to take her own life.

Discussion

This case illustrates the family role of the lost child. The lost child role takes many forms, but the essential theme is a child who appears on the surface to be doing extremely well but who in truth is foundering. The goal of the lost child is to be self-sufficient and not take any energy away from the family—a family that is struggling with other problems (e.g., alcohol/drug abuse and addiction). Unfortunately, the lost child is not dealing with her or his own feelings and can eventually be overwhelmed by them. The lost child is the family member who is at risk for suicide.

As adults, lost children are often high achievers. They affirm the family through their drive to success but often are unable to identify or give voice to their own feelings. This is frequently exhibited in problems with intimacy, empathy, and connection with others.

Other important family therapists—Salvador Minuchin, Theodore Lidz, Lieman Wynne, James Framo, Ron Jackson, and Jay Haley—emphasize a systems approach in their work with families and changing dysfunctional patterns of family communication and interaction. These family therapists have different styles, theories, and methods of working with families. Some see the entire family together in a counseling session. Others may see family members separately or sometimes see the father and son, mother and daughter, or just the children. Family therapists even use a multigenerational approach that includes grandparents, or an expanded family approach of including other relatives. The key element of all of these approaches is looking at the family as a system, a system that is affected and changed by the actions and events in the lives of each of the family members.

Family Roles Played Out at the Dinner Table

The Green family, like many families, had the ritual of having dinner together. When the children were younger, the minor irritations of "spilled milk" (literally and metaphorically) gave rise to Dad's rage. Mr. Green was usually exhausted at dinnertime, stressed out by his job. Mr. Green's father was a mean-tempered, negative, emotionally disconnected, and nasty alcoholic, who didn't model any form of connection or caring toward his children. Mr. Green, like his father, had little patience with his children and would lose his temper easily. As the children got older, the dinner table became a battle zone. The youngest child was the "lost child," the middle child the "scapegoat," and the oldest child the "hero."

The middle child (the scapegoat) would spark the battle by antagonizing his father, challenging him. This son would argue politics, religion, current events, and so on, taking a position that would irritate his father. This son was the brightest child, aware and well read, and would use these skills to mock his father's ignorance on issues.

Mr. Green would soon escalate and explode. The youngest child (lost child) would plead for a truce, which was ignored. She would burst into tears and retreat to her room. The oldest child (the hero) would make jokes and tell the family they were too serious about all this. Sometimes this approach worked, but many times it didn't. Mr. Green would usually explode, grab his dinner plate, and retreat to the den. The oldest child was aligned and enmeshed with his mother. Mom would then sit down by this son and blame the middle child (scapegoat) for causing the conflict.

This is just one scenario of family roles and alliances. The family imbalance is played out night after night at the dinner table.

Five Styles of Managing Anxiety

Harriet Lerner (1997) describes five styles or roles of managing anxiety—underachievers, overfunctioners, blamers, pursuers, and distancers (see Table 5.1). Anxiety about substance abuse in the family often leads to these coping roles.

Enabling Behavior

In an attempt to avoid recognizing problems, the family enables the continued use of alcohol/drugs and other dysfunctional behaviors. Enabling is described as an unhealthy doing-for, or killing with kindness (Table 5.2). Parents may have good intentions in enabling their children. Their lack of insight into the dynamics of the enabling process, however, causes problems to continue and to get progressively worse. (See Case Study 5.2.)

> Protecting one's child is normal and appropriate, but overprotection can cause problems. Enablers overprotect and find it difficult to separate what their child

---

TABLE 5.1

Five Styles of Managing Anxiety

Underfunctioners

- tend to have several areas where they just can't get organized.
- become less competent under stress, thus inviting others to take over.
- tend to develop physical or emotional symptoms when stress is high in either the family or the work situation.
- earn such labels as the "patient," the "frail one," the "sick one," the "problem," the "irresponsible one."
- have difficulty showing their strong, competent side to intimate others.

Overfunctioners

- know what's best not only for themselves but for others as well.
- move in quickly to advise, rescue, and take over when stress hits.
- have difficulty staying out and allowing others to struggle with their own problems.
- avoid worrying about their own personal goals and problems by focusing on others.
- have difficulty sharing their own vulnerable, underfunctioning side, especially with those people who are viewed as having problems.
- may be labeled the person who is "always reliable" or "always together."

Blamers

- respond to anxiety with emotional intensity and fighting.
- have a short fuse.
- expend high levels of energy trying to change someone who does not want to change.
- engage in repetitive cycles of fighting that relieve tension but perpetuate the old pattern.

- hold another person responsible for one's own feelings and actions.
- see others as the sole obstacle to making changes.

Pursuers

- react to anxiety by seeking greater togetherness in a relationship.
- place a high value on talking things out and expressing feelings, and believe others should do the same.
- feel rejected and take it personally when someone close to them wants more time and space alone or away from the relationship.
- tend to pursue harder and then coldly withdraw when an important person seeks distance.
- may negatively label themselves as "too dependent" or "too demanding" in a relationship.
- tend to criticize their partner as someone who can't handle feelings or tolerate closeness.

Distancers

- seek emotional distance or physical space when stress is high.
- consider themselves to be self-reliant and private persons—more "do-it-yourselfers" than help-seekers.
- have difficulty showing their needy, vulnerable, and dependent sides.
- receive such labels as "emotionally unavailable," "withholding," "unable to deal with feelings," from significant others.
- manage anxiety in personal relationships by intensifying work-related projects.
- may cut off a relationship entirely when things get intense, rather than hanging in and working it out.
- open up most freely when they are not pushed or pursued.

SOURCE: *The Dance of Anger* by Harriet Lerner, Ph.D., 1997, HarperCollins.

Case Study 5.2

Enabling Behavior

Jerome

Jerome's marijuana use and related behaviors were driving his family crazy. Mom tried persuasion and pleading to Jerome's sense of "doing the right thing." She picked up after Jerome, believed his stories, denied his abuse of marijuana, and buffered him from his dad's anger.

Dad vacillated from trying to control the situation, to buying and doing things for Jerome. He would "throw money" at the problem and then get angry when Jerome was irresponsible. This cycle continued for quite some time. The family entered family counseling, but most sessions were just "rag on Jerome sessions." Mom and Dad decided to do their own individual counseling, which eventually led to marital counseling. Eventually they stopped blaming each other for Jerome's problems, diminished their enabling behavior, and held Jerome responsible for his behavior. Progress was slow but eventually led to all three of them feeling like they were a more functional and balanced family.

Discussion

Enabling behavior is not the domain of just one family member. Usually both parents, and even siblings, enable in an imbalanced family system. Until all family members can take responsibility for their own enabling behavior, rather than blaming each other, the family will continue to have problems.

Family counseling can be effective if family members work with a therapist who is trained in both family systems and alcohol/drug treatment. Often individual therapy, or some form of individual work (e.g., Al-Anon), is necessary before the family can work together.

needs from what their child wants. The price of overprotection is prolonging the dependency of immaturity and thereby aiding the progression of chemical dependency. (MacDonald 1984)

Enabling behavior has been defined as taking responsibility for someone else's lack of responsibility, or softening the consequences for someone's irresponsibility. Enablers are under the delusion that no one knows about the problems and they can continue to cover them up. The reality is that others are aware of the problems and are directly and indirectly letting the family know they need help. Only the family maintains this denial to the real dimensions of the problem.

✸ Stages in Family Recovery from Substance-Abuse Problems

Families have a wide range and variety of reactions to alcohol/drug problems, yet there are some common, generalizable patterns to a family's response.

TABLE 5.2

Enabling Behavior

Charles Nelson (1988) identified the following four styles of enabling behavior.

Avoiding and Shielding

Avoiding and shielding constitute any behavior by a family member that covers up or prevents the user or the family member from experiencing the full impact of the harmful consequences of the drug use. Enabling behavior includes

- Making up excuses to avoid social contact during drinking and drugging periods
- Side-stepping or avoiding participation in discussions about drugs
- Taking alcohol, sedatives, and/or other drugs to try to lower one's own anxiety or stress about a family member's problems with drugs
- Not standing up for one's rights in fear of the family member going into a binge cycle of drug use
- Cleaning up the family member's vomit after an alcohol/drug episode
- Staying away from home as much as possible to get away from the situation
- Shielding the addict from a crisis that could send her/him into therapy
- Telling the alcoholic to leave until he/she quits drinking but then immediately going out and looking for that family member
- Helping the addict keep up appearances or cover up around relatives, friends, neighbors, or her/his employer

Attempting to Control

Attempting to control is any behavior by a family member that is performed with the intent of taking personal control over the alcoholic/addict's use of the drug. Enabling behavior includes

- Trying to buy things that might divert the addict from drug use (sports equipment, tools, car, house, etc.)
- Spending the night at a hotel or motel to get the user to quit

- Spending the night at a friend's house to get the user to quit
- Screaming, yelling, swearing, or crying in an attempt to get a family member to stop drinking or drugging
- Threatening to hurt oneself in an attempt to get a family member to quit
- Threatening physical violence to get the user to quit
- Checking or measuring the addict's drug stash to determine how much he has been using
- Encouraging the addict to do the drug at home to avoid more problems away from home
- Using or withholding sex as a way to control a partner's alcohol/drug use
- Throwing away, hiding, or destroying the family member's stash or paraphernalia

Taking Over Responsibilities

Taking over responsibilities is any behavior by the family member designed to take over the user's personal responsibilities (e.g., finances, household chores, or employment). Enabling behavior includes

- Cleaning the family member's drug paraphernalia when left out
- Waking the alcoholic in time for work
- Reminding the user to eat at times
- Staying home from work to take care of the family member's problems resulting from drug use
- Preaching to the addict about her failures as a warning about the personal effects of the drug use
- Doing the family member's chores
- Waiting hand and foot on the family member
- Paying all the bills
- Taking a second job to cover the bills piling up after money has been diverted to drugs
- Covering the alcoholic/addict's bad checks

Rationalizing and Accepting

Rationalizing and accepting are any behavior by the family member that conveys a rationalization

(continued on next page)

TABLE 5.2 (continued)	
Enabling Behavior	
or acceptance of the alcoholic/addict's use of the drug. Enabling behavior includes	• Believing and/or communicating that the use of the drugs was safe
• Believing and/or communicating that the family member's episodes of drug use were only isolated instances and not patterns of use	• Believing and/or communicating that the family member's use of drugs increased that person's self-confidence

One model describes the following stages in the family's adjustment to the substance-abuse problem:

1. Denial and minimizing
2. Tension and isolation
3. Frustration and disorganization
4. Attempts to reorganize, shifts in family member alliances
5. Separation in roles, escape
6. Reorganization without the addict/alcoholic
7. Recovery and reorganization with the addict/alcoholic

The application of the stages of grieving can also be used as a model to describe the stages in recovery for the alcoholic/addict and his or her family members.

1. Denial
2. Anger
3. Bargaining
4. Feeling (or depression)
5. Acceptance

Often the stages are positioned differently or combined. Remember, such models are meant to highlight different aspects of the recovery process, not to describe a rigid linear process.

Denial

At the denial stage (see Table 5.3), family members rarely acknowledge that something is wrong, although they sense something might be different about their family. The spouse or family members may seek help in an indirect, nonspecific manner,

TABLE 5.3
Denial Stage in Imbalanced Family Systems
Feelings—embarrassed, humiliated, shamed *Defenses*—minimization, rationalization *Linkage to society*—friends and relatives "maintain the denial" *Motto*—"normal family illusion"

such as talking to friends and/or relatives. Unfortunately, those friends and relatives often reinforce the denial. One such example is the following:

Denial Transaction Between Mary and Her Sister-in-Law, Maureen

Mary: The other night at the party, do you think Harry drank too much?
Maureen: Oh, that happens to everyone once in a while.
Mary: You don't think he has a problem with alcohol, do you?
Maureen: No, of course not. He drinks like most of us in the family, and we certainly don't have a problem. You're overreacting.

In reality, Harry and Maureen grew up in alcoholic family systems and they both have drinking problems.

Anger

Anger is an effective defense to keep family members from talking about issues and feelings that might indicate an alcohol/drug problem in the family. Anger can be expressed as verbal, physical, emotional, and/or sexual threats, abuse, and/or violation. Anger can be actual or threatened rejection and abandonment. Alcoholics/addicts use anger to blame and shame other family members as inadequate and responsible for their predicament. In reality, the anger is a way for the alcoholic/addict to avoid feelings of shame, to control others in the family, and to deny responsibility for problems in the family system.

Once in recovery, many adolescent and adult patients/clients admit that causing a conflict or big fight was a way to get out of the house and use alcohol/drugs. Many clients rationalized that they were already in trouble with the family, so what was the difference if they got into more trouble?

An adolescent patient/client once described her alcoholic/addictive family system as "raging and ragging" (nagging): "Dad is the one who rages around the home, and Mom attempts to control him by ragging at Dad and everyone else. It is no wonder that I don't spend much time at home."

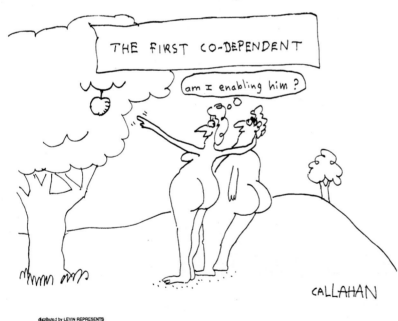

THE FIRST CO-DEPENDENT

am I enabling him?

CALLAHAN

distributed by LEVIN REPRESENTS

The Garden of Eden: Enabling behavior. Callahan, distributed by Levin Represents.

The combined effect is an unsafe, unpredictable family system with underlying feelings of confusion, fear, anxiety, and shame and sometimes immobilizing trauma.

This conflict among family members creates a climate of confusion and a lack of clarity as to what is an appropriate approach to the problem of alcohol/drugs. The result is often a trial-and-error approach. At first, family members try extreme control or rigid threats: "The next time you use alcohol/drugs, I will . . . "(not let you in the house, confine you to your room for one month, get a divorce or separation). When this doesn't work, the next approach might be to let go, or to try to ignore the addictive behavior completely, as if the addict didn't exist. The resulting pattern of control-release is chaotic. This trial-and-error approach creates further anger, confusion, and feelings of hopelessness.

At this stage, the family might go beyond relatives and friends and talk to a minister, priest, rabbi, family physician, or school counselor. The family members may be vague in disclosing the degree to which alcohol/drugs are used. At this stage, family members are still not quite sure they need help and are embarrassed in seeking help. They may start to get help, get frightened, or be resistant to experiencing the pain associated with acknowledging the problem and then back off from getting help. See Table 5.4.

Bargaining

The bargaining stage (see Case Study 5.3) is usually preceded by a major crisis. The family can no longer deny or ignore the problem and cannot cover up the feelings of frustration and anger. The family is essentially saying, "We have had enough of this; it's too chaotic." The family is still not ready to effect change in the system; instead, the goal is to strike some arrangement or bargain. Being held hostage by the addict, the family is willing to pay a ransom to have the addict stop bothering them with outrageous behavior. Unfortunately, the ransom often goes beyond what is reasonable or tolerable, and the family initially agrees to do almost anything to survive in this chaos. Many of the bargains are financial or object-related: "If you stop abusing alcohol/drugs, I'll buy you. . . "

The underlying and false assumption of most bargains is that the addict can stop using. The assumption is that the addict can override the drive and allure of the alcohol/drugs for a reward. Unfortunately, the drive to use alcohol/drugs is stronger than the reward of the bargain, and willpower alone is not strong enough to overcome the drive to use alcohol/drugs.

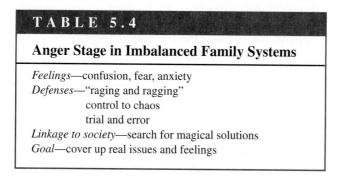

TABLE 5.4
Anger Stage in Imbalanced Family Systems

Feelings—confusion, fear, anxiety
Defenses—"raging and ragging"
         control to chaos
         trial and error
Linkage to society—search for magical solutions
Goal—cover up real issues and feelings

> ## Case Study 5.3
> ### *A Bargain That Doesn't Work*
> #### Marilyn
>
> Marilyn is a very bright, attractive, outgoing 17-year-old. She puts forth minimal effort at school and barely passes her classes, despite her superior intelligence.
>
> She smokes marijuana regularly, drinks alcohol, uses cocaine, and has begun free-basing cocaine. She has been staying out late, and sleeping in every day during the summer. This is the second marriage for her mother, and Marilyn's mother and father are always trying to bribe Marilyn to get her to straighten out. Bribes have included a new car, clothes shopping excursions, and vacations. There have been so many conflicts at home between Marilyn, her mother, and her stepfather, that her real father has agreed to let Marilyn live in the condo on the waterfront for the rest of the summer. It only took a few weeks for the place to be trashed, and the police became regular visitors to Marilyn's parties. Her parents also became aware of Marilyn's freebase cocaine use and took her in for an alcohol/drug evaluation.
>
> ### *Discussion*
>
> Bargaining doesn't work and is a temporary solution. Marilyn was not held accountable for her behavior, school grades, and drug use. The parents were avoiding these issues and related conflicts by blindly hoping that Marilyn would somehow mature and grow out of this stage. They kept on giving her things and buying (no pun intended) her stories.
>
> In the "bargaining" stage, they avoided the reality of feeling what was really going on, and accepted that Marilyn had significant problems. But they avoided the first and biggest problem—her drug abuse.

Some of the bargains are far more subtle. Couples, families, and friends develop lives based on the bargain of maintaining addiction. See Table 5.5. Following are some common bargains related to alcoholism and drug addiction, and their weaknesses:

- *Let's ignore the addict's behavior and it might just stop.* The more you ignore the destructive behavior, the more intense and dramatic the situation becomes.
- *Let's separate or withdraw from the addict temporarily.* Unless there is strong therapeutic and personal support, the addict feeds on the partner's or family members' weaknesses. The individual usually does not have the support to break the codependent dance of addiction. (See Chapter 7.)
- *Avoid making a decision; maybe it will get better with time.* It's very rare that a spontaneous recovery occurs from alcohol/drugs. Chapter 9 discusses alcohol/drug intervention and "raising the addict's bottom" in an attempt to salvage and avoid further damage. Rarely do addicts decide on their own to get help. Sometimes it is so late that scary consequences

TABLE 5.5

Bargaining, Feeling, and Acceptance Stage in Imbalanced Family Systems

Goal—"maintain the chaos of addiction"
Bargains—compromise values
             love/hate—let go/hold on
             avoid making a decision
             confused—doesn't know what is appropriate
Depression/feelings—feelings are experienced
Acceptance

  there is a problem
  on road to recovery

are involved, such as the threat of physical harm, criminal justice and legal problems, job and financial problems, or death.

At the bargaining stage, family members might seek help from experts in the field because their bargains are not working and they need advice and direction. Even when family members are fortunate in finding a counselor who knows about alcohol/drug intervention and treatment, the family members may still not follow through. The attitude at this stage is still a form of bargaining. The therapeutic bargain is to fix the identified patient (the addict) so the bargainer can avoid feeling pain. In some situations, family members may even sabotage counseling to avoid the pain of looking at their roles in the dysfunction. In a distorted sense, the failure of the trained professional validates the failure of the family member: "If the counselor can't help, then I guess we didn't do such a bad job." Many families seeking counseling soon find out that addiction is a family disease and effective treatment involves the entire family.

Feeling

At the feeling stage, family members can no longer deny, cover up with anger, or bargain their feelings away. Many feelings come to the surface and are easily accessed. Family members cry at the slightest provocation, anxious to the point of being hypervigilant (checking things out obsessively) and, in some cases, feeling immobilized. These feelings are undeniable and force the family to seek help.

Acceptance

At the acceptance stage, the family has recognized that they have a problem. They are ready to do the work necessary to heal and develop healthier ways of relating. Recognizing that all the family members are suffering, they have the courage to get help. At this stage, the alcoholic/addict and the family members have begun to work on the problem. This is when treatment and recovery begin.

⚹ In Review

- The alcoholic/drug addict family system is a system in disequilibrium, often trying to counterbalance the extent of the problem with denial. Therefore, instead of *dysfunctional family system,* we can use the term *imbalanced family system.* This term is recommended because it is a more accurate description and avoids the shame connotations of the term *dysfunctional.*
- Families have specific rules, alliances, and patterns of communication.
- There is truly an emotional imbalance in the alcoholic/addict family system. The term *imbalance* gives hope that there is a way to get help and better manage the system. The goal is to establish balance and order by addressing the problems in the family. The term *dysfunctional* implies hopelessness and shame. It is best to avoid using the term.
- Virginia Satir describes unhealthy styles of communication:

    - *Placaters* discount themselves.
    - *Blamers* elevate themselves by discounting others.
    - *Intellectualizers* discount their own feelings.
    - *Distractors* keep others and themselves away from painful feelings; distract and avoid conflict.
    - The alcoholic/addict family system has survival roles—chief enabler, family hero, family scapegoat, lost child, and family mascot.
    - Enabling behaviors include avoiding and shielding, attempting to control, taking over responsibilities, and rationalizing and accepting.
    - During family recovery, the family goes through the stages of grieving—denial, anger, bargaining, depression/feeling, acceptance. However, the family might skip or go back and forth through the stages of grieving.

⚹ Discussion Questions

1. Describe some imbalances in your own family system, and describe the crisis or conflict that may have caused that imbalance.
2. What is your emotional (gut) reaction to using the term *dysfunctional family system* versus *imbalanced family system.* Explain.
3. Identify some family rules in your family of origin, and list the ones you like and those you don't like. If you have children, what are the rules in your family? If you don't have children, what rules do you think would be important if you had children?
4. Please rank your use of these styles of communication, from 1 (least frequently) to 5 (most frequently), and explain.

    - Placater
    - Blamer
    - Intellectualizer
    - Distracter
    - Leveler

5. From the following list, please identify the role you might have played in your family, and the roles that any siblings played. Explain and describe the characteristics and circumstances played out by each role.

- Hero
- Lost child
- Mascot
- Scapegoat
- Chief enabler

⊰ References

Alcohol and Drug Abuse Institute Library, University of Washington, Seattle.

Black, Claudia. 1982. *It will never happen to me!* Denver, Colo.: M.A.C.

Lawson, Ann, and Gary Lawson. 1998. *Alcoholism and the family: A guide to treatment and prevention.* 2d ed. Gaithersburg, Md.: Aspen.

Lerner, Harriet. 1997. *The dance of anger.* New York: HarperCollins.

MacDonald, Donald Ian. 1984. *Drugs, drinking and adolescents.* Chicago: Year Book Medical.

Nelson, Charles. 1988. The style of enabling behavior. In *Treating cocaine dependency,* edited by D. E. Smith and D. Wesson. Center City, Minn.: Hazeldon Foundation.

Satir, Virginia. 1967. *Conjoint family therapy.* Palo Alto, Calif.: Science and Behavior Books.

Satir, Virginia. 1972. *Peoplemaking.* Palo Alto, Calif.: Science and Behavior Books.

Satir, Virginia, et al. 1983. *Helping families to change.* New York: Aronson.

Satir, Virginia, and Michele Baldwin. 1983. *Satir: Step by step—A guide to creating change in families.* Northvale, N.J.: Aronson, Jason.

Wegscheider-Cruse, Sharon. 1976. *The family trap.* Palo Alto, Calif.: Nurturing Network.

Wegscheider-Cruse, Sharon, et al. 1994. *Family reconstruction therapy: The living model.* Palo Alto, Calif.: Science and Behavior Books.

Whitaker, Carl, and Augustus Y. Napier. 1978. *The family crucible.* New York: Harper & Row.

Parenting

Impact on Alcohol/Drug Use and Abuse

Objectives

1. Classify and identify the role parent-child bonding can play in personality and sense of self, and as a risk factor for substance abuse.
2. Identify the six elements of abandonment depression.
3. Identify the impact of early abandonment and lack of nurturing on adult interpersonal relationships.
4. Identify the different temperaments that make children more at risk for substance abuse.
5. Describe the different styles of parenting and the quality of the parent-child relationship as they relate to being a risk factor for substance abuse.
6. Define shame and describe its relationship to imbalanced parenting.
7. Describe the differences between the child growing up in an imbalanced and/or shame-based family system and the child growing up in a balanced, functional family system.
8. Identify the differences between shame and guilt, especially as these feelings relate to sense of self.
9. Classify the escalation of feelings caused by the affect-shame bind.
10. Describe the different domains on which shame has a major impact.
11. Describe parental shame and the many obstacles that make it difficult for parents and family to seek help for substance-abuse problems in the family.
12. Describe the dynamics of rejection sensitivity, fear and difficulty in making decisions, poor frustration tolerance, and defense behaviors as a result of imbalanced parenting and imbalanced family systems.
13. Identify the characteristics of clear boundaries compared with enmeshed boundaries and disengaged boundaries.
14. Define boundary ambiguity.
15. Describe triangulation and the problems related to triangulated communication.
16. Describe the imbalances in family systems throughout the life cycles of the family:
    • Relationships through unattached adults
    • Joining of families through marriage
    • Family and the young adult
    • Family and the adolescent
    • Launching of children
    • Later life
17. Describe the difficulty in engaging fathers in counseling and the role of noble ascriptions.

⚹ Introduction

Some of the parenting variables that influence a child's use and abuse of alcohol/drugs later in life are

- Parent-child bonding
- Temperament of the child
- Parenting styles and the quality of the parent-child relationship
- Parental imbalance and boundary setting
- Parents' use/abuse of alcohol or drugs
- Other family system variables

These factors are the major focus of this chapter.

⚹ Parent-Child Bonding

The parent-child bond is an extremely potent, primary relationship that greatly influences behavior. Maccoby and Martin (1983) describe the parent-child bond as unique among human relationships. Nothing is as powerful as the bonding between parent and child. Extraordinary feats of strength and sacrifice have come to be identified with this strong bond. Examples of the parent-child bond include the incredible adrenaline-induced strength of a father saving a child who is pinned under an automobile, and the dedication and perseverance of a mother who protects her child from the drug- and crime-infested streets of the inner city.

A child's development is often impaired as a result of a poor bond with a parent. Self-concept, social and interpersonal relationships, achievement, and identity are negatively affected by inadequate parent-child bonding.

A positive, caring relationship is essential for healthy development. The effective parent establishes bonding experiences that develop a positive regard for the child and reinforce a positive sense of self. When a parent loses this positive bonding with a child, the child's sense of loss and anger may never be assuaged. This loss is often found in alcoholic/addict family systems.

Often, because of certain circumstances, parents are not available. A variety of conditions may take the parents from the child—death of a parent, a parent away at war, divorce, illness, mental breakdown, criminal-justice problems, financial problems, job relocation (e.g., military), and so on. All of these circumstances prevent bonding between child and parent and are extremely disruptive to the child's life. (See Case Study 6.1.) The child may even suffer depression as a result of times when he or she felt abandoned or rejected.

Certainly, the parent's alcoholism/drug addiction also makes the parent either unavailable or inconsistent in the quality of the parent-child relationship.

Patrick Carnes, author of numerous books on sexual trauma and addiction, describes the importance of developing healthy bonds with caring adults outside of the family system for children who have been sexually violated/traumatized by a family member. In a 1995 interview in *Professional Counselor Magazine,* Carnes states, "One of the things that emerges in trauma literature is why some kids, who have the same identical history of trauma, rebound from that and have resiliency.

Case Study 6.1
Early Bonding—Being Available in the "Now"
Karen

Karen was very young—18 years old—when she had the first of her two children. Over the next few years, she was extremely depressed. Perhaps it was the responsibility of two young children and being tied to the house or the constant conflicts with her husband that caused Karen to decide to leave. It was an extremely difficult decision to leave two toddlers. However, at the time, her own survival seemed more important.

Twelve years later, Karen was in counseling. She was 34 years old and struggling with the fact that her 14-year-old son, Gary, was addicted to alcohol/drugs. Over the past 2 years Gary had been in and out of outpatient counseling programs and was now in his second inpatient alcohol/drug program. Karen needed some support in setting boundaries with Gary. She first needed to talk about her guilt at abandoning him when he was 2 years old. She had left the home, had filed for divorce, and had given custody of both children to Gary's father.

As the counseling proceeded, it became clear that her own alcohol use had contributed dramatically to her problems in those early years in the marriage. It was a few years after leaving the marriage that she acknowledged her own alcoholism. Even though she had been in recovery from alcohol and drugs for several years now and extremely active in Alcoholics Anonymous (AA), she was still experiencing dramatic problems in relationships. Over several sessions, she was able to talk about her own childhood and revealed that her father had sexually violated her. Although she had talked about this several times in previous counseling sessions and during her inpatient alcohol/drug program, she was now able to see that this contributed to her own fears of abusing her own children. She slowly began to accept how her alcoholic behavior prevented her from bonding with her own children. After some time, she was able to accept that she could not recapture those lost years with her children. She could not compensate for the lack of bonding during those formative years, no matter how available she was for Gary and his younger sister today. She began to recognize that her own attempts to compensate for those early years had resulted in her enabling Gary's alcohol and drug use. It took Karen some time to grieve and accept that she missed those early developmental years. She realized that there was a permanent loss in bonding, a loss that could never be recaptured.

Discussion

At age 18, Karen was not really capable of providing adequate nurturing and nourishment to her infant children. Her own depression, alcoholism, and history of sexual violation, along with the developmental reality that she was 18 years old, contributed to her inability to be present with her children. The constant conflicts with her husband made an impossible situation even more difficult.

The guilt of her having "abandoned" her toddlers caused her to indulge her son when they did get reunited. It is important that her therapist not judge Karen but help her work through her issues—the first of which is that she cannot recapture all those lost years—and help her grieve, and accept what she can do to develop a relationship with her son. It is also important to acknowledge the reality that their relationship might not develop, but that she can persevere and maintain her availability to her son "in the now."

As near as I can tell from the literature and what I have seen clinically, the primary factor is the ability of children to have healthy bonds around them that are not traumatic. As an antidote to trauma bonding, you need healthy bonds."

Two prevailing hypotheses regarding parental bonding in adolescent substance abusers are the *overinvolvement hypothesis* and the *functional hypothesis* (Volk et al. 1988). The overinvolvement hypothesis is that one parent (frequently the mother) is overly involved in the adolescent's life to compensate for the lack of availability by the other parent. The functional hypothesis is that the adolescent's substance abuse distracts the family from focusing on other familial problems, such as marital discord, infidelity, and parental abuse of alcohol/drugs.

Abandonment Depression

A young child needs nurturing and connection with a caring parent. James Masterson (1976), in his work with borderline-personality-disordered individuals, identifies an affective (feeling) disorder that he labeled "abandonment depression." Masterson believes that a significant separation stress precipitates abandonment depression (see Table 6.1). It is also likely that this separation occurs early in life, at 18 to 24 months of age. The individual suffering from abandonment depression is metaphorically described as "an egg with the insides removed." All the good stuff—the nutrients, the seed, the juices of life—has been removed, has rotted, or has been destroyed by a lack of nurturing.

The six key elements of abandonment depression are

1. Homicidal rage
2. Suicidal depression

TABLE 6.1
Childhood Experiences of Abandonment and Rejection
• Lack of physical and emotional availability of parents
• Negative blaming; verbal and nonverbal behavior or attacks
• Mixed messages (double binds), saying one thing and meaning something else
• Unreasonably high expectations or standards; ambiguous expectations of behavior, performance, and affect
• Lack of warmth, sensitivity, security, safety, or high regard for feelings, situations, and conflicts
• Discounting of the child's sense of self or physical and psychological boundaries
• Disparaging, blaming, and generally rejecting attitude about the child's difficulty-with developmental tasks
• Disregard, ridicule, blaming, teasing, or other verbal and nonverbal behavior that iseither rejecting or shaming
• Threats to abandon or leave a child in a joking or real manner
• Negative and rejecting statements, actions, and comments about something that is of minor or major importance to the child

3. Panic
4. Feelings of hopelessness and helplessness
5. Emptiness and void
6. Guilt

Perhaps the parent is ill, suffering from depression, or withdrawn due to a personality and/or psychiatric disorder and finds it hard to nurture his or her child. Maybe the parent didn't grow up in a family system that modeled nurturing, caring, and empathetic connection with the children. Masterson (1976) describes three elements that may produce separation stress in children:

1. *Nature:* Possible genetic or constitutional deficiencies such as inability to tolerate separation anxiety or to synthesize positive and negative effects as well as such conditions as attention deficit disorders and developmental disharmonies.
2. *Nurture:* "Maternal libidinal unavailability for the child's move toward separation-individuation or self-activation (i.e., the mother is unable or has difficulty in identifying, acknowledging, and supporting the child's emerging self-activation, experimentation, and exploration). The reasons for maternal libidinal unavailability may be many—death, divorce, physical or emotional illness, etc."
3. *Fate:* "Any accident of fate that impairs the child's ability to separate and/or individuate. On the separation side, events such as death or divorce can prevent the mother from being emotionally available. On the individuation side, events can impair or prevent the child from practicing his emerging individuation. For example, the child may be sickly or in a restricted environment."

Impact of Early Abandonment on Adult Interpersonal Relationships

Individuals suffering from abandonment depression express complaints having to do with intimacy. They have difficulty emotionally entering into healthy relationships and are unable to differentiate their needs from others' needs. They experience difficulty in identifying and communicating feelings or in accepting feelings and communication from others. There is either a fusing of others into self or a fission, causing them to break away emotionally from others.

Masterson (1976) described persons suffering from abandonment depression as experiencing difficulty in establishing intimacy in relationships due to a limited capacity for spontaneity, empathy, and sensitivity. These persons have difficulty in making an emotional commitment to a relationship. Such individuals experience twin fears—the fear of losing (abandonment), which leads to clinging behavior, and the fear of being engulfed (smothered), which leads to feelings of depersonalization, shutting down, distortion of reality, and desensitization (numbing, disconnecting from the body).

At first, using alcohol and drugs to facilitate feeling in interpersonal relationships may seem effective; however, as time goes on, this becomes dysfunctional and destructive. Persons feeling pain also use alcohol/drugs to alleviate the core feeling of abandonment.

Those suffering feelings of abandonment may also choose to enter into dysfunctional and/or alcoholic/addict relationships, or relationships with individuals emotionally and physically unavailable.

The *Diagnostic and Statistical Manual of Mental Disorders* (American Psychiatric Association 1994) lists diagnostic criteria for borderline personality disorder that include the following. These often result from early childhood experiences of abandonment. (See Chapter 10 for more information.)

1. Impulsivity or unpredictability in at least two areas that are potentially self-damaging
2. A pattern of unstable and intense interpersonal relationships
3. Inappropriate, intense anger or lack of control of anger
4. Identity disturbances manifested by uncertainty about several issues relating to identity, such as self-image, gender identity, long-term goals or career choice, friendship patterns, values, and loyalties
5. Affective instability

⚹ Child's Temperament

Each child has his or her own temperament. Temperament is described as a behavioral characteristic that researchers believe is present at birth, within the first few months of life, and during infancy (Garrison and Earls 1987; Kohnstamm, Bates, and Rothbart 1989).

There is emerging evidence that extremes in certain temperament traits, such as high activity level, emotionality, attention span, and sociability, are associated with children of alcoholics. These temperaments also put the child at risk for alcoholism/ drug addiction and other problem behaviors. The parents of these children are faced with challenges beyond the average parenting techniques. Early evaluation and early intervention are essential to address the issues of children with these temperaments. Children who exhibit these genetically determined temperaments may benefit from prevention efforts, which include special educational and counseling programs. Parents also benefit from parenting skills and education in helping these children to cope better.

Aspects of temperament may predict the behavior problems and substance-abuse problems that frequently arise during adolescence. There also appear to be gender differences in temperament that put children at risk for behavior problems and substance abuse. A study by Block, Block, and Keyes (1988) found that nursery school girls who were low in ego resiliency and ego control were using marijuana at age 14, and boys' marijuana use was predicted by low ego control but not by early ego resilience. Masse and Tremblay (1997), in a study of kindergarten boys, found that high novelty seeking and low harm avoidance measured at age 6 predicted early onset of cigarette smoking, drunkenness, and other drug use in adolescence. Dobkin, Tremblay, Masse, and Vitaro (1995), in a study of 755 six-year-old boys, found that disruptive behaviors (fighting, hyperactivity, oppositional behaviors) measured at 6 years of age predicted having been drunk or using other drugs—or both—before age 14.

Some clusters of temperament related to substance use/abuse are labeled as a "difficult temperament"—high activity level, low flexibility and task orientation, mood instability, and social withdrawal (Lerner and Vicary 1984, Ohannessian and Hesselbrook 1995). Tubman and Windle (1999) described a difficult temperament as higher activity level, lower task orientation, inflexibility, a withdrawal orientation, biological arrhythmicity, and low positive mood, as a predictor of higher levels of alcohol problems among adolescents. In a study by Martin, Kaczynski, Maisto, and Tarter (1996) a cluster of temperament traits was a predictor of the number of drugs used by adolescents. That cluster included dispositional traits characterized by heightened negative affect (depressed mood and anxiety) and behavioral undercontrol, reflecting impulsivity, aggressivity, acting out, and sensation seeking.

The research on temperament has primarily been on the traits that predict substance use and abuse and problem behaviors. There are temperament traits that may function as a protective factor, especially for high-risk groups. One such study (Werner and Smith 1999) measured the influence of cuddly, affectionate temperament style in infancy and early childhood. This longitudinal Kauai study of low socioeconomic children of alcohol-abusing parents found decreased risk for alcohol-related and other adverse outcomes in adolescence and adulthood. The explanation was that these children had resiliency as a result of more frequent and stronger social and emotional support.

⚹ Parenting Styles and the Quality of the Parent-Child Relationship

A *supportive* parent with a healthy relationship with her or his child is less likely to have a child who gets involved with alcohol/drugs.

Rollins and Thomas (1979) explained the differences between a supportive and a controlling parent. They defined a supportive parent as possessing "parental behaviors toward the child such as praising, encouraging, and giving physical affection, which indicate to the child that she or he is accepted, approved of, and loved." In contrast, the controlling parent is defined as having "parental behavior toward the child which is intended to direct the child's behavior in a manner acceptable to the parent."

The goal of parenting is to develop a high level of parental support and a moderate level of parental control. Parents who are highly rigid, authoritarian, and controlling tend to have children who are resentful, frustrated, and angry. These children are then prone to problem behaviors, causing them to rebel or passive-aggressively get back at the rigid parent. "Children whose relationships with their parents lacked love, warmth, and closeness and exhibited signs of hostility, have children who exhibit increased levels of substance abuse, delinquency, and dysfunctional coping strategies" (Johnson and Pandina 1991).

The children of parents who are unable to establish moderate control and effective disciplining techniques often experience problem behaviors and associate with other children who have problem behaviors.

The availability of the parent(s) is extremely important in the child's development, as is the quality of the parent-child relationship. Frequently, parents will spend a quantity of time with their children and mislead themselves into thinking they are effectively developing the relationship. The quality of the parent-child relationship is the essential ingredient. The parent needs to be fully present, listening reflectively, and exchanging ideas, while giving full attention to the child. Quality time also involves understanding, touching (hugging), playing, and sharing. Making a genuine, heart-to-heart connection is at the core of a good parent-child relationship.

◈ Shame and Imbalanced Parenting

Shame is a deep-rooted feeling, often a result of traumatic childhood experiences that are excessively shaming (e.g., sexual, physical, and emotional abuse). (See Table 6.2.) Parental imbalance and parenting dysfunction are at the core of these feelings of shame. Merle Fossum and Marilyn Mason (1986) defined shame as "the self looking in on itself and finding the self lacking or flawed." Individuals may feel exposed, vulnerable, and fearful that others know they are feeling inherently bad and inadequate. Shame is more powerful than simple embarrassment, which is a temporary situation with little long-term impact. In shame, people feel that they will never recover from the negative way others see them.

Shame is a feeling that has an integral role in the individual's development. "Shame is a basic, natural human emotion, which in moderation is adaptive, healthy, and absolutely essential for development. We could not eliminate shame even if we wanted to. It's inbred in the species" (Kaufman 1989).

Sigmund Freud used the word *guilt* to describe feelings of shame. Famed family therapist Erik Erikson, in his description of the human life cycle, outlined two developmental stages that focused on guilt and shame: (1) autonomy versus doubt and shame and (2) initiative versus guilt.

Growing up in an alcohol/addict family system or an imbalanced family system creates a foundation of shame. Additional feelings of shame are perpetrated by peers, the school system, other institutions, and other authority figures in the child's life.

TABLE 6.2

Characteristics of Shameful Experiences

1. Unexpected exposure; being judged on a vulnerable aspect of oneself
2. Feeling as if there is a loss of choice
3. Feeling out of place, flawed, defective, or inadequate
4. A threat to the core of one's identity
5. Mistrust in ability to perceive things properly; unsure of self in making decisions or relating to people
6. Trust of self and others is jeopardized; boundaries are distorted; and physical, emotional, and/or sexual violations may occur.
7. Difficulty in assessing what is reality
8. Feeling helpless, powerless, and trapped, with no way out

SOURCE: Fossum and Mason 1986.

These shame-based messages are internalized by children. The result is a vicious pattern of feelings and behavior, which perpetuates the feelings of shame.

Individuals from shame-based family systems often feel that (1) there is no hope for change; (2) shame is inescapable and inevitable; (3) shame is exterior-based, not an internal process; and (4) they are bad, no good, flawed, or worthless as individuals (Fossum and Mason 1986). For these individuals, feelings of shame can include thoughts like these:

No matter what I do, it's never going to be good enough, so why try?

Each time I try, I fail, anyway. The result is always negative.

I must try so much harder than others. It's so much easier for others, so I must be
   inferior and inadequate.

You have to be perfect to be O.K.

Look at _____. Now, if I could only be like them.

It's never going to get any better, no matter how hard I try.

If only others would feel good. Then I would be happy.

Shame is a fascinating topic because it affects us all in some way (see Table 6.3). Most individuals can overcome feelings of shame and grow as a result of it, getting on with their lives. However, some individuals have been shamed dramatically and frequently, especially during early developmental years, and are unable to overcome it. These individuals are at risk for alcoholism and drug dependence or developing relationships with alcoholics/addicts. Too much trauma creates shame, which leads to feelings of hopelessness and helplessness.

There is almost a resignation that life is painfully unfulfilling—not worth trying to change. Expectations and aspirations are only indirectly acknowledged, for fear of reexperiencing rejection and shame. Shame-based individuals perceive themselves as trapped, inescapably destined to again experience the shame message of self-inadequacy and powerlessness. The shame-based orientation is external. The individual's sense of self is formed by others' evaluations and judgments of his or her performance and behavior. The orientation is outside (external world) in versus inside (internal self) out. Three characteristics—no hope, inescapable shame, and an exterior base—are found in shame-based systems and shame-based individuals.

TABLE 6.3

Shame

Definition: self looking in on self, finding the self lacking or feeling exposed—"seen"—in a public way and wanting to cover—feeling hunted

Shame-Based System	Balanced System
1. No hope—hopelessness	1. Hope—choice
2. Inescapable	2. Can make amends
3. Exterior-based	3. Internally based

SOURCE: Fossum and Mason 1986.

In contrast, in a balanced family system, the individual has a much healthier way of approaching life and others. The individual receives feedback from the world and evaluates the feedback. The individual then chooses to make changes or adjustments in decision making, goal setting, and interpersonal communication, based on his or her evaluation of the validity of the feedback. The major focus is on *hope* and *choice*.

In a balanced-system, individuals can recognize their mistakes and not feel that they themselves are the mistake. They can make amends to those who might have been hurt by their mistakes and can learn from their errors. The experience is valued, and there is an opportunity for self-growth. Individuals from a balanced family system have an orientation that is inside out (internal). These individuals relate well to and have empathy for others, balancing their own sense of self with the judgments and reactions of others.

Shame is different than embarrassment. Embarrassment is temporary, one can recover from embarrassment; shame is more long-lasting and deep-rooted. Often, shameful experiences are unresolved and take a very long time and much effort to overcome. For example, finding that your home was burglarized while you were away can elicit feelings of violation and victimization. However, letting someone in to your home, who then robs you at gunpoint, ties you up, and terrorizes you, brings a far greater level of helplessness and horror, which is shattering to your perception of being safe.

Fossum and Mason (1986) make the distinction between shame and guilt. Many people believe the feelings of guilt and shame are the same, but they are very different emotions. Table 6.4 illustrates the differences of shame and guilt as they relate to self. The key point is that shame affects the core of your being, whereas guilt is about things you have done.

The following are ways in which parents can avoid instilling shame in their young children:

1. Provide unconditional love. Let their child know that they really like him or her. Talking, touching with affection, hugging, and, most important, paying attention to the child are some of the ways in which parents express unconditional love.
2. Provide safety, nurturance, security, and care.
3. Communicate clearly with and support their spouse or partner.
4. Resolve conflicts with their spouse or partner (invoking the Alcoholics Anonymous motto "Would you rather be right or happy?").
5. Play with their infants and children.
6. Be available and enjoy the growth and development of their children.
7. Recognize that at times parenting is overwhelming—take a break and get support.
8. Protect their children from others who may hurt, violate, or shame them.
9. When parents "don't like their child's behavior" or are frustrated and annoyed, they need to minimize the impact of those negative feelings.
10. Use appropriate discipline and good judgment in parenting, and learn about parenting by taking classes on parenting and child development.
11. Seek help from teachers, family members, counselors, doctors, clergy, and so on when "shame-based" family issues arise. Do not isolate or deny (minimize

TABLE 6.4

Primary Characteristics of Shame and Guilt

Central Trait	Shame	Guilt
Failure	Of being	Of doing
Involvement of Self	Damage to global sense of self	Damage to active or moral sense of self
Action Tendency	To withdraw; to escape	To confess; to repair damage
Focus	On inadequate self	On impaired relationships
Sense of Self	Inadequate, deficient, defective, worthless, exposed, disgraced	Bad, selfish, evil, remorseful, irresponsible
Key Phrases	I am no good I am not good enough I am unlovable I do not belong I should not be	I have done wrong I have hurt someone It is my fault I must make amends
Primary Response	Strong affective/physical response: eyes down, blush, shrinking, feel small, exposed	Strong cognitive and behavioral response: need to take action
Central Fear	Abandonment: not belonging (not getting in)	Punishment: ostracism (being cast out)
Primary Defenses	Withdrawal, denial, arrogance, exhibitionism, rage, perfectionism	Rationalization, selflessness, paranoia (projection)

SOURCE: Potter-Efron 2002.

or rationalize) these issues, but take early, proactive action, which can prevent a more significant problem later on.

12. Encourage children to express themselves (what they feel and think) in play, verbal and nonverbal communication, and other activities.

Shame and Feelings

Shame-based messages that are internalized have a major impact on feelings. When shame is attached to normal, everyday feelings, it tends to escalate those feelings. For example, when an internalized shame-based message is attached to normal, everyday feelings of frustration or anger, it tends to escalate those feelings to rage (anger + shame = rage). The person feeling shame then directs this rage toward others, blaming and holding them responsible for feelings of anger and frustration. The rage violates others, pushes them away, and creates more of a feeling of isolation, loneliness, and hopelessness with no way out. This out-of-control emotional freight train picks up speed from all the memories of shame experienced in the family of origin. Some may think that the way to slow down this runaway emotional pain is to self-medicate with alcohol/drugs. Unfortunately, this temporary solution may even speed up the emotional turmoil or cause it to be repeated. When people do not deal with feelings of shame, this pattern continues. The next time, even less anger and shame are needed for the escalation to rage. (See Table 6.5.)

One of the largest domains of shame is human sexuality, as evidenced by our society's problems in establishing intimate and caring relationships. Let's look at three areas in particular: adolescent sexual identity, sexual violation, and drugs and sex.

Adolescent Sexual Identity and Shame

The developmental task of exploring and defining one's sexual identity is probably the most difficult task of adolescence. Shame-based messages by parents, schools, institutions, and peers may be devastating to adolescents and delay the development of a secure sense of sexual identity. Shame-based messages include the following:

You are bad if you_____ . (masturbate, are feeling sexual, are aroused, etc.)
Having sexual feelings before marriage is unnatural.
Sex is dirty.
That's all that men want. Men are bad and evil.
Women use sex to manipulate you to get what they want.
Don't watch television; it promotes sexual arousal.
In our family, we don't talk with others about sex.

Sexual Violation and Shame

Sexual violations are common in alcoholic/addict and imbalanced family systems. Children often feel responsible for sexual violation, as if they caused the violation (e.g., I must be responsible for this sexual feeling in others because I am so cute, attractive, shy, or outgoing). Usually, the violation is not talked about or is enabled

TABLE 6.5
Affect-Shame Binds
anger + shame = rage
anxiety + shame = panic
fear + shame = terror
sadness + shame = depression
depression + shame = despair
despair + shame = suicidal thoughts
suicidal thoughts + shame = suicide attempt
hurt + shame = pain
pain + shame = trauma (deep or chronic pain)
trauma + shame = phobia
phobia + shame = loss of reality
unavailability + shame = lack of trust of others
lack of trust of others + shame = paranoia
paranoia + shame = loss of reality

by the mother or, in some cases, the father. When told of the violation, the parent often denies that it happened or that it is possible and rationalizes the action: "Your uncle is that way with everyone. Try to stay away from him." Such parents fail to adequately protect children from future violations. When the behavior is acknowledged by children, usually no one in the family seeks therapeutic help for the victim and/or the perpetrator. Families deny sexual violations for fear of exposing the inappropriate and violating behavior and to avoid familial shame. Instead of families getting help, they maintain denial and scapegoat the victims by not acknowledging the violations or their pain. They take no or limited action to prevent future violations to the victim or to someone else.

Drugs, Sex, and Shame

Cocaine, marijuana, alcohol, methaqualone, and other drugs are often described as sex drugs, or aphrodisiacs. At early stages, alcohol/drugs do reduce inhibitions. This confuses people who define them as aphrodisiacs. In reality, all drugs impair performance, especially at middle and later stages of use.

Under the influence of alcohol/drugs, individuals also experience impaired judgment and may take part in sexual activities in which they would not normally engage if they were sober. The shame of these sexual experiences can be devastating, so they use alcohol/drugs to blot out these feelings of shame. This can become a vicious, negative, addictive cycle. This cycle involves alcohol/drug use, followed by sexual activity, followed by feelings of shame. More alcohol/drug use follows (to numb the feelings of shame), succeeded by sexual activity and more shame and feelings of loss of control.

Parents' Shame

Parents who have not done a good job of parenting may experience feelings of shame. Gomberg (1988) describes this parental shame as falling short of expectations in being a good parent. Jessup (1983) also describes a sense of failure for mothers that is shameful. Eliason and Skinstad (1995) describe the deep sense of identity and self-esteem that many women gain from their children:

> When they perceive failure at meeting the needs of their children, the sense of
> hopelessness that follows can be devastating. The sense of shame . . . about
> mothering in substance using women has been heightened by the media's attention
> to Fetal Alcohol Effects and 'cocaine babies' in recent years. This press is often
> sensationalized and contains blatant mother-blaming implications.

⚹ Other Obstacles to Reaching Parents and Family

One of the major stumbling blocks in getting adolescents into counseling for alcohol/drug problems is parental resistance. Logically, parents want the best for their children, and the parents' intentions are to do the best they can. Parents may deny adolescent substance abuse, because it brings up their own "shame" at being judged "bad parents." This denial can persist as the problems get worse, the adolescent escalates the substance abuse, and the negative consequences increase as well.

TABLE 6.6
Obstacles to Reaching Parents and Family

- Denial
- Skepticism, incongruence
- Assumption that things will be O.K.
- Distorted, depressed view of life
- Fear of being labeled
- Fear of loss of confidentiality
- Narcissism of parents
- Lack of energy/time of parents
- Distrust of the system
- Lack of credible messages—cultural/racial
- Lack of concern/respect for experts
- Lack of awareness of community resources
- Need for services for basic survival
- Cultural mores

Table 6.6 lists the many obstacles that caregivers must overcome to reach parents and family. Parents make the assumption that "things will be O.K." and may have other reasons for not asking for help and resisting taking action. Asking for help, and thereby admitting that a problem exists and that we (parents and family) are not being successful at addressing the adolescent's substance abuse, is a difficult and painful first step for many parents and family members.

Additional Characteristics of Shame and Abandonment

Rejection Sensitivity

Feelings of shame and abandonment can make individuals extremely sensitive to rejection, so much so that they choose not to try to grow and develop. Persons suffering from rejection sensitivity avoid situations that may be potentially shaming for fear of the situation triggering feelings of abandonment or rejection. Healthy individuals can tolerate shame, rejection, or abandonment and respond adaptively to these feelings by making the necessary adjustments and healthy choices in their lives.

Fear and Difficulty Making Decisions

Feelings of rejection, abandonment, and shame result in a variety of fears. Some of these fears are so traumatic that individuals cannot choose to change extremely uncomfortable situations. The fears of failure that may activate or trigger feelings of rejection, abandonment, and shame are so great that individuals choose to maintain self-effacing, even violating situations, instead of choosing healthy, growth-oriented paths.

The fear of success can also bring fears that, once some level of success is attained, it will fall apart and return the individual to previous feelings of failure and rejection. People then sabotage the gains in anticipation of deeper feelings of shame, rejection, and abandonment. What is missing is belief in themselves, their own self-worth, and their emerging talents, skills, and capabilities.

Poor Frustration Tolerance

When goals are blocked, even temporarily, persons who feel abandoned and rejected cannot tolerate this frustration. Such individuals believe there are no alternative choices or solutions to their blocked goals. Poor impulse control and self-destructive thinking may cause people to self-sabotage the progress they have made.

Other Reactions and Defenses

Common reactions and defenses to avoid feelings of abandonment and rejection include being overly defensive, extremely critical, or judgmental; showing rage or distorted thinking; and masking true feelings and emotions. People in pain deny the real issues and feelings by being overly defensive and critical of others. These persons view the world as being similar to the depriving, rejecting, and abandoning mothers and fathers they knew while growing up. Their distorted thinking tells them that the world will respond to them in the same way.

✴ Parental Imbalance and Boundary Setting

In her review of the literature, Carol L. Kempher (1987) identified various factors that contribute to parental imbalance. Often parents are imbalanced as caregivers; sometimes they are overwhelmed by problems of their own. (See Table 6.7.) This prevents them from providing the kind of care, support, structure, and healthy encouragement that children require to develop effectively and grow. Kempher summarized these characteristics of parental imbalance:

1. Increased alcoholism, drug use, and nicotine dependence
2. Increased antisocial or sexually deviant behavior in parents
3. Increased mental and emotional problems, such as depression, personality disorders, or narcissism
4. Increased marital conflict
5. Increased parental absenteeism due to separation, divorce, or death

Parents who are not aware of their own emotional and psychological issues may deny the impact their anger, rage, and physical and emotional unavailability have on their children. Parents play an integral role in the development of their children.

It is natural and essential for parents to set appropriate boundaries with their children. Boundaries act as guideposts for children to bump into as they test their own independence and developmental skills. Good boundaries are a sign of good communication, respectful negotiation, and connection between parents and children. Poor boundaries escalate conflict and frustration, leading to disrespect and poor communication.

T A B L E   6 . 7

Parental Imbalance

Chemically dependent and/or imbalanced parents often

- Lack knowledge and skill in parenting
- Have unrealistic expectations and lack information on what is developmentally appropriate behavior at various ages
- Are insensitive to the special needs of their children
- Have decreased family-management skills
- Have inappropriate disciplining techniques and maintain inconsistent, rigid, or ambiguous boundaries
- Have decreased positive responses to and reinforcement of their children
- Have decreased parental involvement and poor bonding or parent-child attachment

---

It is natural for children to test the limits of parental authority as they explore their own capacity for taking on more responsibility as they grow up. Poor boundary setting causes children to be exposed to situations before they have the developmental skills to handle the situations.

Boundaries are not rules for behavior of children; nor are they processes of limit setting. Boundaries exist between all members of the family, between subsystems, and between the family and society. These are the rules of interaction and the methods of functioning (Lawson and Lawson 1998).

Minuchin (1974) defined three types of boundaries: Clear boundaries are essential to balanced families. Enmeshed and disengaged boundaries are characteristic of imbalanced families.

Clear boundaries allow mutual respect and concern by allowing separateness for each member yet maintaining closeness. Freedom and flexibility in these healthy relationships are developed by clear, direct, and understanding communication. Clear boundaries allow children to develop, grow, and differentiate from the family. Individuation can be accomplished only when clear boundaries are functioning within the family system.

Enmeshed boundaries are inflexible, are unyielding, and leave no room for differences. Differentness or separateness is not tolerated; individuation is not a goal of enmeshed relationships. Families with enmeshed boundaries view differentness as disloyalty and as a threat to the rules of the system. The needs of the individual are subjugated to the needs of the parents or system. Satisfying the parents' definition of unity and sameness is stressed. Individual boundaries are blurred, and the individual is often swallowed up by the system. Individuals discount their own feelings, needs, and desires; they feel smothered and numb. They often use alcohol/drugs to counteract these feelings and the underlying resentment and anger.

Disengaged boundaries are overly rigid, with little or no opportunity for communication. Individuals in families that maintain disengaged boundaries have little sense of belonging, often feeling isolated from one another. The family also isolates from community and society. The parents are emotionally unavailable to each other, to the children, and, for that matter, to anyone else.

Boundary Inadequacy

Boundary inadequacy has been defined as the inability to set consistent and appropriate boundaries in relationships. The three major forms of boundary inadequacy identified by Eli Coleman and Phillip Colgan (1986) are ambiguous, overly rigid, and invasive.

Ambiguous boundary inadequacy involves a pattern of double messages exchanged within the relationship. The double messages create an atmosphere of tension wherein the recipient of the communication can never be sure what can be believed. The inability of the communicator to send clear messages lays the groundwork for the cycle of ambiguity to begin.

Overly rigid boundary inadequacy is characterized by patterns of behavior wherein smooth and efficient functioning is a priority over being responsive and adaptable. Adherence to a preset code of behavior is maintained, regardless of intervening situational variables, wherein roles are played and rules are strictly enforced.

Invasive boundary inadequacy involves patterns of behavior wherein an imbalance of power is used to objectify people. Other people become objects for the person to use in satisfying all needs (e.g., sexual and physical abuse).

Boundary Ambiguity

Boss and Greenberg (1984) use the term *boundary ambiguity* for confusion in family members' perceptions of who is in and out of the family and who is performing various family roles and tasks. The alcoholic family system organizes around the alcoholic or the family member(s) who exhibit dysfunctional behavior. In recovery, the family is challenged to reorganize as a viable system or become dysfunctional with continued boundary ambiguity (i.e., the dry-drunk family).

Ziter (1988) describes the alcoholic/imbalanced family as going through four recovery stages to overcome boundary ambiguity. These stages are very similar to the grieving stages of denial, anger, bargaining, depression, and acceptance described earlier in this chapter.

- *Stage 1—Clustering.* This is described as an early denial stage, when the family members sacrifice in order to maintain family harmony. The family task at this stage is to assure themselves that a family exists and to try to keep the alcoholic in the family system.
- *Stage 2—Conflict.* The reality of the situation is beginning to be understood at this stage. Individual differences are penetrating the denial system, and the family members are experiencing the stress and uncertainty of these ambiguous differences. It is at this stage that anger replaces denial to control family differences.
- *Stage 3—Individuation.* At this stage of family recovery, the family members are able to recognize the individuality of each person. The family's task is to support each other in exploring "self" while negotiating living together. Boundaries are becoming clearer.

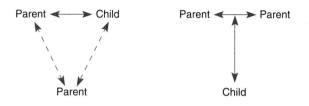

FIGURE 6.1   *Triangulation*

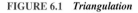

- ***Stage 4***—*Connection.* Family members are making connections with each other. There is a new way of relating that perhaps was not experienced before—an intimate linking. Mutuality emerges, and family members maintain boundaries through their own assertiveness and the respect of other members.

One can see how family members move from a system with imbalance and boundary ambiguity to a balanced system with connection and clarity in boundaries.

Eli Coleman (1987) underscored the importance of setting appropriate boundaries for members of imbalanced families:

> Developing skills at boundary setting is an essential ingredient in the recovery from chemical dependency or codependency. For many it is learning to say "no" to someone's request for physical, sexual, or emotional intimacy. Through saying "no," the individual learns that he or she can have a personal boundary and have it respected. This leads to a clear sense of self-wants and self-desires and it develops a sense of power and control in interpersonal relationships. After learning to say "no," the individual can learn to say "yes," and not lose a sense of individuality.

Triangulation—Another Boundary Issue

Jay Haley, a noted family therapist, defined triangulation (Figure 6.1) as at least two adults involved in an offspring's problem, where the parent-child dyad is pitted against a more peripheral parent, stepparent, or grandparent. The triangle may involve a parent's lover, an estranged parent, or another relative (Haley 1971).

The destructive nature of the triangle is that the parent-child dyad, or alliance, is established at the expense of the peripheral parent. (See Case Study 6.2.) Often the parent-child dyad creates a marital conflict. The parent is overly enmeshed in this alliance, seeking the child's favor despite the reality of the situation.

⚼ Parents' Use/Abuse of Alcohol and Drugs

Kandel and Andrews (1987) postulated that parents can influence their offspring's behavior by modeling actions and defining norms, by controlling the child's susceptibility to the influence of others, and by providing positive attachments.

The modeling of drug use and alcohol use by parents, inadequate supervision of children, and lack of physical and emotional availability are factors that may put children at risk for substance abuse.

Case Study 6.2

Triangulation—It Takes Three or More to Tango

John and Mary and Michelle

John and Mary have significant marital problems. John is the head of the fire department for the county in which they reside and escapes the conflicts at home by spending much of his time with the men at the various fire stations. The couple actively attend community events and act like their marriage is perfect. Their adopted 16-year-old daughter, Michelle, knows the truth. Michelle frequently argues with her mom to the point of hysteria. Mary often gives Michelle reason to be angry by giving her ambiguous, mixed messages (e.g., I want to be close to you, yet I don't trust you because you are stealing my husband, whom I can no longer hold in the marriage). Mary buys Michelle clothes and jewelry but is emotionally cold and unavailable. Mary has no insight into the way she antagonizes Michelle. Michelle is very bright but acts out her frustration with her mom by ditching classes, stealing things from her dresser, and being extremely flirtatious with boys. John and Michelle maintain an enmeshed dyadic alliance. John is frustrated with his wife's coldness, emotional and sexual unavailability, and constant arguments with Michelle and nagging of himself. Michelle makes sexual overtures to young men while with her father and makes other sexually inappropriate remarks. In effect, she is flirtatious with her father; they are acting out their unconscious desires to be intimate with each other. These unconscious conflicts put more pressure on Michelle, and she has begun to use alcohol/drugs excessively and to have sex with numerous young men. At this point, the family has sought counseling, a process that involves unraveling this triangulation and establishing clearer boundaries and lines of communication.

Discussion

All parties in this case are involved quite dramatically in this triangulation. It will take a skilled therapist to unravel the lines of triangulation and prevent any of the family members from permanently sabotaging the process. The therapist must establish a climate of trust, integrity, and competency to help this family. The three family members will not succeed at setting appropriate boundaries unless all of them agree to persevere in the process.

The counselor will need support in this case and might involve other "consultant counselors" who will communicate clearly and directly with the primary counselor. This demonstrates (recapitulates) to the family that members of a system can work together effectively. The counselor must also expect that when issues become uncomfortable, each family member is capable of sabotaging progress and the process. Observing and commenting on that as a natural element of the process of counseling is recommended as a way to reengage family members.

⚹ Other Family System Variables

Grace M. Barnes (1990) describes the three major family system variables necessary to prevent problem behaviors by children: **family cohesion, flexibility,** and **communication clarity.**

Cohesion is defined as the emotional bonding of family members toward each other. Family members respect one another, support each other, and have appropriate boundaries. Cohesion is not possible if family members are enmeshed or disengaged from each other. Instead, there is a balance in roles, tasks, and ability to resolve conflicts.

Flexibility is the family members' ability to alter family roles and rituals in response to situational stress.

Communication clarity is the ability of family members to develop coalitions and to understand each other.

Parental competence is described by Burton White, director of the Harvard Preschool Projects, as the ability and willingness of parents to

- Sensibly design the world of the child
- Serve as a child's personal consultant
- Set limits effectively, for the sake of the child (not the parent) (White, Kaban, and Attanucci 1979)

Interestingly, adolescents in single-parent and stepparent families report more alcohol use than do adolescents in traditional families (Burnside et al. 1986). A study of high school students (Barnes and Nindle 1987) reported a tendency for adolescents living with both natural parents to have fewer alcohol-related problems.

Older siblings can exert a tremendous influence of alcohol/drug use on younger children in the family. Often it is an older sibling who initiates younger brothers and sisters into the rite of alcohol and drug use. The older sibling frequently has better access to alcohol/drugs and is often a more experienced user. Sometimes it is older cousins, stepbrothers/sisters, or friends of the family who initiate alcohol/drug use. Adolescents who have close, quality relationships and good communication with their parents are less likely to be influenced negatively by older siblings or peers.

The adolescent's positive sense of self, attainment of developmental skills, and ability to individuate also minimize negative peer influence. Studies have indicated that the level of closeness and trust in the parent-child relationship determines the choice of positive peer relationships.

Children who grow up in an abstinent family system may also develop alcohol/drug dependence and addiction. People who become alienated from their abstinence backgrounds may use excessive drinking to express their frustration with early rigid familial, religious, and community teachings. Problem drinking or excessive drug use is symbolic of a rebellion or revolt against early family values that became overly rigid. Sometimes alcohol/drug problems skip a generation as well. The child growing up in an alcoholic/addict system decides to "never be like his or her alcoholic/addict dad or mom" and chooses to abstain from any alcohol/drug use as an adult. The genetic predisposition for alcoholism/drug addiction is still passed on to his or her children, who may develop problems with alcohol/drugs, even though they grew up in a household where there was no parental use of alcohol/drugs.

The size of the family may also influence alcohol and drug use by children. As the number of siblings increases, the family becomes more complex in role relationships and tasks. Some children may experience increasing levels of frustration (blocked goals). In very large families, parents may be more controlling/coercive, less available, and less supportive, resulting in problem behaviors by some of the children and perhaps overly responsible (codependent) behaviors by siblings. This is illustrated in Case Study 6.3.

⚹ Imbalanced Life Cycles of Families

Jay Haley (1971) described the following major stages in the family life cycle:

1. Relationships between families through unattached young adults
2. Joining of families through marriage
3. Family and the young child
4. Family and the adolescent
5. Launching of children
6. Later life

As a result of the imbalance in alcoholic/addict family systems, developmental and interpersonal tasks are impaired at each stage of the family life cycle.

Relationships Between Families and the Joining of Families

During the first two stages, the relationships between families are often filled with conflict and tension. Cooperation between families is difficult because the alcoholic/addict family system is trying to deny, minimize, and cover up the family secret of alcoholism/addiction. This results in the families' inability to develop trust and closeness.

Family and the Young Child

At the third stage, the family is either isolated or involved with other families that have similar problems with alcohol/drugs. The child is the innocent victim at this stage. The young child is often embarrassed by his or her parents' unpredictable behavior. As a result, the child frequently prefers playing at other children's homes and rarely invites other children to his or her home. Often, children from alcoholic/addict homes literally adopt their friends' parents. Becoming stepchildren, they spend a great deal of time with their friends' families. (See Case Study 6.4.)

Family and the Adolescent

The fourth stage is the time of most turmoil. Tumultuous even in the balanced family system, adolescence becomes even more dramatic in an imbalanced family system. The adolescent's exploration of a healthy personal identity is incongruent with the imbalanced, unhealthy alcoholic/addict system. The conflict of holding allegiance

Case Study 6.3
Family System Variables
Jane

Jane grew up with four sisters. Dad's alcoholism was denied for most of their childhood. It was Jane's responsibility to take care of Mom emotionally. When Mom experienced chronic fatigue, Jane took care of the other, younger sisters, giving them dinner, getting them to bed, and trying to keep them quiet. Despite her efforts, Mom's physical symptoms increased in frequency. The other sisters didn't seem to be as affected by Mom's pain and Dad's alcohol use. It took Mom's "nervous breakdown" and her being hospitalized for a month in a psychiatric hospital for the other children to recognize the problem. Jane and her next younger sister were now responsible for the house. The middle sister began drinking during this time, and the youngest seemed to spend more time playing quietly by herself.

A few months after Mom returned home, Dad started attending AA meetings. Mom still experienced fatigue and physical pain, but less frequently. Jane went away to college, rarely visiting, immersing herself in studies, and marrying right out of college. The middle sister declared she was gay and went off to school 3,000 miles from home. The youngest and next to oldest stayed close to home, alternating the emotional caretaking of both Mom and Dad.

It was only in later years that the sisters started to share their memories of their painful childhood. Each had sought counseling for various relationship problems. Each had learned about being an adult child of an alcoholic. They were now beginning to heal by talking about their recovery. Mom was now actively pursuing interests outside of the home and spending time on her own. Dad was several years sober now and beginning to communicate more effectively with his daughters.

Discussion

Here is a case where many family system variables affect all family members—the father's alcoholism, the mother's major depression and chronic headaches, a psychiatric hospitalization of the mother that left the children as caretakers and housekeepers, and many other variables implied in growing up in this family system.

A number of good outcomes have occurred over the years, despite these problems. Dad is attending Alcoholics Anonymous; Mom is getting out and her headaches and pain are more manageable; and, probably the most important development, the adult children are talking to each other about their experiences growing up in this family system. There are signs of remarkable resilience in the parents and the children. (For more on the resilient self, see Chapter 7.)

to the family, imbalanced as it is, and exploring self through individuation and differentiation creates tremendous guilt and anxiety for adolescents. If this conflict is unresolved, adolescents can either internalize their own frustration and anger and develop an imbalanced sense of self or act out their anger in a demonstrative and destructive manner. The acting-out behavior often includes problems with alcohol/drugs,

Case Study 6.4
Adopting a Surrogate Family
Steve

At the age of 8, Steve was always with his friend Joe's family. He would have breakfast and dinner with them and spend most of his free hours playing with Joe and talking with Joe's parents. When Steve had problems, concerns, or conflicts, he would talk to Joe's parents and not discuss the issues with his own family.

Discussion

One could make a calculated guess that Steve adopted his friend's family because there were problems/imbalances in his own family. Often children will go elsewhere to find the support, nurturance, and comfort they do not have in their own immediate family. Sometimes an aunt, a grandmother, a teacher, a counselor, a clergyman, or some other significant person becomes a mentor or surrogate parent.

---

sexual promiscuity, problems in school and with authority figures, and criminal-justice problems. The internalized anger is sometimes more subtly manifested in the need for constant approval from peers, a poor self-concept, insecurity, or fears of abandonment and rejection.

Launching of Children

During the fifth stage, when the children are launched, the parents' alcohol and drug use usually intensifies. The empty-nest syndrome forces the parents to look at the dissatisfaction in their own marital system. The usual way to avoid the issues of marital imbalance is to increase the use of alcohol/drugs.

Of course, adult children of alcoholics/addicts are at risk for creating imbalanced relationships with their partners and for recapitulating the family of origin by developing imbalanced family systems as well. If there is no help, the result is the repetition of the same imbalanced system from generation to generation.

Later Life

In the sixth stage, the issues intensify in an alcoholic/addict family system. Consciously or unconsciously, the adult recognizes the imbalanced patterns of relating during childhood. Adult children of alcoholics/addicts enter treatment as they notice the imbalances in their own lives. Contacts with their parents in these later years may bring highly emotionally charged conflict to the forefront, making it difficult to have caring or effective relationships with their parents. If the parents are still using alcohol/drugs, this even further intensifies the difficulty in maintaining or developing better relationships. Working through the stages of grief and accepting the painful limitations of these imbalanced relationships are other developmental tasks for adult children. Healing may occur before the parents die. Perhaps the legacy of alcoholism/addiction will not be passed on to the next generation.

How does a counselor get resistant family members to participate in counseling? Alcoholic/addict families are among the most difficult families to get into treatment, whether the setting is inpatient, residential, or outpatient treatment. Families often abdicate responsibility for the alcoholic/addict's problems. It is too difficult for them to admit their feelings of embarrassment, shame, and personal feelings of inadequacy in trying to control family members' abuse of alcohol/drugs. Mason (1958) reported that, of 1,000 eligible parents of alcoholics/addicts, only 30 to 40 would appear at monthly parent-staff meetings and almost none of these attended more than three times.

Not only are family members resistant to attending sessions, but also the alcoholics/addicts themselves often sabotage family involvement. Alcoholics/addicts are often self-protective of their families, not wanting them to experience more pain. Alcoholics/addicts may even feel a sense of betrayal in assisting counselors to get the rest of the family involved. This would be disloyal to the rules of the imbalanced, enmeshed family system.

For many alcoholics/addicts, having their spouses or other family members involved in treatment might blow their cover. Alcoholics/addicts may have lied or deceived counselors in giving inaccurate or distorted information about their alcohol/ drug use, family interactions, or other information. There is also fear that counselors would blame, criticize, or shame other family members; then these family members would get back at the alcoholics/addicts.

❧ Fathers of Alcoholics/Addicts— Dealing with Resistance

The fathers of alcoholics/addicts are by far the most difficult family members to get into family sessions. A large percentage of these fathers have alcohol/drug problems themselves and don't want this brought to the attention of the counselor (the same may hold true for mothers). The father is difficult to engage in the process of family therapy because he has generally been unavailable to the drug user and other family members. The father is often angry and defensive.

I have heard many fathers say, "Since nobody ever listened to me or allowed me to follow through in what I thought would work in the first place, I am angry and don't want to get involved." The truth is that most fathers are frightened by the emotional content of counseling and profess not to believe in counseling. They see therapists as invading the family systems the fathers have tried to control. Fathers are also trying to avoid their own emotional pain and issues.

In an attempt to engage fathers in treatment, Labate (1975) recommends a kind of romancing of the father by acknowledging the positive intentions that the father possesses, emphasizing that the father's participation in treatment is needed to make treatment successful. Labate suggests the following:

1. Reassuring the father that he is important
2. Pointing out that changes depend on his participation

3. Making the father aware that he has the power to sabotage treatment
4. Noting that the father has choices, such as transferring to another counselor, who might work with him individually
5. Placing responsibility for change squarely on the father's shoulders
6. Getting the father to consider realigning his priorities (e.g., choosing his family's happiness over acquisition of more material goods)

Labate's strategies can be used on any family member of the alcoholic/addict—the spouse, brothers, sisters, or other family members—who may have the same resistance to family treatment.

⚹ Noble Ascriptions to Counteract Defensiveness

"Anyone working with addicts' families for the first time is impressed with the tremendous defensiveness that most of them show. It sometimes seems as if they are just waiting for the therapist to cast even a minor aspersion so they can protest or perhaps abort therapy prematurely" (Stanton et al. 1982). In approaching alcoholics/ addicts and family members in treatment, it is essential that the counselor's style be nonpejorative, nonjudgmental, sensitive to the patient's issues of shame, and in no way blaming. Duncan Stanton suggested that the treatment be put in the context that each family member's intentions were and are noble and that there is a good reason or adaptive function for even the most destructive behavior. For example, anger, frustration, and generally attacking behavior can be relabeled as "a concern that is painful to tolerate," rather than "You are really angry for no reason" or "There he goes again, using anger to hurt and control us." Destructive enabling behavior can be nobly ascribed as "It is difficult to see your child in pain, pain that you would prefer that the child not go through."

"Simply defining problems as interactional or familial stumbling blocks serves to have them viewed as shared, rather than loading the blame entirely on one or two members—'we're all in this together'" (Stanton et al. 1982). This approach does not abandon the therapist's role in challenging the thoughts, beliefs, and behaviors that might hinder the family from becoming more functional. Instead, the counselor expresses perspectives and viewpoints in a human, caring, and nonshaming manner, facilitating trust in the therapeutic alliance. The ascribing of noble intentions or characteristics takes the shame out of the therapeutic work—shame that would inevitably cause one or more family members to sabotage treatment.

Teaching and Modeling Compassion

One way to counter shame and anger is to teach and model compassion in children. Parents, teachers, siblings, even other children can help teach and model compassion. If compassion is learned at young ages, it becomes a natural personality trait as an adult.

Compassion is the practice of recognizing and being sensitive to others' suffering, as well as one's own. Compassion is a heartfelt emotion that includes understanding, sensitivity, tolerance, support, and care.

TABLE 6.8
10 Steps of Compassion

Compassion involves:

1. being sensitive to others' suffering, as well as your own suffering
2. being reflective (gentle) instead of reactive
3. changing critical attitudes (greed, hatred, and delusion) into caring attitudes (generosity, love, and awareness)
4. being truthful, helpful, kind, and appropriate
5. not blaming (taking responsibility)
6. not complaining
7. invoking "right speech"
8. "cherishing" others
9. avoiding and reducing criticism, contempt, defensiveness, and stonewalling in relationships
10. and having the grace to love and be loved

SOURCE: Richard Fields, PhD. 2008. *Minestrone for the mind: Awakening to mindfulness,* Health Communications.

Compassion is a cornerstone of Buddha's teaching (dharma). The Dalai Lama, along with noted authorities in the psychology/counseling field, has been conducting large public conferences (2008) focusing on helping parents teach children to be more compassionate.

Shame, aggression, emotional and physical violations can be quite traumatic. Children are sometimes shaming, bullying, and violating their peers. By teaching respect and compassion, we can counter the peer culture from hurting and harming one another.

The ultimate goal of teaching compassion is to help establish safety and trust in relationships—a trust that promotes peace, cooperation, and well-being between peoples in our communities and our world. (See Table 6.8.)

✵ In Review

- A poor bond between parent and child can often impair the child's development. Self-concept, social and interpersonal relationships, achievement, and identity are negatively affected by inadequate parent-child bonding. A positive, caring relationship is essential for healthy development.
- Two prevailing hypotheses regarding parental bonding in adolescent substance abusers are the *overinvolvement hypothesis* and the *functional hypothesis.* The overinvolvement hypothesis is that one parent (frequently the mother) is overly involved in the adolescent's life to compensate for the lack of availability by the other parent. The functional hypothesis is that the adolescent's substance

abuse distracts the family from focusing on other familial problems, such as marital discord, infidelity, and parental abuse of alcohol/drugs.

- The individual suffering from abandonment depression is metaphorically described as "an egg with the insides removed." All the good stuff—the nutrients, the seed, the juices of life—has been removed, has rotted, or has been destroyed by a lack of nurturing.

  The six key elements of abandonment depression are
  1. Homicidal rage
  2. Suicidal depression
  3. Panic
  4. Parental imbalance and boundary setting
  5. Parents' use/abuse of alcohol and drugs
  6. Other family system variables

- Individuals suffering from abandonment depression often have difficulty in affect (feeling) regulation, which impairs interpersonal relationships.

- The child's temperament is described as a behavioral characteristic present at birth, or within the first few months. Certain temperaments put the individual more at risk for substance abuse. A so-called difficult temperament puts the individual at risk for problem behaviors, including substance abuse. A difficult temperament includes high activity level, low flexibility, task orientation, mood instability, and social withdrawal.

- The goal of parenting is to develop a high level of parental support and a moderate level of parental control. Parents who are highly rigid, authoritarian, and controlling tend to have children who are resentful, frustrated, and angry. These children are then prone to problem behaviors, causing them to rebel or passive-aggressively get back at the rigid parent. "Children whose relationships with their parents lacked love, warmth, and closeness and exhibited signs of hostility, have children who exhibit increased levels of substance abuse, delinquency, and dysfunctional coping strategies" (Johnson and Pandina 1991).

- The children of parents who are unable to establish moderate control and effective disciplining techniques often experience problem behaviors and associate with other children who have problem behaviors.

- Shame plays a major role in devastating the parent-child relationship. Shame is a deep-rooted feeling that results from traumatic childhood experiences. Shame is defined as the self looking in on itself and finding itself lacking, flawed, or inadequate. When shame attaches to feelings, those feelings are usually escalated (e.g., anger + shame = rage).

  Many metaphors can be used to describe shame: It is the archer out there, ready to shoot you in a public domain; it is a flash flood of emotion that wipes out the interpersonal emotional bridge to other people.

- Parents who use/abuse alcohol or drugs model the same behavior in their offspring. Conversely, family cohesion, flexibility, and communication clarity can positively influence a child against using/abusing alcohol or drugs.

- Individuals from shame-based family systems often feel that (1) there is no hope for change; (2) shame is inescapable and inevitable; (3) shame is exterior-based, not an internal process; and (4) they are bad, no good, flawed, or worthless as individuals (Fossum and Mason 1986).

- Some of the obstacles to engaging parents to seek counseling or help for their children who have substance abuse problems are

> Denial
> Skepticism
> Assumption that things will be O.K.
> Distorted, depressed view of life
> Fear of being labeled as bad parents
> Fear of loss of confidentiality
> Narcissism of parents (for more, see Table 6.6)

- Parental imbalance is defined as parents who lack knowledge and skills in parenting. These parents have unrealistic expectations of their children and are insensitive to the needs of their children.
- Imbalanced families often have difficulty in setting appropriate boundaries. Boundary inadequacy is defined as the inability to set consistent and appropriate boundaries in relationships, as evidenced by ambiguous, overly rigid, and invasive boundaries. Triangulation is another form of boundary inadequacy, in which the parent-child affiliation is established at the expense of the peripheral parent. Frequently, these problems in boundary setting lead to physical and sexual violations and emotional and psychological abuse. This is especially true in alcohol/addict family system.
- Jay Haley, a noted family therapist, defined triangulation (Figure 6.1) as at least two adults involved in an offspring's problem, where the parent-child dyad is pitted against a more peripheral parent, stepparent, or grandparent. The triangle may involve a parent's lover, an estranged parent, or another relative (Haley 1971).
- Noble ascriptions: Duncan Stanton suggested that the treatment be put in the context that each family member's intentions were and are noble and that there is a good reason or adaptive function for even the most destructive behavior. For example, anger, frustration, and generally attacking behavior can be relabeled as "a concern that is painful to tolerate," rather than "You are really angry for no reason" or "There he goes again, using anger to hurt and control us." Destructive enabling behavior can be nobly ascribed as "It is difficult to see your child in pain, pain that you would prefer that the child not go through."

✳ Discussion Questions

1. Rank in order from most influential to least influential the parenting factors that may contribute to substance abuse. Then explain the rationale for your ranking.

> _____ Parent-child bonding
> _____ Child's temperament
> _____ Parenting styles

_____ Shame and imbalanced parenting
_____ Parent's shame
_____ Parental imbalance in boundary setting

2. Give examples and describe incidents of shame at various ages. Explain how the incidents fit the definition of shame.
3. Give examples and describe a situation where shame attached to a feeling and escalated that feeling. Explain the sequence and why this occurred.
4. Describe and illustrate the "life cycle" of your own family.

⚹ References

American Psychiatric Association. 1994. *Diagnostic and statistical manual of mental disorders.* 4th ed. Washington, D.C.: Author.

Barnes, Grace M. 1990. Impact of the family on adolescent drinking patterns. In *Alcohol and the family,* edited by R. Collins et al. New York: Guilford Press.

Barnes, Grace M., and M. Nindle. 1987. Family factors in adolescent alcohol and drug abuse. *Pediatrician* 14: 13–18.

Block, J., J. H. Block, and S. Keyes. 1988. Longitudinally foretelling drug usage in adolescence: Early childhood personality and environmental precursors. *Child Development* 59(2): 336–55.

Boss, P., and J. Greenberg. 1984. Family boundary ambiguity: A new variable in family stress theory. *Family Process* 23: 535–46.

Burnside, M. A., et al. 1986. Alcohol use by adolescents in disrupted families. *Alcoholism: Clinical and Experimental Research* 10: 274–78.

Carnes, Patrick. 1995. Patrick J. Carnes: Riding the tides, navigating counseling's turbulent waters [Interview]. *Professional Counselor Magazine,* December, pp. 47–52.

Coleman, Eli. 1987. *Chemical dependency and intimacy dysfunction.* New York: Haworth Press.

Coleman, Eli, and Phillip Colgan. 1986. Boundary inadequacy in drug dependent families. *Journal of Psychoactive Drugs* 18: 21–30.

Dobkin, P. L., R. E. Tremblay, L. C. Masse, and F. Vitaro. 1995. *Child Development* 66: 1198–1214.

Eliason, M. J., and A. H. Skinstad. 1995. Drug/alcohol addictions and mothering. *Alcoholism Treatment Quarterly* 12(1): 83–95.

Fields, Richard. 2008. *Minestrone for the mind: Awakening to mindfulness. 10 steps for positive change.* Deerfield Beach, Fla.: Health Communications (July).

Fossum, M., and M. Mason. 1986. *Facing shame: Families in recovery.* New York: W. W. Norton.

Garrison, W. T., and F. J. Earls. 1987. Temperament and child psychopathology. *Developmental Clinical Psychology and Psychiatry* 12.

Gomberg, E. S. L. 1988. Shame and guilt issues among women alcoholics. *Alcoholism Treatment Quarterly* 5: 139–55.

Haley, Jay. 1971. *Changing families: A family therapy reader.* New York: Grune & Stratton.

Jessup, M. 1983. *Chemically dependent women in San Francisco: A status report.* San Francisco: California Department of Public Health, San Francisco Community Substance Abuse Services.

Johnson, Valerie, and Robert J. Pandina. 1991. Effects of the family environment on adolescent substance use, delinquency, and coping skills. *American Journal of Drug and Alcohol Abuse* 1(17): 71–88.

Kandel, D. B., and K. A. Andrews. 1987. Processes of adolescent socialization by parents and peers. *International Journal of Addiction* 22: 319–42.

Kaufman, E. 1989. The psychotherapy of dually diagnosed patients. *Journal of Substance Abuse Treatment* 6(1): 9–18.

Kempher, Carol. 1987. Special populations: Etiology and prevention of vulnerability to chemical dependency in children of substance abusers. In *Youth at high risk for substance abuse,* edited by B. S. Brown and A. R. Mills. NIDA monograph. Washington, D.C.: U.S. Department of Health and Human Services.

Kohnstamm, G., J. Bates, and M. K. Rothbart. 1999. In *Alcohol use among adolescents,* edited by M. Windle. Thousand Oaks, Calif.: Sage.

Labate, K. 1975. Pathogenic role rigidity in fathers: Some observations. *Journal of Marriage and Family Counseling* 1: 69–79.

Lawson, Ann W., and Gary W. Lawson. 1998. *Alcoholism and the family: A guide to treatment and prevention.* 2nd edition. Gaithersburg, Md.: Aspen.

Lerner, J. V., and J. R. Vicary. 1984. Difficult temperament and drug use: Analyses from the New York longitudinal study. *Journal of Drug Education* 14(1): 1–8.

Maccoby, E., and J. A. Martin. 1983. Socialization in the context of the family: Parent-child interaction. In *Handbook of Child Psychology,* vol. 4, edited by E. M. Hetherington. New York: Wiley.

Martin, C. S., N. A. Kaczynski, S. A. Maisto, and R. E. Tarter. 1996. Polydrug use in adolescent drinkers with and without DSM-IV alcohol abuse and dependence. *Alcoholism, Clinical and Experimental Research* 20(6): 1099–1108.

Mason, P. 1958. Mother of the addict. *Psychiatric Quarterly Supplement* 32: 189–99.

Masse, Louise C., and Richard E. Tremblay. 1997. Behavior of boys in kindergarten and the onset of substance use during adolescence. *Archives of General Psychiatry* 54(1): 62–68. Available at http://archpsych.ama-assn.org/

Masterson, James F. 1976. *Psychotherapy of the borderline adult: A developmental approach.* New York: Brunner/Mazel.

Minuchin, Salvador. 1974. *Families and family therapy.* Cambridge, Mass.: Harvard University Press.

Ohannessian, C. M., and V. M. Hesselbrock. 1995. *Journal of Studies on Alcohol* 56(3): 318–27.

Potter-Efron, Ronald. 2002. *Shame, guilt, and alcoholism: Treatment issues in clinical practice,* 2nd edition. New York: Haworth Press.

Rollins, B. C., and D. L. Thomas. 1979. Parental support, power, and control techniques in the socialization of the child. In *Contemporary theories of the family,* vol. 1, edited by W. R. Burr et al. New York: Free Press.

Stanton, Duncan M., et al. 1982. *Family therapy of drug abuse.* New York: Guilford Press.

Tubman, J., and M. Windle. 1999. In *Alcohol use among adolescents,* edited by M. Windle. Thousand Oaks, Calif.: Sage.

Volk, R. J., et al. 1988. Family systems of adolescent substance abusers. *Family Relations* 38: 266–72.

Werner, Emmy E., and Ruth S. Smith. 2001. *Journeys from childhood to midlife: Risk, resilience, and recovery.* Ithaca, N.Y.: Cornell University Press.

Werner, R. J., and C. A. Smith. 1999. In *Alcohol use among adolescents,* edited by M. Windle. Thousand Oaks, Calif.: Sage.

White, B., B. Kaban, and J. Attanucci. 1979. *The origins of human competence: The final report on the Harvard Preschool Project.* Lexington, Mass.: Lexington Books/D. C. Heath.

Ziter, MaryLou Politi. 1988. Treating alcoholic families: The resolution of boundary ambiguity. *Alcoholism Treatment Quarterly* 5: 221–33.

Growing Up in an Alcoholic Family System

Objectives

1. Describe and define what we mean by adult children of alcoholics.
2. Identify the basic facts about children of alcoholics that the National Association of Children of Alcoholics developed in its charter statement in 1983.
3. Identify at least seven characteristics of adult children of alcoholics.
4. Compare the symptoms of post-traumatic stress disorder (PTSD) to growing up in an alcoholic family system.
5. Identify the behaviors of children in alcoholic family systems.
6. Identify and describe how role-reversal, unpredictability, unavailability, and social isolation impact the child in the alcoholic system.
7. Describe the dimensions of the family disease model and the impact of alcoholism/drug addiction on the marriage.
8. Describe adult children of alcoholics (ACA) in adult relationships.
9. Define and describe codependency and some "codependent dances."
10. List characteristics and thoughts of both the overattached and the overseparated individual.
11. Describe the various modalities and methods for recovery for adult children of alcoholics.
12. Describe and give some examples of second-order change and second-order communications.
13. List the eleven curative factors of group psychotherapy, and describe them for recovery of adult children of alcoholics.

❧ Introduction

This chapter focuses on children of alcoholics. In the 1980s this was an emerging issue that shifted the focus away from the alcoholic/addict to the children in the alcoholic/addict family system.

Alcoholism is a family disease that includes codependency, enabling behavior, and marital discord. The children in an alcoholic system, much like the nonalcoholic spouse, compensate to keep the system in homeostasis. The family is organized around the alcoholic's behavior and drinking. The alcoholism is the central organizing principle around which the family focuses.

Children growing up in an alcoholic/addict family system experience traumas, which result in specific adult behavioral characteristics and developmental disabilities. Adult children of alcoholics (ACA) have trouble establishing effective boundaries in relationships and are often either overseparated or overattached in partner relationships. Recovery for adult children involves dealing with unresolved feelings of childhood grief and working through feelings of shame, abandonment, and rejection.

By understanding the healing and recovery process for adult children, perhaps this pattern of imbalance can be broken for the next generation.

⋇ The Adult Children of Alcoholics Movement

In the 1980s, one of the most significant alcohol/drug issues brought to the attention of the general public was the awareness of the characteristics of adult children of alcoholics. Children who grew up in alcoholic families are now adults, hence the term *adult children of alcoholics*. These adults report difficulties in establishing effective, intimate, interpersonal relationships.

The talent and dedication of people such as Timmen Cermak, Claudia Black, Stephanie Brown, Janet Woititz, Sharon Wegscheider-Cruse, Robert Ackerman, and Lori Dwinell created an awareness of the trauma of growing up in an alcoholic family system. Because of this awareness, our society not only has recognized but today is dealing with how the imbalanced aspects of alcoholism affect all family members.

In 1979, a *Newsweek* article about adult children of alcoholics reported the early work of Claudia Black (1982) and Stephanie Brown, who both described and labeled the characteristics of ACA. Brown (1988) described the reaction after the *Newsweek* article as "a prairie fire of interest." The proliferation of articles, materials, books, general information, workshops, and speakers on ACA issues was dramatic from 1979 to the late 1980s. Adult children of alcoholics were finally recognized as a treatment population that had generally been ignored for years. This explosion of interest was in direct proportion to the neglect and oversight that occurred as professionals focused myopically on the alcoholics, while ignoring the children who grew up in alcoholic families. In 1983, the National Association for Children of Alcoholics (NACOA) was formed. Timmen Cermak, one of the founders, was its first president. Numerous planning meetings established the NACOA as a central organizing force in disseminating information, providing direction, and developing resources for adult children of alcoholics. The NACOA organized national conferences to provide a forum for the dissemination of ACA treatment information for both professionals and the lay public.

In 1983, the NACOA developed some basic facts about children of alcoholics in its charter statement:

- An estimated 28 million Americans have at least one alcoholic parent.
- More than half of all alcoholics have an alcoholic parent.
- Children of alcoholics are at the highest risk of developing alcoholism themselves or marrying someone who is alcoholic.
- In up to 90 percent of child abuse cases, alcohol is a significant factor.
- Children of alcoholics are frequently victims of incest, child neglect, and other forms of violence and exploitation.

The popularity of the ACA movement also brought with it some concerns for overgeneralization and a lack of clinical foundation. Appropriately, this point is made by Stephanie Brown (1988), one of the pioneers of the movement.

> Like many social movements, the sudden recognition, widespread interest, and emotional intensity have been powerful and helpful for many children and adults. However, there continues to be a lack of a solid clinical research and theoretical foundation on which to base important decisions for intervention, education, prevention, and treatment.

⚹ Characteristics of Adult Children of Alcoholics

Following are some of the behavioral characteristics of ACA:

1. Fear of losing control
2. All-or-none, black-or-white thinking
3. Fear of experiencing feelings
4. Overdeveloped sense of responsibility or irresponsibility
5. Difficulty with intimacy and with asking for what is wanted or needed
6. Flashbacks of childhood but many memory gaps
7. Feelings of being little, or like a child, when under stress
8. Unreasonable loyalty
9. Addiction to excitement
10. Difficulty relaxing
11. Feelings of guilt, abandonment, and/or depression
12. Tendency to confuse love with self-pity
13. Backlog of shock and grief
14. Compulsive behaviors
15. Living in a world of denial
16. Guessing at what is normal
17. Tendency toward physical symptoms (e.g., headaches, gastrointestinal problems)

⚹ Growing Up in an Alcoholic Home as Post-Traumatic Stress Disorder

Timmen Cermak (1984) stated that the effect of growing up in an alcoholic family system is analogous to the post-traumatic stress disorder (PTSD) (see Case Study 7.1) of war veterans or survivors of the Holocaust because the same coping mechanisms are used. The soldier who helplessly watches as a buddy is shot and killed shuts down his own emotions to survive the trauma, which can later be reexperienced in a safe environment. This same reaction of shutting down emotionally occurs in the children of alcoholics. After these children become adults, they reexperience feelings of childhood traumas and suffer chronic symptoms of acute anxiety, depression, sleep disturbances, and nightmares, as well as an inability to work or function effectively at daily activities.

The following major symptoms of PTSD are similar to symptoms experienced by ACA:

1. Reexperiencing the trauma, as evidenced by

    a. Nightmares
    b. Recurrent obsessive thoughts
    c. Sudden reemergence of survival behavior in the face of events that resemble the original trauma
    d. Emotional overload

2. Psychic numbing, as evidenced by

    a. A sense of depersonalization
    b. A sense of not fitting into one's surroundings
    c. A feeling of emotional anesthesia
    d. Constriction of emotions, especially in situations demanding intimacy, tenderness, or sexuality
    e. Lack of feelings during times of stress
    f. Sudden experience of a wall between the self and the feelings
    g. Confusion instead of having feelings
    h. A lump in the throat instead of allowing feelings to emerge, or pressure and tightness in the jaw, shoulders, or other parts of the body
    i. Feelings that emotions will be overwhelming if one gets in touch with them

3. Hypervigilance, as evidenced by

    a. Inability to relax
    b. Frequent startle responses
    c. Chronic anxiety
    d. Panic attacks

4. Survivor guilt, as evidenced by

    a. Chronic depression
    b. A sourceless sense of guilt

5. Intensification of symptoms by exposure to events that resemble the original trauma

In order to constitute post-traumatic stress disorder, the trauma must be significant. Severe emotional or physical abuse and/or sexual violation can be so traumatizing to the child that symptoms of PTSD might occur. Unfortunately, the diagnosis of PTSD has frequently been used too loosely, without evidence of significant trauma. Just growing up in an alcoholic family does not mean one suffers from PTSD. Cermak is using PTSD as a model to understand the symptoms of ACA, not as a generalized label.

⚹ Childhood in an Alcoholic Home

Children in alcoholic families learn to distrust their own observations (what they see and hear) and feelings (what they sense), and they feel powerless to change the family system. They cannot speak out and cannot trust their feelings because the rules in an alcoholic family system are don't talk, don't feel, and don't trust. Because these

Case Study 7.1
The ACA and Post-Traumatic Stress Disorder
Joe

Joe was a client who had experienced both the trauma of growing up in an alcoholic family system and post-traumatic stress as a result of military service in Vietnam. Joe was referred to me by a colleague, who was counseling Joe's 12-year-old daughter.

Joe came home drunk one evening, went to his daughter's bedroom to kiss her good night, and began crying and talking about how unhappy he was. Although there was no sexual violation, the daughter was extremely upset by her father's behavior. She was frightened and concerned about his drinking and his deep emotional sadness.

Joe was one of those patients for whom I initially had very little hope; he turned out to be a case that reinforced my belief in the inherent goodness in people. He was 25 minutes late for his first counseling session. He insisted that his lateness was due to a business appointment and wondered why I was so concerned with time. He believed that his only problem was his business. Joe said, "If I could only get out from under the financial pressure, everything would be back to normal." He agreed to come back for counseling to help with stress management although he felt that his daughter needed assistance, not him.

Gradually, I was able to establish a therapeutic bond with Joe. Once I got to know him, I soon realized that he had the heart of a puppy dog and he had suffered significant disappointments and trauma in his life.

Joe's alcoholic father, who was well read and extremely bright, owned his own business. His dad spent most of his time drinking at the office and the local bar while discussing many topics with his customers and friends; he was well versed in politics, philosophy, religion, physics, even psychology. Although he was a friendly and entertaining drunk with his friends, he was emotionally unpredictable at home. At times, Joe's dad was maudlin about his childhood and his father's death when he was 8. At other times, he raged around the house, screaming resentments for his need to work so hard to support his wife and children. Once Joe was so angry with his father that he took a baseball bat and was going to smash him in the face.

Sometimes Joe felt sorry for his father and put him to bed after a drinking binge; when things got to be overwhelming, Joe just ran out of the house. On those evenings, Joe frequently went down to the school and threw rocks at the classroom windows. This and similar aggressive behavior kept him in trouble throughout his childhood. Joe was extremely bright and, despite his aggressive behavior, pulled good grades in high school. Because he spent more time drinking than studying in college, in 1968 his military deferment was revoked.

In the service, Joe was put through training for military intelligence and could have avoided Vietnam if his alcoholism and aggressive anger hadn't gotten him into trouble with his top sergeant. In Vietnam, Joe's major job was to fly to battle zones after conflicts and get a body count for Vietnamese and American soldiers.

Joe felt sadness for the Vietnamese children; he described them stealing, cheating, and manipulating the GIs to survive. It reminded him of his own childhood anger and aggressive behavior. In counseling sessions, Joe initially denied the emotional trauma of his experiences in Vietnam. He insisted that he had had it good, compared with others. Joe suffered from this traumatic exposure as well as from survivor's guilt. He

(continued on next page)

Case Study 7.1 (*continued*)
The ACA and Post-Traumatic Stress Disorder
Joe

experienced all the traditional signs of post-traumatic stress: sleep disorders and nightmares, night sweats, inability to concentrate, hypertension, disorientation, and explosive temper. All of these symptoms were complicated by his alcoholism.

After a year and a half of individual counseling, followed by group counseling with other ACA, Joe was able to maintain sobriety, grieve the loss of his father, and grieve his experiences in Vietnam. After some time in counseling, Joe and some other group members visited the Vietnam War Memorial in Washington, D.C. This was an important event in his painful journey to recovery.

Discussion

This case illustrates the many layers of pain that are often covered up by denial, alcohol/drugs, anger, and withdrawal. Joe was very unhappy and depressed, and he felt shame and guilt about his own behavior. Although he initially couldn't admit or ask for help, he did continue to come back. For many clients like Joe, it is important to recognize that it is hard for them to ask for help, admit their vulnerability or pain to themselves and others, and see that recovery is possible.

Joe is one of those rewarding and remarkable stories that validate the need for the counselor to hang in there, not abandon him, not get angry with him, but hold him responsible for his behavior and recognize that progress is slow.

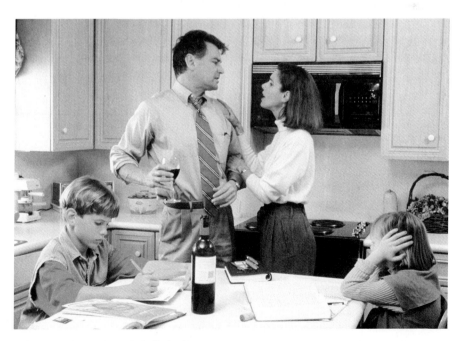

Children growing up in an alcoholic family.

children distrust their own observations and feelings, they must wonder or guess at what is normal. At a time when most functional families are providing structure, discipline, and natural consequences for their children's behavior, alcoholic families provide control, rigidity, fear, irresponsibility, immaturity, and, most important, *unpredictability*. Children in alcoholic families try to control the behavior of the alcoholic parent and the codependent spouse by becoming super-responsible and trying to do everything correctly to obtain the parent's approval. They soon find out that, despite their best efforts to be perfect, the parent always finds fault with something. While desperately trying to predict or control the behavior of their parents, children do not realize that alcoholism and drug addiction is a disease that results in unpredictable behavior.

✴ Identification of Children of Alcoholic Families

Robert Ackerman (1978) described various behavioral characteristics of children of alcoholics, including the following:

- Being superachievers or perfectionists or exhibiting efforts that go far beyond the reasonable criteria of every task
- Exhibiting an inordinate need to control their environment and therefore becoming anxious with the slightest threat to their security (e.g., a teacher's comment on homework or an unusually low grade may provoke emotional upset)
- Displaying social disengagement from or excessive attention to the peer group (as an isolated loner or a class clown)
- Exhibiting signs of physical neglect (untidiness, soiled clothing, poor hygiene) and/or physical abuse (bruises, cuts, etc.)
- Being unable to concentrate and sometimes showing marked variations in academic performance, especially when parents are in a binge pattern of alcohol use or in codependent conflict

✴ Denial of Feelings in an Alcoholic Family

The alcoholic family swears an allegiance to the family secret of alcoholism. Family members dedicate themselves to denying that Dad and/or Mom is out of control. The children hope that perhaps their family secret will change and continually explore ways to make it change.

Sometimes this becomes an almost magical quest by the children to find that special way of being or ritualistic behavior that can make Dad and/or Mom change. Children give up their own sense of self in their search for the key that will change their parents' dysfunctional behavior.

A friend tells this story illustrating how children's feelings are discounted: When the alcoholic dad falls down, drunk, and spends the night on the front lawn, still in his work clothes, does the child really believe Mom's explanation? "You know your dad loves astronomy; he came home late last night, lay down to gaze at the stars, and, since he was tired from working late, just fell asleep, gazing at the constellations."

Children must maintain the *illusion of normalcy,* the illusion that their families are normal. The child defensively maintains the belief that this is what other families go through.

Howard Clinebell (1985) reported that the following factors produce damage in the lives of children of alcoholics:

1. *Role reversal:* Children may undertake parental duties because the parent is unable to be responsible or because the parent forces responsibilities on the children. The alcoholic may be treated as a child and, in return, act helpless. In incestuous families, the daughter and mother often switch roles.
2. *Unpredictability:* An inconsistent and unpredictable relationship with the alcoholic emotionally deprives the children.
3. *Unavailability:* The nonalcoholic, inadequate parent is struggling with major problems; because this parent's own needs are unmet, he or she is unable to attend to the needs of the children.
4. *Social isolation:* The damaging factor is the social isolation of the family, as protection from further pain and suffering, due to embarrassment.

Even periods of parental sobriety have negative effects on the children in alcoholic families. This is due primarily to the inconsistency and shattered hope that this time it will be different. The alcoholic father "inspires the natural love of his offspring, who build there from an ideal father image of omnipotence and loving kindness. This disillusionment of the drunken episode is shattering to the frail superego structure of the child who is subjected to alternating experiences of exalted hopes and blighting disappointments" (Newell 1950).

✖ Perspective of the Child in an Alcoholic Family

M. Cork (1969) interviewed 115 children living in alcoholic families in an attempt to understand the child's perspective. Cork found that the children react to the alcoholic family system in a number of common ways. The interviewed children in alcoholic families

1. would not go to a friend's house because they would not dare reciprocate and invite friends to their homes due to the unpredictability and embarrassing behaviors of their parents.
2. were angry at everybody.
3. were preoccupied at school with worry about what would happen when they returned home.
4. envied their friends who seemed to have fun with their families.
5. felt alone when they were only children.
6. felt neglected when both parents were drinking.
7. felt they had to be parentlike, especially if the mother was drinking.
8. worried about each parent's loneliness if the parents were separated; wished for their parents to reunite, even if their home was calmer during the

TABLE 7.1

Problems of Children in Alcoholic Families

Physical Neglect or Abuse	Acting-Out Behaviors	Emotional Reaction to Alcoholism and Chaotic Family Life	Social and Interpersonal Difficulties
Serious illness Accidents	Involvement with police and courts Aggression Alcohol and other drug abuse	Suicidal tendencies Depression Repressed emotions Lack of self-confidence Lack of life direction Fear of abandonment Fear of future	Family relationship problems Peer problems Adjustment problems Feeling different from norm Embarrassment Overresponsible Feeling unloved and unable to trust

SOURCE: G. Lawson, James S. Peterson, and Ann Lawson, *Alcoholism and the Family: A Guide to Treatment and Prevention,* Aspen Publications, 1983. Reprinted by permission of G. Lawson.

separation; seemed to feel an even deeper loss if the alcoholic parent moved out of the house.

9. were unable to separate and individuate from their parents as adolescents; it was difficult to break away from somebody with whom they had no ties; one child poignantly said, "I want to be somebody, but I feel like nobody."
10. excused the alcoholic's behavior and often condemned the nonalcoholics for being hostile and angry; children could deduce from this that love and caring would come from alcoholics; research, unfortunately, indicates that many ACA do marry alcoholics to try out their hypothesis.
11. experienced multiple separations and reunions of their parents and learned not to expect any state to continue consistently.
12. continued to have problems, even when the alcoholic stopped drinking. See Tables 7.1 and 7.2 for lists of these problems.

⚮ Family Disease Model

Just as alcoholism is classified as a disease (i.e., it has a known etiology, progressive nature, and known outcome), the alcoholic family is often described in the context of a "family disease." The family members are described as suffering from alcoholism, codependency, and enabling behavior, perpetuating both the alcoholism- and alcohol-related problems. The family is organized around the alcoholic's drinking and the consequences of that drinking. The central organizing principle of the family is focused around the alcoholic's behavior (e.g., Is she drinking? Will she drink? How much will she drink? When and with whom will she drink? Will she get drunk?). The family responds to the alcoholic in a codependent (giving up of self) fashion or enables both alcoholic behavior and drinking. The family disease model describes

TABLE 7.2		
Problems of Alcoholic Families Affecting More Than One Person		
Marital	*Parental*	***Cross-Boundaries—*** ***Parent and Child Relationships***

Marital instability
Prolonged separation
Divorce
Death of a spouse
Physical abuse of a spouse
	Inadequate parenting
	Lack of structure
	Inconsistencies
	Emotional neglect of
	    children
	Inability or unwillingness
	    to perform parental
	    duties
		Physical and sexual abuse of children
		Parentification of children (child becomes the
		    parent)
		Role reversal
		Family conflict
		Isolation of family from society
		Isolation of individual family member within
		    the family
		Incongruent communication (mixed messages)
		Lack of trust between family members
		Family secrets

SOURCE: G. Lawson, James S. Peterson, and Ann Lawson, *Alcoholism and the Family: A Guide to Treatment and Prevention*, Aspen Publications, 1983. Reprinted by permission of G. Lawson.

the family as trying to maintain homeostasis, compensating for the disequilibrium of the alcoholic's behavior and drinking. This results in family members' disconnecting from their own feelings, distorting their perceptions, and invoking the "no-talk, no-feel, no-trust" rule.

✻ Alcoholism/Drug Addiction—Impact on Marriage

Marriages are at risk when there is a substance-abuse problem. Feelings of betrayal, continuous conflict, chaos, loss, resentments, and pain are constant parts of the marital cycle when one partner is alcoholic/drug-addicted. Ironically, some studies indicate that if spouses drink together and with approximately equal patterns and amounts of use, it may not initially create a problem. However, problems will arise when one partner goes out to drink with friends, or a partner cuts back his or her drinking, enters into treatment, or voluntarily seeks sobriety.

Sexual problems related to substance abuse are very common, confounded by problems of intimacy. John Gottman, author of *Why Marriages Fail* (1995), describes the four horsemen of the apocalypse of marriages—criticism, contempt (nonverbal), defensiveness, and withdrawal. The codependent dance of couples where there is an alcohol or drug problem frequently involves an "in the marriage," "out of the marriage," and "on the fence" attitude toward the marriage and each other. Frequently, all four horsemen are present. There is also a strong ambivalence that the wife of an alcoholic has toward her husband. There is a vacillation between being supportive and understanding and feeling hopeless and withdrawn.

Certainly, recovery not only involves treatment for alcoholics/addicts or problem users but also involves treatment for the spouse.

> Behavioral marital therapy focuses on teaching partners how to communicate with each other, solve problems together and resolve their conflicts. Husbands and wives look directly for ways to break the cycle of criticism, denial and blame that characterizes a chemically dependent family and develop new roles and new ways of interacting that will support recovery. ("After Drug Treatment" 1999)

✴ ACA in Relationships

ACA Define Self Through Others

ACA define their sense of identity by the impressions others have of them. ACA have a strong, often imbalanced need for affirmation from others that they are indeed worthwhile. They approach their world from the outside in versus the inside-out stance of self-confident people.

Even though many of my ACA patients have been extremely successful in their professional lives, they still feel inadequate and don't trust their talents, skills, and accomplishments. Many feel that they are charlatans and will be exposed as inadequate persons. They fear that at any time their professional abilities may all be taken away from them. Then they will relive their ultimate fear of being all alone, helpless, abandoned, and rejected; the fears they felt growing up will be played out again. Successful careers and stylish and attractive lifestyles camouflage their poor sense of self, and they are surprised when others don't see through their disguises.

The Disengaged ACA

Growing up in alcoholic families with parents who are unavailable, children often develop patterns of interpersonal disengagement. ACA may maintain this pattern of disengagement in most interpersonal relationships. Cermak (1984) describes disengaged ACA as having the following behaviors:

1. Hard-driving, workaholic; always preoccupied by projects and things that have to be done; rarely satisfied with accomplishments; in denial of feelings, relationships take a back seat
2. Defensive, fearful of closeness to others; plays cards close to the vest; unable to deal honestly on an emotional level; longing for relationships; chronic anger
3. Overwhelmed by feelings, buffeted by emotional storms; desperately trying to get other people to behave properly; often unable to work effectively.

Disengaged ACAs exhibit behaviors that on the surface make them seem self-sufficient and self-actualized; in actuality, they are depressed and suffering from deep emotional pain.

Atypical Depression

Another diagnostic category recently associated with ACA and others who grew up in imbalanced family systems is atypical depression. Atypical depression is an impairment in interpersonal and social skills due to an extreme sensitivity to rejection. Because these individuals are highly sensitive, they overreact, thinking others' remarks, opinions, and/or actions are personal attacks. Many individuals suffering from atypical depression report that this sensitivity began in early childhood and have histories of physical, emotional, and/or sexual violation.

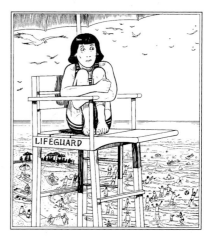

Codependency

Timmen Cermak quotes a metaphor from Charles Alexander: that codependency is "like being a lifeguard on a crowded beach, knowing that you cannot swim, and not telling anyone for fear of a panic." This is the sense of desperation that ACA feel as they guess at what is normal.

Codependency is "like being a lifeguard on a crowded beach, knowing that you cannot swim, and not telling anyone for fear of a panic."

Cermak, himself an adult child of an alcoholic, defined codependency in diagnostic terms in the hope that codependency would be recognized as a psychiatric disorder. The following are diagnostic criteria for codependent personality disorder:

1. Continual investment of self-esteem in the ability to influence or control feelings and behaviors in the self and others in the face of obvious adverse consequences
2. Assumption of responsibility for meeting others' needs to the exclusion of acknowledging one's own needs
3. Anxiety and boundary distortions in situations of intimacy and separation
4. Enmeshment in relationships with personality-disordered, drug-dependent, and impulse-disordered individuals
5. Maintenance of a primary relationship with an active substance abuser for at least 2 years without seeking outside support and/or exhibiting three or more of the following characteristics:

   a. Constriction of emotions with or without dramatic outbursts
   b. Depression
   c. Hypervigilance
   d. Compulsions
   e. Anxiety
   f. Excessive reliance on denial
   g. Substance abuse
   h. Recurrent physical or sexual abuse
   i. Stress-related medical illnesses

An individual who has all five criteria of codependency would be diagnosed as having codependent personality disorder. A personality disorder affects all aspects of one's life because pervasive personality traits become inflexible and maladaptive.

The results are significant subjective distress and social and occupational impairment. Treatment for codependent personality disorder often involves extensive education, counseling, therapeutic interventions, and sometimes medication to deal with major anxiety and depression.

If you find yourself identifying with some of the diagnostic criteria for codependent personality disorder but not all of them, you might have some codependent traits but not a full-blown disorder. If these codependent traits result in significant difficulties in establishing effective, caring, and intimate relationships, they probably need to be investigated.

Boundary Inadequacy

Boundary inadequacy is the inability to set consistent and appropriate boundaries. The result is vascillating or ambiguous boundaries, overly rigid boundaries, and invasive boundaries. As a result, ACA have difficulty in relationships; often they choose an alcoholic, addict, or a generally dysfunctional partner, or develop codependent relationships. If one were to ask persons with strong codependent traits and difficulties in setting appropriate boundaries to choose persons they were interested in from 100 people—90 of whom are fairly functional and stable—their choices would probably come from the 10 dysfunctional people.

For ACA, boundaries are often distorted in interpersonal relationships; sometimes they are excessively involved (overattachment) or excessively detached (overseparation).

Overattachment and Overseparation

In their work on chemical dependency and intimacy dysfunction, Eli Coleman and Philip Colgan (1987) focused on overattachment and overseparation in men who grew up in alcoholic families. They identified thoughts, feelings, and behaviors common to both the overseparated and the overattached individuals. Table 7.3 lists these thoughts, feelings, and behaviors.

The thoughts of the overattached and overseparated sound like common lyrics to country-western songs. These codependent lyrics include "You should be grateful," "I want so little," "You don't care," "What am I doing wrong?" and "I'm nobody without you." Many people identify strongly with either the overseparated or the overattached column in Table 7.3; others cross over, having both overattached and overseparated characteristics. Overseparated individuals tend to develop relationships with overattached individuals and vice versa. Frequently, ACA duplicate the kind of relationship their codependent parents had. Just as the disease of alcoholism and drug addiction progresses from generation to generation, so do the patterns of inadequate boundary setting and codependent relationships.

Codependent Dances

The most traditional codependent dance is between alcoholics/addicts and their codependent partners. Alcoholics/addicts and their partners are both codependent;

TABLE 7.3	
Overseparation and Overattachment	
Overseparation	*Overattachment*
Thoughts	
You're not good enough.	I'm not good enough.
They want so much.	I want so little.
They give so little.	I give so much.
I'm ambivalent.	You don't care.
If only they would . . .	What am I doing wrong?
I am a rock.	I'm nobody without you.
You should be grateful.	I'm so unappreciated
Feelings	
Fear, smothering	Fear, abandonment
Self-controlled	Out of control
Indifferent	Needy, burdened
Unsafe with others	Unsafe alone
Trappedt	Shut out
Numb	Desperate
Behaviors	
Is self-protective	Is self-sacrificing
Controls others	Pleases others
Acts to guard feelings	Acts contrary to feelings
Denies	Explains
Is compulsively independent	Is compulsively dependent

SOURCE: Eli Coleman and Philip Colgan, "Chemical dependency and intimacy dysfunction" in *Journal of Chemical Dependency*, Vol. 1 (1), 1987. Copyright © 1987 by the Haworth Press, Inc. For copies of the complete work, contact Marianne Arnold at The Haworth Document Delivery Service (Telephone 1-800-3-HAWORTH; 10 Alice Street, Binghampton, NY 13904). For other questions concerning rights and permissions contact Wando Latour at the above address.

alcoholics/addicts need partners who enable them to continue to use drugs/alcohol and not suffer the full impact of their addiction. Their partners need alcoholics/ addicts to avoid their own fears of abandonment and depression. Both of them fear feelings of loneliness, isolation, anxiety, and depression.

The fear of abandonment and rejection is so strong for ACA that they choose not to develop an individual sense of self. This neglect of oneself while preoccupied or obsessed with changing the partner is codependency. The codependent dances these couples perform have some common features: (1) shame-based styles of communicating and interacting; (2) a denial by at least one partner of dysfunctional and/or codependent behavior; (3) a relationship of bargaining, not an intimate partnership; and (4) shame-based litany of the past. Each partner holds on to unresolved conflicts and continues to use them to shame the other.

⚹ Recovery for Adult Children of Alcoholics

An ACA's prognosis for treatment is directly related to the severity of the parental alcoholism and the levels of abuse, violation, and trauma experienced while growing up in the alcoholic/addict family system. The onset of the alcoholism is also a factor in the ACA's recovery. The earlier the alcoholism in the family, and the younger the child when exposed to direct or indirect consequences of the parents' alcoholism, the more extensive the damage, and therefore the deeper the wounds. Impact at early ages can have dramatic developmental consequences (Brown 1988).

Inherited Family Belief Systems

A major recovery issue at the heart of all ACAs' problems is their core belief system. The "process of recovery involves challenging the deepest core beliefs about others and the self that were constructed to preserve core attachments" (Brown 1988). As discussed earlier in this chapter, these core beliefs serve to deny the ACAs' feelings and maintain the illusion of their parents' normalcy. ACA avoid exploring these holes in their belief systems for fear that their swiss cheese system might fall apart. When ACA can acknowledge how the belief systems acquired from their parents have prevented them from attaining what they want, recovery can begin.

In *Struggle for Intimacy,* Janet Geringer Woititz (1985) devotes an entire chapter to some of the misconceptions, or inappropriate beliefs, that ACA have when it comes to establishing intimate relationships.

Overview of ACA Recovery

Once ACA are aware that their belief systems are not serving them, and are preventing, blocking, or sabotaging the development of effective relationships, the next step is to develop a more reality-based belief system.

The first step in developing this reality-based belief system is to recognize the dysfunction and trauma of the past and unlock the feelings denied by this dysfunctional belief system.

A trusting therapeutic alliance with a counselor/therapist allows ACA to feel the loss, grief, and trauma of the past. This difficult process involves (1) giving up the old defense mechanisms and dysfunctional beliefs, (2) feeling, and (3) choosing to honor and integrate those feelings in a new more functional belief system.

Eventually ACA loosen their defensive controls and develop the ability to respond to different situations and circumstances with flexibility. ACA can now establish effective boundaries in relationships, stop engaging in dysfunctional behavior and relationships, and establish a core belief system that allows for effective choicemaking and change.

Powerlessness in the Alcoholic Family System

Just as alcoholics/addicts must first admit they are powerless over drugs/alcohol, so must ACA admit that as children they were powerless to change the alcoholic family system. They were innocent children whose feelings were ignored while living in unhealthy imbalanced situations. Recognizing that as children they were not responsible for their parents' disease of alcoholism frees ACA to honor their own feelings.

Feeling Awareness

For ACA who have spent a major portion of their lives denying feelings, the most difficult task of recovery is recognizing and integrating feelings in making decisions, resolving conflicts, and developing interpersonal relationships.

Jerry, a patient of mine who is a recovering alcoholic and an ACA, quizzically and candidly commented, "Feelings, I am not quite sure what you mean when you ask 'What do you feel?' I don't know what you mean or want from me. When you ask me if I feel sad, or I sound angry, I don't recognize that I am experiencing those feelings until you mention it."

Many ACA have similar reactions. Unaware of what they feel, they are equally inexperienced in recognizing what others feel. This makes it difficult to effectively communicate with others—especially family members—and to establish sensitive, caring, and intimate relationships.

Identifying Feelings for ACA

Jael Greenleaf, an ACA counselor in Los Angeles, describes ACA as having an emotional learning disability. (See Case Studies 7.2 and 7.3.) ACA have learned not to trust their feelings; thus they make decisions based on what they think is appropriate, without integrating what they feel. Feelings are what make us, or define us as, human. The famous television series *Star Trek* gave us Mr. Spock, the cognitive logical unemotional alien, and in the later version of the series, Data, a robot with extensive computer capabilities. Data was often fascinated by and marveled at human feelings and emotions and tried to understand them. Mr. Spock does not understand human emotions that may override the logic of a decision. The captains of the *Enterprise* remind Spock and Data that human emotions are essential and part of the human equation in approaching life.

By being sensitive to what we feel, we can begin to understand our feelings (affective self) and integrate them with what we know (cognitive self). When our affective self is congruent with our cognitive self, the application (whatever action we take) is often more successful. Decisions become easier to make when feelings are balanced with the cognitive side, and there is an interplay of these two sides of our self. Our decisions become more fulfilling, our goals more attainable, and our relationships more effective, when we integrate our feelings. The struggle for the ACA begins with identifying, understanding, and integrating feelings.

A good technique to help ACA access their feelings is journaling, or writing a feeling diary. Often a counselor asks the ACA to buy a special notebook and keep it nearby—in the car, at work, and at home. Whenever the ACA is aware of an emotional reaction, thought, or feeling, he or she writes about it in the journal. By writing rather than thinking, ACA soon find that they are accessing feelings that they may not have been aware of previously.

Case Study 7.2
Rejection Sensitivity
Frank

A colleague, old friend, and workshop training partner of mine tells a story of his fear of rejection. Growing up in an imbalanced, alcoholic family system, Frank learned how to defend against shame by being likable and by avoiding conflict. He figured that if everyone liked him and he avoided conflict, he would not be subject to rejection, attack, or shame. Unfortunately, his likable quality put him in a real dilemma back in the third grade.

As Frank tells the story, his classmates really liked him and nominated him for third-grade class president. Normally, he would be just likable enough, but not too popular, because that would bring the unwanted attention he feared. That year, there were no outstanding choices for class president, and his likable, nonaggressive style became the qualities that the class wanted in its president. His classmates reacted to the nomination with genuine acceptance and encouragement. Frank felt this put him in a lose-lose position. Frank thought that if he ran and lost, he would experience tremendous feelings of rejection and shame. If he ran and won, he would disappoint his classmates by being an inadequate class president, unable to meet the responsibilities of the office. Ultimately, this would lead to the same feelings of rejection and shame. Either way, Frank felt he would be rejected and shamed. His only choice was to reject the nomination for office. He did this rather adroitly by taking the nomination as an opportunity to lend his support to another, more popular classmate. "Thanks for the nomination," he said, "but my support goes to Larry. He would make a far more capable class president than me, and he was the one I had intended to nominate." Unfortunately, Frank missed out on the opportunity to grow from experiencing what it is like to run for office and perhaps the opportunity to be class president.

Discussion

This case illustrates how growing up in an alcoholic family can cause the ACA to choose to avoid the attention of others (public domain) and to not take positive risk that can produce growth. For Frank, the fear of losing the election was much bigger than if it were "just an election." A loss would rekindle in Frank waves of rejection and strong feelings of personal inadequacy and shame. So Frank played it safe by deflecting the attention and supporting another person. This was a life pattern that would later cause him to regret the decisions he had made. A healthier response would have been to run in the election, gain the experience, sort out the results, and move on.

Another method of feeling awareness involves ACA verbalizing and communicating what they feel directly to others. One method would be using the statement:

"I feel _____, when I_____." For example:

"I feel upset when I notice you haven't taken the garbage out, after you said you would."

"I feel confused, and both sad and angry, when I don't get a present for Valentine's Day."

Case Study 7.3
Difficulty in Making Decisions
Norman

Norman, 29, is an adult child of an alcoholic. He grew up in an extremely abusive and physically violating dysfunctional family system. During one alcoholic rage, Norman's dad shoved his mom's head through the front window of their living room. Another time, his mom hid his dad's car keys in the garbage because his dad was drunk. They both struggled with the garbage, and she severely cut her hand on the jagged edge of a coffee can. Later, two tall police officers came to quiet them down during another domestic dispute. These were just a few of Norman's memories.

His parents' fighting had a far-reaching impact on Norman and the other children in the family. The fear of abandonment, shame, and rejection caused Norman to act out during his childhood in many destructive ways. He did not achieve at school, despite being very bright and capable.

One day in individual counseling, Norman talked about a trip he took to Reno, Nevada. This trip was a metaphor for his fear of making a career change. After watching for some time at the roulette table with his wife and a friend, he decided to place his bet. Norman placed a two-dollar bet on the red and a two-dollar bet on the black. He surmised that this was a secure bet. He smiled to himself smugly as the roulette wheel spun and the ball bounded around from number to number. When it landed on a red number, the croupier just pushed his two dollars from the black spot to the red spot, and Norman collected his bet. Despite the odd looks from the croupier, and his friend's efforts to explain why this was a stupid bet, Norman continued to play two dollars on black and two dollars on red simultaneously. After several spins, he stopped betting. He felt entertained and justified that he had played roulette. I didn't hesitate to point out to Norman that the numbers zero and double zero on the roulette wheel are green. If either of those numbers had come up, he would have lost both bets.

This was analogous to what Norman was doing in his conflict about his career. He was betting on his current job for security, but not actively putting himself on the line to find a more fulfilling job. The longer he waited to take action, the more time he was wasting, and the more likely it was that zero or double zero would come up, in the form of either losing his current job due to his dissatisfaction projected to the work setting or not being able to motivate himself to find a better job because he was suffering from feelings of rejection, shame, and abandonment.

Even with this therapeutic insight, Norman waited several months to take any direct action. After a great deal of work, he eventually landed a new job in the field that he really wanted. That job didn't work out but it led to another job. After 2 years of struggle, Norman found himself in a career position that was consistent with his feelings of entitlement and accomplishment; his job affirmed his skills and capabilities.

Discussion

This is a good example of how "playing it safe" for too long can result in significant negative consequences. Norman grew up in a household that was extremely abusive physically, verbally, and emotionally. Norman, like many ACA, did not act on his passion or feelings. He knew he was unhappy in his job, and he also knew what kind of

(continued on next page)

> ### Case Study 7.3 (*continued*)
> *Difficulty in Making Decisions*
> **Norman**
>
> job, he wanted, but he waited too long to take action or make a decision. Change often involves knowing what you feel, knowing what you want, but also having a plan and taking action. Norman was immobilized by fear over negative "what-ifs." What if he couldn't find a new job? What if he got a job and he didn't like it? What if he got fired from his new job? And on and on. This fearful negative cycle of thinking caused him to avoid making a decision, and to stay in an abusive working situation, much like the abusive family he grew up in.

"Right now, I am not feeling close and caring toward you. I do not want to have sex. I am still feeling hurt by the fight we had earlier today. I would prefer talking about it tomorrow when our emotions are not running so deep."

Therapists help ACA identify and explore a wide variety of feelings (shame, rejection, abandonment, loss, loneliness, isolation, and grief) that were experienced growing up in an alcoholic family system. ACA therapists use various treatment methods to access feelings, including guided imagery, gestalt exercises, art therapy, role plays, workbooks, and books and articles on ACA issues (bibliotherapy).

Grief Work

Children who grow up in alcoholic families experience loss, violation, and trauma growing up in imbalanced alcoholic family systems. Many never have an opportunity to mourn what they have lost or missed out on. Mourning is a process of allowing feelings of loss to come to the surface, to be felt, and to be grieved.

An analogy is the improper healing of a cut. In the child's case, an emotionally damaging cut or violation of self has occurred. The cut has healed over but was not cleaned out first; the dirt (leftover unresolved issues and feelings) was not removed. The result is a numbing pain, which is tolerated and denied for years and is thought to be quite normal. Grief work involves going back and cleaning out this wound by gently and sensitively removing the dirt. By avoiding the feelings and pain accompanying proper healing of this infected wound, individuals are unable to function to a fuller potential. Once their wounds are cleaned, true healing allows ACA to make more effective choices.

Grief work requires the help of a professional therapist trained and experienced in ACA recovery. The counselor/therapist must be sensitive to the patient's ego strength, general level of functioning, underlying psychiatric issues, and support system. Attempting to do ACA grief work without an experienced professional may cause unnecessary emotional harm by going too deep, too quickly into traumatic issues of the past. A professional trained and experienced in ACA recovery recognizes the pace and depth of the work to be done and shows appropriate judgment in helping patients through this work.

Choice Making

Changing old, imbalanced patterns is possible only if individuals feel they have choices. Discouraging voices of doom and gloom need to be quieted for recovery efforts to be implemented. Self-pity, victim roles, and the poor-me syndrome prevent ACA from even entertaining a choice to change. The old familial belief system whispers in the ACA's ear: "Change is not possible, so why even try? You'll just waste time and energy and fail, anyway, just as you always have in the past."

Changes involve integration and congruency with feelings and choosing not to respond in dysfunctional, codependent ways. There is the acknowledgment that change is difficult, takes time, may involve pain, and requires support. Sometimes small changes and positive choices can establish the foundation for more significant growth-related choices later.

A variety of therapeutic issues must be explored before the ACA can improve interpersonal relationships. Some of the cognitive and affective therapeutic themes are these:

- Family-of-origin issues (beliefs, roles, rules, and thoughts about relationships)
- Sense of self, or self-concept, and interpersonal interaction, choosing relationships, and maintaining dysfunctional imbalanced relationships
- Boundary setting and decision making in interpersonal situations
- Self-sabotage or destructive behavior, poor impulse control, poor anger and frustration tolerance, and an inability to set and maintain healthy long-range goals

Second-Order Change

Second-order change is a cognitive-behavioral technique to change the way one traditionally responds to situations and interpersonal interactions. Many interactions are mechanical, automatic, even rhetorical. These are first-order interactions. Individuals can choose to respond differently to the first-order cues in communication and interaction. This new response or new order of interaction is second-order change. The following examples illustrate a very common first-order interaction and one possible second-order change. The meta-message, or the underlying true feeling message, is in parentheses. (See Case Study 7.4.)

First-Order—Phone Call from Mom

Mom: Why haven't you called? (Shame on you for not caring about your mom. You probably don't like me. I know I'm just a bother now that I am old.)

Adult child: Well, Mom, I have been very busy with my new job and everything. (Please give me a break, Mom. I'm not in the mood for

Case Study 7.4

Letter to Parents from a Recovering Alcoholic and ACA about the Parents' Alcoholism

Dear Mom and Dad,

It's hard to write a letter like this, so I guess I'll just get right to the point. I'm writing because I'm concerned that you both continue to drink a lot despite the fact that you have both been in ill health recently. And I'm sure that you, Dad, have been warned more than once by doctors that to continue to drink threatens your health.

I've wanted to talk to you both about your drinking for years, but so far I have never been able to break the silence and tell you how truly worried I am about it.

Only you can make a decision to stop drinking. But I feel very strongly that I must tell you both, with love and compassion, how concerned I am, and how much it hurts me to see you continue to damage yourselves through drinking.

I am sure that in your hearts you know that you have a problem, for I have seen you both struggle with it; seen your efforts to control what and when you drink; seen your efforts to cut back. I know I rejoiced during that period when you sobered up entirely for a few months, and you found renewed health and happiness together.

I am also sure you are both aware that the stakes are high; that you are endangering your health as you mix alcohol and various prescription medication, and that drinking can only worsen your struggles with heart disease, diabetes, and the effects of aging.

You know what you have to do. It's so simple, and yet I know from experience how hard it can be. You both so desperately need to stop drinking now, throw out all the booze in the house (even the supply reserved for guests), and get some help staying sober, for you have proven by slipping back into drinking that you cannot do it by yourselves.

I suspect getting help will be the hardest part; it certainly was for me. But it's really the most necessary part of getting better and infinitely better than struggling alone.

Getting help could mean any of the following: Telling Dr. Green that you know you have a problem with alcohol and are tired of struggling with it; that you want to get some counseling or get into a treatment program. Calling AA and attending a meeting together; the nearest AA meeting is right down the street on Maple Rd. Calling the local drug/alcohol helpline and getting a referral to a counselor, social worker, or therapist experienced in working with alcoholics who want to recover.

This letter is not meant to blame or shame or accuse you; it is merely a plea for you to help yourselves for your own sakes, and for the sake of our family. It is an effort to tell the truth about the problem that our whole family has struggled with for so many years.

The truth hurts sometimes. The truth is that all of us have begun to insulate ourselves from your drinking, to control the time and length of our visits, to arrange sober holidays in our own homes, as my sister did this Christmas. We have all shied away from confronting you because it is so painful to see you both caught in this awful disease.

I hope that this letter has not made you angry or resentful. If it has, so be it; but I want you to know that I love you both, and that I want to help you, if there is any way in the world that I can. If you want to talk about this letter, please call me; if not, if it makes you too upset or uncomfortable, we need never discuss it.

(continued on next page)

Case Study 7.4 *(continued)*

Letter to Parents from a Recovering Alcoholic and ACA about the Parents' Alcoholism

Ultimately, there may be an element of selfishness in this letter; because, in the end, I want to be able to look into my heart and say "I tried to help. I told them the truth and encouraged them to get help and save their own lives." For me, it's an important step in dealing with my past and working on my own sobriety.

Please, for your own sake and the sake of us all, share this letter with each other, and talk about it openly together. I pray that you both will find the strength to quit drinking and get some help together.

Your loving son,

Epilogue

The parents who were sent this letter both got sober. Unfortunately, the mother died shortly thereafter. The son spent some quality time with her during the months before she passed away. The father has been in recovery for a number of years now and has remarried. Father and son have quality time together when they visit.

Discussion Questions

Would you write a letter like this to one of your parents about a family issue?
Would you send a letter like this?
What are the "real" healing elements of this exercise?
Suggestion: Write a letter and then identify what the depth and breadth of the problem is.

---

	shame right now. I feel overwhelmed, considering the new job, and other adjustments I am going through. I don't need this right now.)
Mom:	Well, I guess your job is more important than your mother. (Double shame on you for not making your mother number one in your life.)
Adult child:	Mom, it's not that my job is more important than you. I just didn't get around to calling because I've been so busy at work. (Let me explain. Please, please, understand.)
Mom:	You haven't asked me how my back is. (More shame—I don't care about your silly job. I want you to be more concerned with my ailments.)
Adult child:	Now, Mom, that isn't fair. You didn't even give me a chance to ask you how you were. (I'm beginning to get angry and lose patience with you. Here we go again. I can't even talk with you without getting angry—self-shame.)
Mom:	Now, don't get so upset, dear. (Watch it. This is your powerful supermom, able to abandon and hurt you with the slightest provocation.)

Adult child:	[Change in tone] How are you feeling, Mom? I have been worried about you. (I don't want to fight or be abandoned. I'll just give her what she wants. I'm feeling like a helpless child again.)
Mom:	Well, you know those doctors want me to come in for some more tests. But I don't think they know what they are talking about. I just don't have any way to get into the hospital, with my back hurting the way it does. (I am helpless. I want you to come home and be with me and take care of me. If you don't, I'll just punish you by suffering.)
Adult child:	Mom, can't you get Aunt Joanie to take you in for the tests? (I am worried. I can't come. Maybe I can fix it for you by getting you some help.)
Mom:	Oh dear, don't worry about me; I'll be all right. (Worry about me. Shame on you for not coming right away. You ungrateful daughter, I'll just suffer alone.)

This dialogue need not be carried out in this first-order manner. The anger, resentments, and shame do not have to be responded to in this traditional codependent dance. The following second-order change occurs after the adult child has done some therapeutic work on the underlying issue of her mother's not wanting to let go of her, for fear of having to work on her (mom's) own issues of loneliness and abandonment.

Second-Order—Change

Mom:	Why haven't you called? (Shame on you for not caring about your mom.)
Adult child:	Mom, boy, I've been wondering about you. How are you doing? (I'm not going to respond to the shaming question. I'll change the focus to you and your reason for calling.)
Mom:	Well, I'm surprised that you asked. Most of the time you're too busy with your job to even call me. (I'll try some more shaming to see if I can get you angry, because I am angry that your job comes before your dear old mom.)
Adult child:	Mom, it's unfortunate that I had to move out of town for this job promotion. I know it's hard on you. By the way, how is Aunt Joanie? (I had to take care of myself. I recognize that you feel abandoned and would prefer that I stay at home, but we all have to let go sometime. Why can't you understand like Aunt Joanie?)
Mom:	She's fine. But you know my back has been killing me. The doctors want me to go to the hospital for some more tests, but I hurt too much, and I don't know how I can get there. (Poor me, won't you please come home and help me?)
Adult child:	I know your back has been a problem for quite some time now. It would be nice to find out what the problem is. (I'd like to see you get in for the tests, but I can't help you get to the hospital. If you want some results, you'll have to figure out transportation.)

Mom:	So would I. But I need someone to help me, and Aunt Joanie doesn't drive. (Please, won't you come back home and help?)
Adult child:	Well, there are other ways for you to get a ride to the hospital. I hope you can figure out a way. (I'm not coming, just for this. There are other solutions to the problem and you are capable of figuring it out.)
Mom:	Well, I just don't know if I can do it myself. (Poor me. Shame on you for not helping your poor old mom.)
Adult child:	Well, Mom, I'm sure you'll be able to figure it out. You were always pretty resourceful when we were growing up. I love you. I'll talk to you soon. (You must take care of this yourself. You were very capable raising three children practically on your own, considering Dad's alcoholism. I'm not jumping in to help. I still love and admire you. I am ending this conversation and not giving you an opportunity to feel sorry for yourself.)

You can see the difference in the second-order change. The adult child avoided the shame-based messages and did not get emotionally hooked by displaying anger, rage, or lack of emotional control. Instead, in the second-order model, she focused on the real issues and stayed balanced and in emotional control while maintaining appropriate boundaries.

Changes in Interactions with Family

Robert Ackerman (1978), a noted author, speaker, and counselor specializing in ACA work, tells a story that illustrates the difficulty in changing interactions with family: After working with Ackerman for a few months, one of his patients felt she had made enough progress to share her new therapeutic awareness with her family. She was going home for Christmas (an emotional time for most families, especially alcoholic families) and wanted to talk to her parents about her new insights. Ackerman suggested that she think about what her goal was in sharing her insights. Essentially ignoring his advice, on returning home she told her parents all about her childhood pain resulting from growing up in an alcoholic family and described how this had affected her relationships with men. Initially, her parents were actively listening and seemed to understand. However, the next few days the family returned to the traditional dysfunctional arguments, escalated emotions, and shame-based communications of the past. The daughter had to spend the next few days at a friend's home to survive the rest of the holiday.

At her next therapy appointment, the patient expressed surprise that her parents could engage her in the old dysfunctional dances. She asked, "Why were they still able to push all of my buttons?" Dr. Ackerman, in the wisdom of his years of experience, matter-of-factly said, "They installed the buttons."

The same struggle goes on for most ACA who interact with their families. Some of these families have members still actively using alcohol/drugs or maintaining dysfunctional behavior. It might be necessary for ACA to let their parents know how they feel about their continued use of alcohol/drugs. In some situations, with the help of their therapists, patients have decided to send a letter to their parents who are still using alcohol/drugs. The goal of the letter is to assist ACA in healing and accepting their parents' disease. It is a way for ACA to get in touch with their feelings about their parents' continued use of alcohol/drugs. Patients decide for themselves whether the letter is appropriate for the goal they have in mind, and whether they want to send the letter.

Many ACA must ultimately let go and accept that their parents may never choose to stop using alcohol/drugs. Each patient continues to struggle with personal recovery issues in an ongoing process of self-discovery, supported by others in recovery. At times, it is a process of two steps forward, one step backward, but the process and progress continue.

Group Psychotherapy

Group psychotherapy is the next step once ACA have worked through some of the previously described core issues. Group psychotherapy is a dynamic process in which each group member gets feedback from other group members. Members share their perceptions, feelings, and insights into each other's behavior.

Irvin D. Yalom (1975) describes the following eleven curative factors that make group psychotherapy such an effective process. (See Case Study 7.5.)

1. *Instilling hope.* ACA group members see firsthand the growth of other group members. Continued contact with other group members who have improved while doing their work in the group gives ACA hope for their own recovery and confidence in the group process.
2. *Sharing universality.* ACA realize that they are not alone and that others share common problems. Group therapy reveals that ACA characteristics are universal to those who grew up in alcoholic/addict family systems, as well as imbalanced family systems. ACA no longer suffer in social or interpersonal isolation. There is the opportunity for affirmation by other group members, who understand them and identify with the issues they have in common.
3. *Imparting information.* Group therapy provides information, education, and training on ACA issues, including family systems, alcoholism/addiction, codependency, and boundary setting in relationships. Both the therapist and other group members offer suggestions, advice, and direct guidance about life problems.
4. *Fostering altruism.* Altruism is the act of giving to others and caring about others' life situations. The group is a place for support, reassurance, encouragement, insight, and sharing, all of which help both the giver and the receiver to grow.
5. *Recapitulating the primary family group.* Recapitulation offers an opportunity for the group to act as a functional family with positive corrective capabilities. Early familial conflicts can be acted out. With the help of the group, ACA can resolve these conflicts in a functional manner, rather than the previously dysfunctional and rigid manner of the family of origin.
6. *Developing socializing techniques.* Socializing is an obvious curative factor of group therapy. ACA can explore maladaptive social behavior through

Case Study 7.5
Interpersonal Relationships
Naomi

Naomi was a very attractive, young, and active director of marketing for a major retail clothing manufacturer. She grew up in an alcoholic family and compensated by being extremely successful in all endeavors. She described her mom's sense of self as being directly related to all of Naomi's accomplishments. Unfortunately, Naomi approached interpersonal relationships outside of the family in the same manner and tended to attract friends who mirrored her accomplishments back to her. In group therapy, Naomi began to use this same interpersonal dynamic of trying to control others so they reflected a positive mirror image of her success back to her. Initially, she was worried that the group would ask her to leave when they began to see her self-centeredness. Instead the group was able to make her aware of her imbalanced need for affirmation. The group gave her permission to explore her issues and be herself, while not having to look good all the time. In fact, they enjoyed the Naomi who wasn't always on and saw this aspect of her personality as more relaxed, fun loving, vulnerable, available, present, and worth getting to know.

Discussion

One way to avoid being vulnerable is to be "in control" of most interpersonal interactions. A way to avoid being shamed or criticized is to be "perfect." Naomi was so into control, perfectionism, and image management (e.g., looking good) that pursuing achievement and others' affirmation of her achievements was the dominant way for her to interact with others.

Group therapy reflected back to Naomi this style of interpersonal interaction. Naomi soon realized how lonely she was and began to be more vulnerable in group. She realized that her interpersonal relationships would improve as she became more present and authentic. She began to listen to others and to value relationships for what they were, rather than for the role the other person played in completing a task or achieving a goal.

honest and caring feedback from group members. Alternative social choices and techniques can be developed with the feedback of the group. ACA are particularly vulnerable to choosing dysfunctional relationships and maintaining codependent interactions in relationships. The group can alert ACA who try to return to codependent ways of interaction and dysfunctional choice making.

7. *Imitating behavior.* By seeing the reactions and behaviors of others, ACA have numerous new models of behavior.

8. *Sharing interpersonal learning.* The group is a social microcosm of the real world. ACA tend to duplicate the way they approach the real interpersonal world in their therapy group. Insights into adult children's interpersonal behavior and corrective emotional strategies can be explored in the safe environment of the group setting.

9. *Developing group cohesiveness.* The bonding that occurs in therapy groups results in a cohesive understanding, which makes the group a safe place to go with stressful problems, interpersonal conflicts, difficult decisions, and other issues. The group develops a functional interpersonal cohesiveness, allowing members to pull for and struggle with the difficult issues in their lives.

10. *Sharing catharsis.* The group is a place where ACA feel safe in expressing feelings not safely expressed in other settings. Fears, insecurities, destructive thoughts, suicidal ideation, rage, shame, and other emotions are safe to express in the group.

11. *Exploring existential factors.* The group helps its members explore meaning in their lives. Issues of attachment in relationships, congruency in work efforts, and spirituality are all safe for each group member to explore and develop. In other words, the functional therapy group explores the human condition.

In summary, group therapy is a dynamic process that has a tremendous potential for ACA recovery, especially after ACA have spent time exploring their issues in individual counseling.

⋈ In Review

- In 1983, the NACOA developed some basic facts about children of alcoholics in its charter statement:
  - An estimated 28 million Americans have at least one alcoholic parent.
  - More than half of all alcoholics have an alcoholic parent.
  - Children of alcoholics are at the highest risk of developing alcoholism themselves or marrying someone who is alcoholic.
  - In up to 90 percent of child abuse cases, alcohol is a significant factor.
  - Children of alcoholics are frequently victims of incest, child neglect, and other forms of violence and exploitation.
- Alcoholism affects the children of alcoholics, not just the alcoholic and spouse. Adults who were children in alcoholic family systems (adult children of alcoholics) are vulnerable to having feelings and behaviors that are characteristic of post-traumatic stress disorder.
- Children of alcoholics tend to distrust their own feelings and to deny reality.
- Following are some of the behavioral characteristics of ACA:
  - Fear of losing control
  - All-or-none, black-or-white thinking
  - Fear of experiencing feelings
  - Overdeveloped sense of responsibility or irresponsibility
  - Difficulty with intimacy and with asking for what is wanted or needed
  - Flashbacks of childhood but many memory gaps
  - Feelings of being little, or like a child, when under stress
  - Unreasonable loyalty
  - Addiction to excitement
  - Difficulty relaxing

- Feelings of guilt, abandonment, and/or depression
- Tendency to confuse love with self-pity
- Backlog of shock and grief
- Compulsive behaviors
- Living in a world of denial
- Guessing at what is normal
- Tendency toward physical symptoms (e.g., headaches, gastrointestinal problems)

- Howard Clinebell (1985) reported that the following factors produce damage in the lives of children of alcoholics:
  - *Role reversal:* Children may undertake parental duties because the parent is unable to be responsible or because the parent forces responsibilities on the children. The alcoholic may be treated as a child and, in return, act helpless. In incestuous families, the daughter and mother often switch roles.
  - *Unpredictability:* An inconsistent and unpredictable relationship with the alcoholic emotionally deprives the children.
  - *Unavailability:* The nonalcoholic, inadequate parent is struggling with major problems; because this parent's own needs are unmet, he or she is unable to attend to the needs of the children.
  - *Social isolation:* The damaging factor is the social isolation of the family, as protection from further pain and suffering, due to embarrassment.
- Codependency is defined in this chapter as continual investment of self-esteem in the ability to influence or control feelings and behaviors in the self and others in the face of obvious adverse consequences.
- Alcoholism is a family disease, where the family is centrally organized around the alcoholic's behavior and/or drinking. Codependency and enabling behavior, plus denial, end up perpetuating both the alcoholism and the alcohol-related problems. The marriage is also at risk, with sexual and intimacy problems.
- One of the results of growing up in an alcoholic system is that interpersonal relationships are often imbalanced in the form of overattachment, overseparation, and codependent dances.
- Grief is a feature of recovery from growing up in an alcoholic system. Second-order change is one technique to change family interaction.
- The eleven curative factors of group therapy (Yalom 1975) are outlined as a way for adult children of alcoholics to pursue recovery:
  - Instilling hope
  - Sharing universality
  - Imparting information
  - Fostering altruism
  - Recapitulating the primary family group
  - Developing socializing techniques
  - Imitating behavior
  - Sharing interpersonal learning
  - Developing group cohesiveness

- Sharing catharsis
- Exploring existential factors

⚹ Discussion Questions

1. Rate your own level for each of the ACA behavioral characteristics below, from 1 (hardly ever an issue) to 10 (almost always an issue). Then discuss these in small group discussion.
   - Fear of losing control
   - All-or-none, black-or-white thinking
   - Fear of experiencing feelings
   - Overdeveloped sense of responsibility or irresponsibility
   - Difficulty with intimacy and with asking for what is wanted or needed
   - Flashbacks of childhood but many memory gaps
   - Feelings of being little, or like a child, when under stress
   - Unreasonable loyalty
   - Addiction to excitement
   - Difficulty relaxing
   - Feelings of guilt, abandonment, and/or depression
   - Tendency to confuse love with self-pity
   - Backlog of shock and grief
   - Compulsive behaviors
   - Living in a world of denial
   - Guessing at what is normal
   - Tendency toward physical symptoms (e.g., headaches, gastrointestinal problems)

2. Tim Cermak, M.D., defined codependency using the following diagnostic criteria. Give examples for each criterion and explain why you think it meets the codependency criteria.
   - Continual investment of self-esteem in the ability to influence or control feelings and behaviors in the self and others in the face of obvious adverse consequences
   - Assumption of responsibility for meeting others' needs to the exclusion of acknowledging one's own needs
   - Anxiety and boundary distortions in situations of intimacy and separation
   - Enmeshment in relationships with personality-disordered, drug-dependent, and impulse-disordered individuals
   - Maintenance of a primary relationship with an active substance abuser for at least two years without seeking outside support and/or exhibiting three or more of the following characteristics:
     a.   Constriction of emotions with or without dramatic outbursts
     b.   Depression
     c.   Hypervigilance
     d.   Compulsions

e. Anxiety
f. Excessive reliance on denial
g. Substance abuse
h. Recurrent physical or sexual abuse
i. Stress-related medical illnesses

3. Rank the eleven curative factors of group psychotherapy in order of most to least important and explain your rationale.

Instilling hope
Sharing universality
Imparting information
Fostering altruism
Recapitulating the primary family group
Developing socializing techniques
Imitating behavior
Sharing interpersonal learning
Developing group cohesiveness
Sharing catharsis
Exploring existential factors

❧ References

Ackerman, Robert J. 1978. *Children of alcoholics: A guidebook for educators, therapists, and parents.* Holmes Beach, Fla.: Learning.

After drug treatment: What happens to the marriage. 1999. *Springbrook Northwest Newsletter,* summer.

Black, Claudia. 1982. *It will never happen to me.* Denver, Colo.: M.A.C.

Brown, Stephanie. 1988. *Treating adult children of alcoholics: A developmental perspective.* New York: Wiley.

Cermak, Timmen. 1984. Children of alcoholics and the case for a new diagnostic category of co-dependency. *Alcohol, Health, and Research World* 8: 38–42.

Clinebell, Howard J., Jr. 1985. *Understanding and counseling the alcoholic through religion and psychology.* Nashville, Tenn.: Abingdon Press.

Coleman, Eli, and Philip Colgan. 1987. Chemical dependency and intimacy dysfunction. *Journal of Chemical Dependency Treatment* 1: 75–91.

Cork, M. 1969. *The forgotten children.* Toronto: Addiction Research Foundation.

Newell, Nancy. 1950. Alcoholism and the father image. *Quarterly Journal of Studies on Alcoholism* 11: 92–95.

Yalom, Irvin D. 1975. *The theory and practice of group psychotherapy.* New York: Basic Books.

Prevention, Intervention, and Treatment

Prevention of Substance-Abuse Problems

Objectives

1. Describe early prevention approaches (i.e., scare tactics, coverting approaches, drug-specific approaches) and explain why they were ineffective.
2. Describe "alternative activities" and explain why they need to be acceptable, attractive, and attainable.
3. Explain the shift in prevention efforts in the 1980s and list the kinds of skills that were emphasized.
4. Define primary, secondary, and tertiary prevention.
5. Describe elements of various school-based prevention curricula.
6. Explain the key components of prevention:
   • Addressing community needs
   • Including youth in the planning process
   • Promoting proactivity
   • Developing a long-term plan
7. Describe the "social stress model," including the coping track and the abuse track.
8. Explain the importance of targeting prevention efforts for at-risk youth.
9. Identify and describe the at-risk factors for youth.
10. Define and describe resiliency and resilient factors.
11. Define and describe emotional intelligence and emotional intelligence factors.
12. Identify and describe the forty developmental assets.
13. Identify why there is a need for prevention efforts for special populations, including people of color and minorities, older adults, young older-adults, and the family.

⚘ Introduction

Alcohol/drug prevention has often been a misunderstood and neglected aspect in addressing the American drug problem. This chapter provides a foundation so that you can apply prevention efforts at home, in school systems, and in the community. Prevention efforts have shifted from scare tactics (dangers and evils of drugs) to emphases on the worth of people and the coping skills needed to avoid a destructive pattern of alcohol/drug dependence. Specific prevention skills outlined in this chapter include goal setting, decision making, and conflict resolution. The goal of prevention, outlined in this chapter, is to develop active, involved, empowered, and capable young people.

⚜ Early Prevention Approaches

For years, society has searched for easy ways to prevent drug dependence and addiction. Frightening movies and horror stories of drug abuse failed to make young people too scared to use drugs. Early efforts to prevent drug use focused primarily on providing the following:

- Information on the dangers of specific drugs
- Warnings of physical, social, and psychological harm
- Punishments for sale, use, and possession

Scare tactics proved to be an ineffective prevention strategy. Much of the information was invalid, exaggerated, and overgeneralized, causing young people to question the credibility of the program.

Similar programs were developed and labeled by drug educator Walter M. Mathews (1975) as **converting programs.** These programs used the following tactics to attempt to dissuade young people from using drugs:

1. *Directing:* Teacher tells students what they must believe, value, and do.
2. *Preaching:* This was similar to directing, with an added appeal to the students' duty to a vague external authority.
3. *Convincing:* Teachers appealed to logic where lecturing was the method used.
4. *Scaring:* Teachers emphasized the dangers of drug use.

Additional converting approaches emphasized admonishment, indoctrination, persuasion, distortion, and fear.

Adolescence is a time of questioning and exploration. The information provided in these approaches was not geared to the sensitivity of young people; it insulted their individuality and ability to make decisions. Adults in authority told them what to do, rather than talking with them. These propaganda approaches did not emphasize communication and open discussion.

The failure of these approaches led to a new prevention strategy of providing factual information about drugs, or **drug-specific approaches.** These approaches emphasized each drug and its pharmacological properties and assumed young people would make responsible decisions about drug use if they knew the negative effects. Inadvertently, these drug-specific approaches heightened curiosity and caused the opposite, alleviating fears of drugs. Many students acquired the knowledge to better attain desired levels of intoxication.

As a result of the failure of scare tactics and drug-specific approaches, the government's Special Action Office on Drug Abuse Prevention (SAODAP) declared a 6-month moratorium in 1973 on all prevention materials development, prevention program implementation, and prevention activities. The moratorium allowed further review of research and determined that scare tactics and drug-specific information did not significantly deter drug use and were therefore ineffective. In 1974, Robert DuPont, then the director of the National Institute on Drug Abuse (NIDA), surveyed drug education programs and concluded that the educators and students believed that the majority of school-based drug education programs were ineffective and should be abolished. In a review of research on school-based drug education programs, Michael

Goodstadt (1975) concluded that "there is an almost total lack of evidence indicating beneficial effects of drug education, very few educational programs have been evaluated and almost none have shown any significant improvement in anything other than levels of knowledge; attitudes and drug use have generally remained the same."

In 1974, the prevention branch of NIDA initiated a nationwide, 14-month planning process to develop a national strategy for primary prevention. This planning process involved over 400 prevention specialists in a series of nine planning conferences. In 1975, the institute published the resulting recommendations in *Toward a National Strategy for Primary Drug Abuse Prevention.* The report defined primary drug abuse prevention as "a constructive process designed to promote personal and social growth of the individual to full human potential and thereby inhibit or reduce physical, mental, emotional, or social impairment which results in or from the abuse of chemical substances."

The report established three basic themes for primary prevention: (1) primary prevention must be understood as the development and reinforcement of positive behaviors; (2) primary prevention programs must be responsive in both design and operation to the needs of those they are intended to serve or support; and (3) primary prevention should, wherever possible, use collaborative efforts to utilize the already available capacities and resources of existing human service institutions.

The result of SAODAP's moratorium and prevention planning meetings was a major shift in focus from drugs to the young people and from pharmacological effects to healthy children.

In 1977, NIDA and other agencies developed an interagency report entitled *Recommendations for Future Federal Activities in Drug Abuse Prevention.* This report outlined three major goals for prevention activities:

1. Reducing the percentage of frequent use of the three gateway drugs (tobacco, alcohol, and marijuana) by 15 percent among 8- to 20-year-olds.
2. Reducing the destructive behavior associated with alcohol and other drug abuse by 20 percent among 14- to 20-year-olds, as evidenced by a reduction in overdose deaths, emergency room visits, drug arrests, and other alcohol/drug-related incidents.
3. Retraining attitudes concerning the use of psychoactive substances, especially the gateway drugs, by maintaining current levels of awareness regarding the addictive nature of heroin and alcohol and raising awareness of the addictive nature of tobacco by 50 percent.

✹ Alternative Activities as a Prevention Approach

In Chapter 1, we examined the primary function of alcohol/drugs as serving our natural innate drive to alter our sense of consciousness. Ronald Siegal, in his book *Intoxication,* describes altering one's consciousness as the fourth drive, after hunger, thirst, and sex. The primary goal of alternative activities is to teach people that they are capable of altering their consciousness in a meaningful, longer-lasting, lifeenhancing, and satisfying way that is incompatible with alcohol/drug use.

The late 1970s saw a strong movement toward alternative activity programs for young people. The programs usually involved wilderness activities, requiring teamwork, challenge, and risk that developed feelings of competence, skill, and self-worth. Today, many adolescent and adult inpatient and residential chemical dependency treatment programs are including alternative activity program elements as a natural part of the clients' recovery program. This can include rope courses, climbing structures, and even what one program calls "equine therapy" (i.e., working with horses).

Alan Cohen (1972), a strong advocate of alternative activities, defines alternatives as pursuits that are valued and truly preferred by individuals and seen as incompatible with drugs. Cohen emphasizes that alternatives are not just a substitution for drugs; they are an integrated and valued part of the person's life.

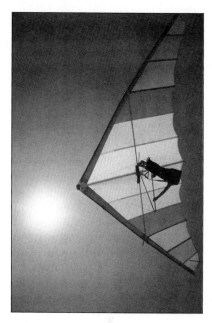

Hang glider against a blue sky.

Alternatives Are Actively Pursued by the Individual

Cohen felt that for an alternative to be successful, the process of searching for the alternative should be a potent alternative in itself. Individuals are encouraged to find other activities they can develop, persevere through to mastery, and enjoy. The process of being able to choose ways to get high naturally through one's own interests is truly empowering. It follows that alternatives are more effective if they call for activity, assertion of will or will power, and effort and commitment. Alternatives are less successful if individuals are passive recipients of the activity. This is consistent with the function of drug dependence and alcoholism as a rather passive activity. All alcoholics/addicts have to do is sit back and passively wait for the alcohol/drug to take effect.

Cohen (1972) illustrates this in the example of listening to music: "Passively listening to music is not necessarily a promising alternative to drugs, since one could be passively stoned at the time. Training in active listening and deep study of music is more likely to be frustrating to drug use since the clarity of one's senses and cognition become important in successful completion of the task."

Alternatives Are Acceptable, Attractive, and Attainable

Alternatives must be acceptable and attractive. Any alternative offered must be realistic, attainable, and meaningful. Alternatives must also help people understand themselves and improve their self-image and personal awareness. Dohner (1972) outlined the following characteristics of positive alternatives:

1. They must contribute to the individual's identity and independence.
2. They must offer active participation and involvement.
3. They must offer a chance for commitment.
4. They must provide a feeling of identification with a larger body of experience.
5. Some of the alternatives must be in the realm of the noncognitive and the intuitive.

Alternatives Use Mentors and Role Models

Another essential feature of alternatives is a successful role model or mentor—someone who can guide, facilitate, and encourage the successful attainment of the alternative skill. This person could be a positive parent model, a coach, a teacher, a peer, or anyone else who understands and respects the boundaries in the development of the alternative skill.

Alternatives Integrate Self-Concepts

Alternative activities are effective as preventive tools if they enhance the development of skills associated with improving one's sense of self. Table 8.1 lists Allan Cohen's categories for various alternative activities based on personal attributes and attraction.

TABLE 8.1

Motives for and Alternatives to the Use of Drugs

Level of Experience	Corresponding Motives	Alternatives to Drugs
Physical	Desire for physical satisfaction, physical relaxation, relief from sickness, more energy, maintenance of physical dependency	Athletics, dance, exercise, hiking, diet, health training, carpentry, or outdoor work
Sensory	Desire to stimulate sight, sound, touch, taste; need for sensual-sexual stimulation; desire to magnify the brain's sensoriums	Sensory awareness training, sky diving, experiencing sensory beauty of nature (lovemaking, swimming, running, mountaineering), *skiing, surfing, massage
Emotional	Relief from psychological pain, attempt to solve personal perplexities, relief from bad mood, escape from anxiety, desire for emotional insight, liberation of feeling, emotional relaxation	Competent individual counseling, well-run group therapy, instruction in psychology of personal development (sensitivity training), *self-help meetings, *emotional support system
Interpersonal	To gain peer acceptance; to break through interpersonal barriers; to communicate, especially nonverbally; defiance of authority figures; cement two-person relationships; relaxation of interpersonal inhibition; solve interpersonal hangups	Expertly managed sensitivity and encounter groups, well-run group therapy, instruction in social customs, confidence training, social-interpersonal counseling, emphasis on assisting others in distress via education, marriage, *participation in organizations and community activities within personal interests
Social (including sociocultural and environmental)	To promote social change; to find identifiable subcultures to tune out intolerable environmental conditions	Social service; community action in positive social change; helping the poor, aged, infirm, young; tutoring handicapped; improving the

(continued on next page)

TABLE 8.1 (continued)

Motives for and Alternatives to the Use of Drugs

Level of Experience	Corresponding Motives	Alternatives to Drugs
		environment; *Peace Corps work with the homeless, hungry, impoverished, and oppressed
Political	To promote political change; identify with antiestablishment subgroup to change drug legislation out of desperation with the sociopolitical order; to gain wealth or affluence of power	Political service; political action; nonpartisan projects such as ecological lobbying; fieldwork with politicians, and public officials
Intellectual	To escape mental boredom; out of intellectual curiosity to solve cognitive problems; to gain new understanding in the world of ideas; to study better; to research one's own awareness for science	Intellectual excitement through reading, discussion; creative games and puzzles; self-hypnosis; training in concentration; synectics training in intellectual breakthroughs; memory training; *seminars, workshops, and conferences; study or discussion groups; work with computers; writing a book or article
Creative-aesthetic	To improve creativity in the arts, to enhance enjoyment of art already produced, to enjoy imaginative mental productions	Nongraded instruction in producing and/or appreciating art, music, drama, crafts, handiwork, cooking, sewing, gardening, writing, singing
Philosophical	To discover meaningful values, to grasp the nature of the universe, to find meaning in life, to help establish personal identity, to organize a belief structure	Discussions, seminars, courses in the meaning of life; study of ethics, morality, the nature of reality; relevant philosophical literature; guided exploration of value systems
Spiritual, mystical	To transcend orthodox religion, to develop spiritual insights, to reach higher levels of consciousness, to have divine visions, to communicate with God, to augment yogic practices, to get a spiritual shortcut, to attain enlightenment, to attain spiritual powers	Exposure to nonchemical methods of spiritual development; study of world religions, introduction to applied mysticism, meditation, yogic techniques; *attending churches with recovery orientation; all activities that enhance spiritual awareness (nature, human connectedness, and activities that deal with existential despair)
Miscellaneous	Adventure, risk, drama, kicks, unexpressed motives, pro-drug general attitudes	Outward Bound survival training; combinations of preceding alternatives; pronaturalness attitudes; brainwave training; meaningful employment

* This author's additions are indicated by asterisks.
SOURCE: Allan Y. Cohen, "The Journey Beyond Trips: Alternative to Drugs" in David E. Smith and Dr. George R. Gay, eds., *It's So Good, Don't Even Try It Once: Heroin in Perspective.* Copyright © 1972 Prentice-Hall, Inc., Englewood Cliffs, N.J.

Use the worksheet shown in Table 8.2 to list your motives and preferred alternatives to alcohol/drug use. Also, identify the steps and resources necessary to implement each alternative.

⚔ Prevention Approaches of the 1980s

In the 1980s, the prevention strategy shifted from drugs to people, emphasizing the following:

- Educational information
- Coping skills

TABLE 8.2

Alternatives Worksheet

Level of Experience	Corresponding Motives	Steps and Resources to Implement Alternatives to Alcohol/Drugs
Physical		
Sensory		
Emotional		
Interpersonal		
Social		
Political		
Intellectual		
Creative-aesthetic		
Philosophical		
Spiritual, mystical		
Miscellaneous		

- Personal competence
- Decision making
- Refusal skills
- Alternative activities

The goal of these programs was to develop capable young people able to make responsible decisions about alcohol/drugs. The focus changed to understanding the impact of drugs on individuals, rather than understanding the pharmacological properties of alcohol/drugs. The affective aspect focused on the individual's needs, feelings, and emotions about alcohol/drugs.

These prevention programs worked toward developing the following skills:

- Clarifying personal values and ethics
- Improving self-concept
- Learning effective decision making
- Understanding and listening to each other's viewpoints
- Communicating about alcohol/drugs with peers, parents, and others
- Being involved in social and interpersonal activities
- Dealing effectively with feelings of anger, depression, and anxiety
- Having the ability to relax, play, and enjoy daily activities
- Developing and exploring ways to alter one's sense of consciousness through alternative activities

Agencies originally focused on prevention in secondary schools for adolescents 12 to 17 years of age. It quickly became apparent that in many cases it was already too late to provide preventive education to adolescents. This group required more intervention, skill building, and treatment-related approaches.

As a result, alcohol and drug curricula and primary prevention activities shifted to kindergarten through sixth grade. Agencies also developed secondary and tertiary prevention approaches for grades seven to twelve.

A definition of prevention covers three basic categories:

1. **Primary prevention** assumes that the individual has never tried drugs or alcohol and enforces a no-use norm by building positive self-esteem, developing good coping and refusal skills, and providing information on alcohol and drugs.
2. **Secondary prevention** assumes that the individual is in the early stages of use but does not regularly use drugs. Secondary prevention/intervention strategies try to stop drug use by providing drug information, developing decision-making and refusal skills, and improving family communication; it may also include individual counseling.
3. **Tertiary prevention** assumes that the individual is regularly using drugs but has not become a habitual user. Tertiary prevention/intervention includes counseling, drug education, and family therapy. There is a very fine line between the tertiary level of prevention and intervention and treatment services.

⍒ School-Based Prevention Curricula

In 1983, the U.S. Department of Health and Human Services monograph *Drug Abuse Prevention Research* outlined four dimensions of prevention:

1. Course content centers on mental health, drug information, human development, nutrition, ethics, and chemical safety; these courses usually fit into regular social studies, language arts, science, and other subject area curricula.
2. Courses on values clarification, problem-solving and decision-making skills, communication skills such as reflection and confrontation, alternative means for meeting needs, group process skills, role-playing, and dramatization
3. Courses that include competencies in human development, interpersonal relationships, personal autonomy, self-esteem, identity, decision-making skills, personal accountability, and accurate attributions of causality
4. Courses that also include general knowledge, conceptual frameworks, implicit assumptions and perspectives that define and describe the way each individual perceives the meaning of self, the nature of the world external to self, and the interrelatedness of things

Empowerment

A term often used in prevention programs is *empowerment*. Many prevention programs emphasize the empowering of the individual. The basic goal of prevention is to empower individuals and prevent the destructive passive choice of alcohol/drug dependence and addiction. Empowerment is a feeling that is developed by being able to

- Say no when that is what one feels and wants.
- Establish the core aspects of a sense of self.
- Be aware of what one feels and integrate and communicate those feelings to others in establishing goals and making decisions.
- Establish and set boundaries, especially in interpersonal and intimate relationships.
- Establish integrity in relationships and a healthy, nondestructive, nonsabotaging approach to life.

These prevention programs are usually targeted at the general school population, rather than the high-risk students who have already exhibited problem behaviors in and outside of school.

Goal Setting

A model lesson for goal setting would include lessons on (1) setting goals, (2) ranking priorities, (3) making decisions in relation to the goals, (4) persevering in the face of difficult situations, and (5) maintaining effort (motivation) until goals are attained or modified.

Capability Development

Other prevention lessons involve developing capabilities. I had the good fortune many years ago to work with Stephen Glenn at the National Drug Abuse Center in Washington, D.C. Today, Glenn lectures throughout the United States on the family prevention theme of developing capable people. His model for developing capable children includes fostering the following in children:

1. Identification with viable role models
2. Identification with and responsibility for family process
3. Faith in personal resources to solve problems
4. Adequate development of intrapersonal skills (responsibility)
5. Adequate development of interpersonal skills (communication)
6. Well-developed situation skills (demand skills)
7. Adequately developed judgment skills (application)

⊰ Key Components of a Prevention Program

Address Community Needs

Alcohol/drug prevention should address itself to the needs of the community and interface with community leaders, agencies, and the people. Edward M. Brecher knew community was important when he wrote the following in *Licit and Illicit Drugs* (1972): Stop viewing the drug problem as primarily a national problem to be solved on a national scale. In fact, as workers in the drug scene confirm, the drug problem is a collection of local problems. The predominant drugs differ from place to place and from time to time. Effective solutions to problems also vary; a plan that works now for New York City may not be applicable to upstate New York and vice versa. With respect to education, . . . the need for local wisdom and local control is particularly pressing. Warning children against drugs readily available to them is a risky business at best, requiring careful, truthful, unsensational approaches.

Include Youth in Prevention Planning

A prevention program must take into account the consumer of that program. To develop prevention programs in a vacuum, or from a strictly theoretical base, does not take into account the most important variable—the needs of youth.

Promote Proactivity

A core theme in prevention is to teach young people to move from being passive to being active, or proactive. Being proactive involves taking initiative, anticipating potential problems, and integrating your feelings. Too many young people spend excessive time in passive activities (e.g., watching television, playing computer games).

Parents can teach and model active behaviors and encourage activities that help young people develop a capable, positive sense of self. Proactive choices help develop the child's coping skills and ability to overcome setbacks.

Develop a Long-Term Perspective

Prevention is a long-term strategy. Longitudinal studies over 5 to 10 years are necessary to determine the effects of prevention. Unfortunately, most prevention programs have short-term funding, which limits the evaluation of their true effectiveness. Currently, we focus on the short-range perspective of drug enforcement and interdiction without the balance of a comprehensive prevention strategy to deal with the demand side of alcohol/drugs with youth. Our true hope is that the prevention and family approaches used with 3- to 10-year-olds—the next generation—may break this cycle of problems with dependence and addiction to alcohol/drugs.

In summary, an effective substance-abuse prevention strategy should do the following:

Emphasize cognitive and affective skills that help young people accept responsibility and motivate them to make wise decisions about alcohol and drugs.

Focus on people, not pharmacology, emphasizing educational information, coping skills, personal competence, decision making, refusal skills, and alternative activities.

Develop prevention programs that provide information plus communication, establish credibility, and meet community needs.

Take into account the needs of youth and develop prevention approaches cooperatively with young people in the community.

Develop primary efforts (those who have never used alcohol/drugs), secondary efforts (those in early stages of alcohol/drug use), and tertiary prevention efforts (those in regular stages of alcohol/drug use).

Develop longitudinal commitment to long-term prevention efforts.

Table 8.3 presents additional guidelines for making prevention programs more effective.

⚹ Programs Aimed at At-Risk Youth

Clinicians and researchers have identified a variety of factors that are predictive of later substance abuse by young people. Antisocial behaviors and aggressiveness can predict, as early as the first grade, early alcohol/drug initiation and later substance abuse. Family imbalance, parental problems with alcohol/drugs, and parental dysfunction are also predictive of children having problems with alcohol/drugs.

At-risk youth require a more intensive and modified prevention program than students with no real social and interpersonal problems, who are supported by fairly functional family systems.

Often, teachers and parents cooperatively identify at-risk youth appropriate for the program. Sometimes, key school personnel—teachers, coaches, dean of students, school-nurse, counselor, psychologist—develop a team approach with parents in identifying students at risk for alcohol/drug problems.

The number of young people who are high risk for developing substance abuse problems is astounding. (See Table 8.4.)

TABLE 8.3

Guidelines for Making Prevention Programs More Effective

- **Blend school-based and community prevention efforts to effect environmental change.** Community-wide approaches that involve broad participation of all sectors in the development of prevention efforts, including individually focused and environmental and policy focused, are needed.

- **Link prevention programs with the primary mission of schools: academics.** Prevention efforts at schools need to be more fully integrated with academic curricula. The case needs to be made that time spent in schools on prevention programs contributes to academic success.

- **Integrate prevention resource systems to support prevention efforts.** A more integrated approach that crosses disciplines and agencies is needed to maximize available resources. A less categorical approach to prevention is needed in order to address common risk factors. Prevention is about systems and strategies, not more discrete programs.

- **Forge agreement on what is to be prevented as a foundation for program design.** Standards for definitions and terms across prevention disciplines need to be developed in order to avoid contributing to confusion in those looking for guidance.

- **Employ new technologies to support prevention.** Technologies are now available to both reach individuals with prevention messages as well as disseminate information on evidence-based prevention to help communities develop prevention efforts.

- **Increase funding, training, and support for prevention researchers and practitioners.** Prevention works, but questions remain about both what works best in prevention and how communities can implement effective prevention activities.

- **Learn what practitioners, including teachers, are doing at ground level.** Because of the likelihood that practitioners consider program components to be fungible, it is important to know more about which components are essential and in what combinations.

SOURCE: Robert Wood Johnson Foundation, *Prevention 2000* (2000).

High-risk youngsters are hard to reach because they resist traditional authority, often have a low literacy level, and may be on the streets instead of in school or in structured community settings.

Their self-efficacy makes them less likely to respond to appeals based on caring about self, such as "take care of your health" or "don't take unnecessary risks that may hurt you." Also, these youth are already drinking and, in some cases, using multiple drugs at early ages. It is too late for refusal skills (saying no). Other obstacles include the following (Office for Substance Abuse Prevention 1988):

- Rejection of help because of fear and lack of trust or perhaps bravado
- Feelings of ambivalence and confusion about alcohol as a result of the many conflicting messages about alcohol use in U.S. society
- Fear by children and youth of being rejected again

TABLE 8.4

American Youth—High Risk for Alcohol-Related Problems

Alcohol Is the #1 Drug of Choice for Children and Adolescents

1. Before the age of 18, approximately one in four children is exposed to family alcoholism or addiction, or alcohol abuse.

2. Children of alcoholics are significantly more likely to initiate drinking during adolescence and to develop alcohol use disorders.

3. Persons who first drank alcohol before age 15 were more than five times as likely to report alcohol dependence or abuse in the past year than were persons who first drank at age 21 or older.

4. Almost 74% of persons aged 21 or older reported that they started drinking alcohol before age 21.

5. 36.4% of ninth-grade students reported having consumed alcohol before they were age 13.

6. Among eighth-graders, students with higher grade point averages reported less alcohol use in the past month.

7. Among eighth-graders, higher truancy rates were associated with greater rates of alcohol use in the past month.

8. High school students who use alcohol or other drugs frequently are up to five times more likely than other students to drop out of school.

9. Among high school students who reported riding with a driver who had been drinking, 80% were frequent drinkers and only 14% never drank.

10. In 2003, 1.5 million youth ages 12 to 17 needed treatment for an alcohol problem. Of this group, only 95,000 (6.3%) of them received any treatment at a specialty facility, leaving an estimated 1.4 million youths who needed but did not receive treatment.

11. Of all children under age 15 killed in vehicle crashes in 2003, 21% were killed in alcohol-related crashes.

SOURCE: Excerpts from *How Does Alcohol Affect the World of a Child?* NIH Publication No. 99-4670 PDF updated March 2005.

- Hopelessness by young people in inner cities about the possibility of ever having a worthwhile future with a decent job and a chance of achieving the American Dream
- The presence in some inner-city neighborhoods of an open, accessible drug culture without apparent social sanctions and of large sums of money for youth who deal in drugs

Often, the special relationship with a parent, a family member, a teacher, a minister, a coach, or others is what keeps some children on the road to a sober and successful life. Strong religious training is an example of a family ritual that also may save many young people from the streets.

One example of a school-based program for at-risk youth is *Interpersonal Problem Solving.* The program's major focus is on effective problem solving and effective interpersonal skills. Program topics include

- Dealing with authority figures
- Developing empathy
- Standing up for one's rights
- Resisting peer pressure
- Improving behavior in school
- Getting along better with family members

⋊ Risk Factors for Substance Abuse

In the early years of alcohol/drug prevention, efforts were primarily focused on generic prevention programs. The thinking was "this is a good thing to promote; maybe it will prevent substance abuse" (e.g., good health habits). These programs were global and aimed at the entire school population. Prevention in the new millennium is targeted at specific at-risk populations, communities of high risk, while focusing on specific risk factors.

J. David Hawkins, Richard E. Catalono, and Janet Y. Miller, in their 1992 study "Risk and Protective Factors for Alcohol and Other Drug Problems in Adolescence and Early Adulthood: Implications for Substance Abuse Prevention" (see Appendix D [available for download at www.mhhe.com/fields6e]), outline seventeen risk factors for substance abuse and accompanying interventions:

1. Laws and norms
2. Availability
3. Extreme economic deprivation
4. Neighborhood disorganization
5. Physiological factors
6. Family drug behavior
7. Family management practices
8. Family conflict
9. Low bonding to family
10. Early and persistent problem behaviors
11. Academic failure
12. Low commitment to school
13. Peer rejection in elementary grades
14. Association with drug using peers
15. Alienation and rebelliousness
16. Attitudes favorable to drug use
17. Early onset of drug use

Table 8.5 presents factors associated with risk behaviors. Table 8.6 presents factors associated with healthy behaviors.

TABLE 8.5
Factors Associated with Risk Behaviors
Demographic
Less education Low income Unemployment
Psychosocial
High level of stressful life events Poor social support[a] Poor ethnic identity[b]
Ecological
Exposure to community and interpersonal violence[c] Poor interactions with health care workers[d]
Individual
Psychological status (e.g., alienation,[e] powerlessness, depression,[f] or post-traumatic   stress disorder) Perceptions of levels of stress Experiences of racism

[a]Neighbors and Jackson, 1984; Gombeski et al. 1982.
[b]Bullough 1967; Abrams, Allen, and Gray 1993; Carter 1991; Munford, 1994.
[c]Sanders-Phillips 1994a, 1994b, 1996a; Cohen et al. 1991.
[d]Freimuth and Mettzger 1990; Harrison and Harrison 1971; James et al. 1984; Perez-Stable 1987; Webb 1984;
Makuc, Fried, and Kleinman 1989; Sanders-Phillips 1996a; Balsheim 1991; Farris and Glenn 1976.
[e]Bullough 1972; Cohen et al. 1982; Hibbard 1985; Morris, Hatch, and Chipman, 1966; Seeman and Evans 1962;
Seeman and Seeman 1983.
[f]Cohen et al. 1991; Leftwich and Collins 1994.

⚓ Resiliency

Steven Wolin, M.D., a professor at George Washington University, and his wife, Sybil Wolin, Ph.D., a developmental psychologist, are co-authors of *The Resilient Self: How Survivors of Troubled Families Rise Above Adversity* (1994) and developers of Project Resilience, Washington, D.C.

The Wolins define resiliency as an internal protective factor and the ability to bounce back. In their research on adult children of alcoholics, they found that some children of alcoholics grow up free of drinking because they

- Build on their own strengths
- Develop their own lifestyle and values, which are an improvement over those of their parents
- Establish healthy "rituals" in their own family

Applying this knowledge, the Wolins worked with adolescents and young adults from the inner city who grew up in dysfunctional and abusive, alcoholic/addict family systems. They applied their "challenge" model of resiliency, helping these young

---

TABLE 8.6

Factors Associated with Healthy Behaviors

Demographic

High education level
High income
Employment
Positive marital status[a]

Psychosocial

High level of social support[b]
   Emotional support
   Information sharing
   Provision of tangible goods and services
Church participation

Individual

Internal locus of control
Greater self-efficacy regarding the prevention of disease
Positive perceptions of health status
Greater knowledge and positive attitudes about health-promoting behaviors

[a]Cohen et al. 1991; Gottlieb and Green 1984; Rakowski 1988.
[b]Gottlieb and Green 1984; Neighbors and Jackson 1984; Shumaker and Hill 1991.
SOURCE: Meyer D. Glantz and Christine R. Hartel. *Drug Abuse: Origins and Interventions,* 1999. Washington, D.C.: American Psychological Association.

---

people realize their own resiliency in attaining healthy growth. They called this "survivor's pride"—a sense that you have been tested and that you have prevailed. (See Figures 8.1 and 8.2.)

Resiliency is described by the Wolins as not getting stuck in the "damage model" but, instead, challenging yourself and celebrating your survival and growth. Resiliency work is about reframing the damage, uncovering strength in a damage- or deficit-oriented story. In the damage model, the individual is seen as helpless, fragile, passive, and trapped. The Wolins emphasize that you need to help the individual understand the damage, express the anger, grieve the past, and move to resiliency.

Resiliency involves deliberation (making a plan). In many abusive family situations, it is a "getaway plan," creating distance from unhealthy situations. Resiliency skills also involve eventually choosing a spouse who is healthy and is developing healthy rituals.

They also describe how, too frequently, therapists perpetuate the victim's trap by

- Maintaining the myth that family problems will inevitably be perpetuated from one generation to the next
- Having the patients deplete themselves by continually blaming their parents for hurting them

RESILIENCY

Resiliency is defined as:

- Mastering your painful memories rather than compulsively rehashing the damage you have suffered

- Accepting that your troubled family has left its mark and give up the futile wish that your scars can ever disappear completely

- Getting revenge by living well instead of squandering your energy by blaming and fault-finding

- Breaking the cycle of your family's troubles and putting the past in its place

FIGURE 8.1
SOURCE: Wolin and Wolin 1994.

RESILIENT ACTIONS

Resilient Actions:

- Find and build on your own strengths

- Improve deliberately and methodically on your parents' lifestyles

- Marry consciously into strong, healthy families

- Fight off memories of horrible family get-togethers in order to establish healthy family times, routines, vacations, celebrations, and rituals in your own generation

FIGURE 8.2
SOURCE: Wolin and Wolin 1994.

Instead, the Wolins describe a more positive therapeutic goal of helping patients get revenge by seeking resiliency: by living healthy, productive lives rather than blaming and finding fault.

They describe seven resiliency factors (Wolin and Wolin 1994):

1. Insight—the habit of asking tough questions that pierce the denial and confusion in troubled families
2. Independence—emotional and physical distancing from a troubled family, which keeps survivors out of harm's way
3. Relationships—fulfilling ties to others that provide the stability, nurturing, and love that troubled families do not give
4. Initiative—a push for mastery that combats the feelings of helplessness troubled families produce in their offspring
5. Creativity—representing one's inner pain and hurtful experiences in art forms; "building a new world on the ruins of the old"
6. Humor—the ability to minimize pain and troubles by laughing at oneself
7. Morality—an informed conscience, which imbues the survivor surrounded by "badness" with a sense of his or her own "goodness"

✖ Emotional Intelligence

In 1995, Daniel Goleman, in his book *Emotional Intelligence,* made a case for a new kind of intelligence, or IQ—an IQ that goes beyond the traditional verbal and performance scales of most IQ tests and redefines what skills make up a successful person. Goleman labels this new IQ *emotional intelligence* and defines it as abilities such as

- Being able to motivate oneself and persist in the face of frustration
- Being able to control impulse and delay gratification
- Being able to regulate one's mood and keep distress from swamping the ability to think
- Being able to empathize and hope

The characteristics of emotional intelligence make one more successful at work, at relationships, at parenting, at coupleship, and at life in general. As we see increases in domestic violence, abuse, physical violence, and alcohol/drug abuse in homes, schools, community, our nation, and throughout the world, we see the importance of emotional intelligence. Managing anger and other moods (depression, fear, worry, and anxiety) is one of the key components of emotional intelligence.

"Of all the moods . . . anger is the mood people are worst at controlling. . . . Anger is the most seductive of the negative emotions, the self-righteous inner monologue that propels along filling the mind with the most convincing arguments to vent rage" (Goleman 1995).

The goals of the emotionally intelligent individual are optimism, motivation, perseverance, and self-efficacy.

✖ Domains of Prevention

Schools, religious and voluntary organizations, the media, the private sector, law enforcement, and health care are the secondary line of defense against drug and alcohol abuse by young people (see Figure 8.3). Families can make a real difference. Secondary approaches have little effect if the home and family environment are not involved and supportive of prevention efforts.

In conducting alcohol/drug educational and skill activities for parents over the past 20 years, I have found that the parents who don't need the information and are already effective parents are the ones that come to every event. The parents who need help are either in denial, too embarrassed or ashamed, or too out of control to attend. Until we develop programs that can get these parents to participate, we are fighting an uphill battle.

✖ Prevention Programs and Prevention Emphasis in the New Millennium

Developmental Assets Model

The Search Institute of Minneapolis has developed a research-based framework of developmental assets, or factors that are critical for young people's successful growth

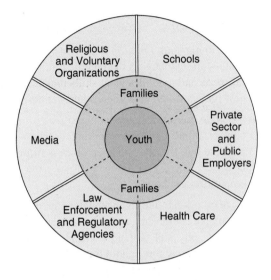

FIGURE 8.3   *A Conceptual Model for Preventive Approaches to Alcohol and Drug Abuse*
SOURCE: Attorney General John Van De Kamp's Commission of Drug and Alcohol Abuse, 1986, Sacramento, CA.
Reprinted by permission of California Attorney General's Office.

and development. The institute's *Healthy Communities—Healthy Youth* programs are part of a national initiative to "motivate and equip individuals, organizations, and their leaders to join together in nurturing competent, caring, and responsible children and adolescents." The institute has identified and measured forty developmental assets (see Table 8.7). These assets are the foundation that children and adolescents from many cultural backgrounds need to be responsible, successful, and caring human beings.

"These assets are more than just nice ideas. Research on youth in hundreds of communities finds that these assets are powerful influences on behavior [see Figure 8.4]. Yet, the average 6th- to 12th-grade student experiences only 18 of the 40 assets" (Search Institute 1999). The application of education and skill development of these developmental assets takes place in the schools, with parents and other adults, with young people, with youth serving organizations, in neighborhoods, in communities, in business and industry, in local government, in congregations, in the juvenile justice system, in community care systems, and in community organizations.

⚹ High-Risk Youth and CSAPs

The National Cross-Site Evaluation of High-Risk Youth Program (NIDA 2002) found that the rate of substance use for high-risk youth participating in their CSAP (Community Substance Abuse Programs) was 12 percent lower at completion of the program than for comparison youth. They also found that this effect lasted—the rate of use for these youth was 6 percent below the rate for the comparison group

TABLE 8.7

Forty Developmental Assets

Type	Asset Name and Definition
Support	1. **Family support**—Family life provides high levels of love and support.
	2. **Positive family communication**—Young person and his or her parent(s) communicate positively, and young person is willing to seek parents' advice and counsel.
	3. **Other adult relationships**—Young person receives support from three or more nonparent adults.
	4. **Caring neighborhood**—Young person experiences caring neighbors.
	5. **Caring school climate**—School provides a caring, encouraging environment.
	6. **Parent involvement in schooling**—Parent(s) are actively involved in helping young person succeed in school.
Empowerment	7. **Community values youth**—Young person perceives that adults in the community value youth.
	8. **Youth as resources**—Young people are given useful roles in the community.
	9. **Service to others**—Young person serves in the community one hour or more per week.
	10. **Safety**—Young person feels safe at home, at school, and in the neighborhood.
Boundaries and Expectations	11. **Family boundaries**—Family has clear rules and consequences, and they monitor the young person's whereabouts.
	12. **School boundaries**—School provides clear rules and consequences.
	13. **Neighborhood boundaries**—Neighbors take responsibility for monitoring young people's behavior.
	14. **Adult role models**—Parent(s) and other adults model positive, responsible behavior.
	15. **Positive peer influence**—Young person's best friends model responsible behavior.
	16. **High expectations**—Both parent(s) and teachers encourage the young person to do well.
Constructive Use of Time	17. **Creative activities**—Young person spends three or more hours per week in lessons or practice in music, theater, or other arts.
	18. **Youth programs**—Young person spends three or more hours per week in sports, clubs, or organizations at school and/or in community organizations.
	19. **Religious community**—Young person spends one or more hours per week in activities in a religious institution.
	20. **Time at home**—Young person is out with friends, "with nothing special to do," two or fewer nights per week.
Commitment to Learning	21. **Achievement motivation**—Young person is motivated to do well in school.
	22. **School engagement**—Young person is actively engaged in learning.
	23. **Homework**—Young person reports doing at least one hour of homework every schoolday.
	24. **Bonding to school**—Young person cares about his or her school.
	25. **Reading for pleasure**—Young person reads for pleasure three or more hours per week.

(continued on next page)

T A B L E 8 . 7 (*c o n t i n u e d*)

Forty Developmental Assets

Type	Asset Name and Definition
Positive Values	26. **Caring**—Young person places high value on helping other people.
	27. **Equality and social justice**—Young person places high value on promoting equality and reducing hunger and poverty.
	28. **Integrity**—Young person acts on convictions and stands up for his or her beliefs.
	29. **Honesty**—Young person tells the truth, even when it is not easy.
	30. **Responsibility**—Young person accepts and takes personal responsibility.
	31. **Restraint**—Young person believes it is important not to be sexually active or to use alcohol or other drugs.
Social Competencies	32. **Planning and decision making**—Young person knows how to plan ahead and make choices.
	33. **Interpersonal competence**—Young person has empathy, sensitivity, and friendship skills.
	34. **Cultural competence**—Young person has knowledge of and comfort with people of different cultural/racial/ethnic backgrounds.
	35. **Resistance skills**—Young person can resist negative peer pressure and dangerous situations.
	36. **Peaceful conflict resolution**—Young person seeks to resolve conflict nonviolently.
Positive Identity	37. **Personal power**—Young person feels he or she has control over "things that happen to me."
	38. **Self-esteem**—Young person reports having a high self-esteem.
	39. **Sense of purpose**—Young person reports that "my life has a purpose."
	40. **Positive view of personal future**—Young person is optimistic about his or her personal future.

SOURCE: Search Institute 1999.

---

18 months later. These prevention programs work and produce lasting results despite the fact that these youth face multiple risk factors in their communities. Connections with positive social environments—schools, family, peers, community, and society—appeared to be important factors in preventing substance abuse. Figure 8.5 depicts this "Web of Influence."

✷ Prevention and Special Populations

People of Color and Other Minorities

A variety of factors put people of color and other minorities at risk for substance-abuse problems. Minorities as a group have more unemployment, have less prestigious occupations, and live in poverty and lower socioeconomic conditions. Thus, they experience more feelings of frustration, anger, resentment, and powerlessness.

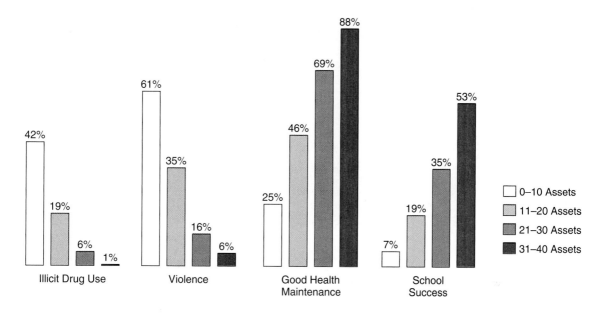

FIGURE 8.4 *The Power of Developmental Assets* The more assets young people experience, the less likely they are to engage in a wide range of risky behaviors, and the more likely they are to engage in positive behaviors.
SOURCE: Based on Search Institute's study of almost 100,000 youth in 312 towns and cities across the United States during the 1996–1997 school year.

Inadequate education, housing, income, and other factors create additional stress and pressure, which may lead to problems with alcohol/drugs.

For people of color, prevention must go beyond the approaches previously described. One of the biggest problems facing people of color is the crack epidemic in the inner cities, the increase in young cocaine and heroin addicts' giving birth to cocaine- and heroin-addicted babies, and the rise in methamphetamine use.

Prevention for people of color and other minorities must be community based. Residents must conceptualize the problem and jointly develop appropriate strategies.

Community-based prevention programs also must emphasize a systemic strategy to uproot the factors in the system that oppress people of color, such as prejudice and racism, and to implement training in diversity and methods of accessing the system.

College Students

During their first year of college, most students dramatically increase their alcohol/drug use. The MTV spring break party illustrates the pervasive "let loose and get loaded" attitude of young college students.

Alcohol/drug use and abuse is a glamorized way of escape from the pressures of school. The newly acquired freedom of being away at college allows students more opportunities to use alcohol/drugs. The anxiety of adjusting to college and living

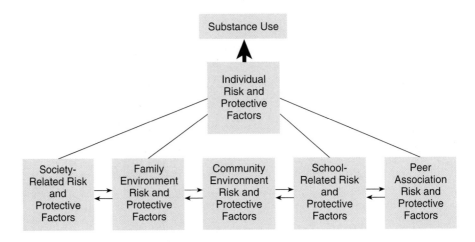

FIGURE 8.5   *The "Web of Influence" on Substance Use*
SOURCE: NIDA 2002.

away from home can result in escalated alcohol/drug use. The functions of alcohol/drugs on college campuses are many—to party, to stay up late and study, to explore a personal sense of self and identity, to facilitate social and interpersonal relationships, and so forth.

Older Adults

Older adults are often forgotten or ignored when it comes to prevention efforts. The lack of any true role experienced by some elders leads to feelings of loneliness, boredom, frustration, rejection, abandonment, anxiety, fear, and depression. When elders complain about these feelings, sometimes the response is to prescribe medication.

Prevention efforts with elders frequently involve training and educational projects to assist them to keep accurate records of their medications or to develop methods to have someone monitor their medication. Elders need to be approached with individuality and dignity. They need to be empowered to develop their own advocacy. Pharmacists, physicians, and other health providers must act in cooperation and be sensitive to each individual case. Drug dosages and regimens must meet individual needs and be sensitive to the elders' ability to maintain their treatment plans.

Monitoring and educating the elder population are necessary prevention strategies. Advocacy for alternatives to medication are also essential, as well as the expansion of senior services. The more active and involved the lifestyles of elders, the healthier are the later years of their lives.

Prevention with elders also involves proactive approaches to healthy activities that promote physical movement (health permitting), interpersonal interaction, and a sense of value and worth. In the years to come, a majority of the population will be elders. Prevention programs and services need to be further developed now to meet the needs of this ever-expanding population.

Prevention and the Family

Unfortunately, prevention activities take place almost exclusively in school systems. We expect the school systems to prevent this epidemic of alcohol/drug use. The reality is that the families are the real first line of defense against alcohol/drug use by young people.

⚹ In Review

- The early prevention approaches focused primarily on supplying information on the dangers of specific drugs; on warnings of physical, social, and psychological harm; and on punishment for sale, use, and possession. These scare tactics were ineffective, as were other converting programs, which tried to direct, preach, or convince young people not to use drugs. The information presented in these early prevention approaches was often invalid, exaggerated, and overgeneralized, causing young people to question the credibility of the prevention efforts.
- The next prevention efforts focused on drug-specific information in the hope that young people would make wise decisions about drugs. Unfortunately, these approaches heightened curiosity and alleviated fears, leading to an increase in drug experimentation, rather than the intended decrease.
- The ineffectiveness of scare tactics and drug-specific approaches led to a moratorium on prevention efforts by the government and a review of those features of a prevention program that were effective.
- In Chapter 1, we examined the primary function of alcohol/drugs as serving our natural innate drive to alter our sense of consciousness. Ronald Siegal, in his book *Intoxication,* describes altering one's consciousness as the fourth drive, after hunger, thirst, and sex. The primary goal of alternative activities is to teach people that they are capable of altering their consciousness in a meaningful, longer-lasting, life-enhancing, and satisfying way that is incompatible with alcohol/drug use.
- Alternative activities are successful if they are acceptable, attractive, and attainable.
- In the 1980s, the thrust of these new prevention strategies shifted from drugs to people, emphasizing educational information, coping skills, personal competence, decision making, refusal skills, and alternative activities.
- Credibility is a basic premise for the effectiveness of any alcohol/drug prevention program.
- The key components of a prevention program are
    - Addressing community needs
    - Including youth in prevention planning
    - Promoting proactivity
    - Developing a long-term perspective
- Jean Rhodes and Leonard Jason (1988) developed a model that emphasizes the development of **attachments, competence,** and **coping skills** to minimize

risk for substance abuse. The more stress the child experiences—without appropriate and strong bonding to parents, attachment to drug-free role models, access to models with a strong sense of self, and good coping skills and resources—the higher the risk of substance abuse.

- Current prevention programs should be aimed at at-risk youth and people of color and other minorities and should be community-based.
- Hawkins, Catalono, and Miller (1992) outlined seventeen risk factors for substance abuse:

> Laws and norms
> Availability
> Extreme economic deprivation
> Neighborhood disorganization
> Physiological factors
> Family drug behavior
> Family management practices
> Family conflict
> Low bonding to family
> Early and persistent problem behaviors
> Academic failure
> Low commitment to school
> Peer rejection in elementary grades
> Association with drug using peers
> Alienation and rebelliousness
> Attitudes favorable to drug use
> Early onset of drug use

- Steven Wolin and Sybil Wolin developed a challenge model of resiliency. They define resiliency as an internal protective factor and the ability to bounce back. In their research on adult children of alcoholics, they found that some children of alcoholics grow up free of drinking because they
  - Build on their own strengths
  - Develop their own lifestyle and values, which are an improvement over those of their parents
  - Establish healthy "rituals" in their own family
- The Wolins describe seven resiliency factors:
  - Insight—the habit of asking tough questions that pierce the denial and confusion in troubled families
  - Independence—emotional and physical distancing from a troubled family, which keeps survivors out of harm's way
  - Relationships—fulfilling ties to others that provide the stability, nurturing, and love that troubled families do not give
  - Initiative—a push for mastery that combats the feelings of helplessness troubled families produce in their offspring
  - Creativity—representing one's inner pain and hurtful experiences in art forms; "building a new world on the ruins of the old"

- Humor—the ability to minimize pain and troubles by laughing at oneself
- Morality—an informed conscience, which imbues the survivor surrounded by "badness" with a sense of his or her own "goodness"

- Daniel Goleman introduced the concept of emotional intelligence. Goleman labels this new IQ *emotional intelligence* and defines it as abilities such as

  - Being able to motivate oneself and persist in the face of frustration
  - Being able to control impulse and delay gratification
  - Being able to regulate one's mood and keep distress from swamping the ability to think
  - Being able to empathize and hope

- The Search Institute of Minneapolis has developed a research-based framework of developmental assets, or factors that are critical for young people's successful growth and development. The developmental assets model describes forty developmental assets in the areas of support, empowerment, boundaries and expectations, constructive use of time, commitment to learning, positive values, social competence, and positive identity.
- The forty developmental assets are

  Support

  1. family
  2. positive family communication
  3. other adults
  4. caring neighbors
  5. caring school climate
  6. parent involvement in school

  Empowerment

  7. community values youth
  8. youth as resources
  9. service to others
  10. safety

  Boundaries and expectations

  11. family
  12. school
  13. neighborhood
  14. adult role models
  15. positive peer
  16. high expectations—parents and teachers

  Constructive use of time

  17. creative activities
  18. youth programs
  19. religious community
  20. time at home

Commitment to learning

21. achievement motivation
22. school engagement
23. homework
24. bonding to school
25. reading for pleasure

Positive values

26. caring
27. equality and social justice
28. integrity
29. honesty
30. responsibility
31. restraint

Social competencies

32. planning and decision making
33. interpersonal competence
34. cultural competence
35. resistance skills
36. peaceful conflict resolution

Positive identity

37. personal power
38. self-esteem
39. sense of purpose
40. positive view of personal future

⊁ Discussion Questions

1. The media ad that shows eggs frying in a pan, as a metaphor for how your brain looks on drugs, has been a controversial prevention approach. Do you think this is an effective prevention strategy? Why or why not?
2. Design a prevention advertising approach that you believe will be effective with young people, based on your reading of Chapter 8.
3. Discuss a prevention effort that had impact on you while you were growing up.
4. Describe an effective "community prevention" approach and describe what elements you think are essential.
5. Rank the seventeen risk factors for substance abuse outlined by Hawkins, Catalano, and Miller in terms of most important to least important and explain your rationale.

⊁ References

Botvin, G. J., and T. A. Wills. 1985. Personal and social skills training: Cognitive-behavioral approaches to substance abuse prevention. NIDA Research Monograph Series 63: 8–49.
Brecher, Edward M. 1972. *Licit and illicit drugs.* Boston: Little, Brown.

Cohen, A.Y. 1972. *Alternatives to drug abuse: Steps toward prevention.* Rockville, Md.: National Institute on Drug Abuse.

Dohner, V.A. 1972. Alternatives to drugs—A new approach to drug education. *Journal of Drug Education* 2(1): 3–22.

Drug abuse prevention research. 1983. Monograph No. 33. Washington, D.C.: U.S. Dept. of Health and Human Services.

Glantz, Meyer D., and Christine R. Hartel, eds. 1999. *Drug abuse: Origins and interventions.* Washington, D. C.: American Psychological Association.

Goleman, Daniel. 1995. *Emotional intelligence: Why it can matter more than IQ.* New York: Bantam Books.

Goodstadt, Michael. 1975. Evaluating drug prevention programs. In *Balancing head and heart: Sensible ideas for the prevention of drug and alcohol abuse,* edited by E. Schaps et al. Lafayette, Calif.: Prevention Materials Institute Press.

Harrington, N. G., and L. Donohew. 1997. Jump Start: A targeted substance abuse prevention program. *Health Education and Behavior* 24(5): 568–86.

Hawkins, J. D., R. Catalano, and J. Miller. 1992. Risk and protective factors for alcohol and other drug problems in adolescence and early adulthood. *Psychological Bulletin* 112(1): 64–105.

Kumpfer, K. L. 1996. Effectiveness of a culturally tailored, family-focused substance abuse program: The Strengthening Families program. In National Conference on Drug Abuse Prevention Research, September 19–20, 1996, Washington, D. C. *Putting research to work for the community: Presentations, papers, and recommendations.* Rockville, Md.: National Institute on Drug Abuse, 1998, pp. 101–24.

Mathews, Walter M. 1975. A critique of traditional drug education programs. *Journal of Drug Education* 5(1): 57–64.

National Institute on Drug Abuse [NIDA]. 2001. *Substance use among older adults.* Washington, D.C.: NIDA, Substance Abuse and Mental Health Services Administration.

National Institute on Drug Abuse [NIDA]. 2002. *The National Cross-Site Evaluation of High-Risk Youth Program: Preventing substance abuse: Major findings.* Washington, D.C.: NIDA, Substance Abuse and Mental Health Services Administration.

National Institute of Health [NIH]. March 2005. *How does alcohol affect the world of the child?* NIH Publication No. 99–4670.

Office for Substance Abuse Prevention. 1988. *Communicating about alcohol and other drugs: Strategies for reading populations at risk.* Monograph 5. Rockville, Md.: Author.

Prevention 2000: Moving effective prevention programs into practice. 2000. St. Michaels, Md.: Robert Wood Johnson Foundation.

Rhodes, Jean E., and Leonard A. Jason. 1988. *Preventing substance abuse among children and adolescents.* New York: Pergamon Press.

Schinke, S. P., and L. D. Gilchrist. 1983. Primary prevention of tobacco smoking. *Journal of School Health* 53: 416–19.

Search Institute. 1999. *Ideas for asset building poster.* Search Institute, 700 South Third Street, Suite 210, Minneapolis, Minn. 55415.

Spivak, G., and M. Shuve. 1979. *The social adjustment of young children.* San Francisco: Jossey-Bass.

Spoth, R., and C. Redmond. 1996. Illustrating a framework for rural prevention research: Project Family Studies of rural family participation and outcomes. In *Preventing childhood disorders, substance abuse, and delinquency.* Edited by R. D. Peters and R. J. McMahon. Thousand Oaks, Calif.: Sage, pp. 299–328.

Substance Abuse and Mental Health Services Administration [SAMHSA]. 2003. More older Americans will need substance abuse treatment by 2020. *SAMHSA News* XI(1): 19.

Thompson, C. K. 1997. A community outreach project in a rural school district in Pennsylvania. In *Bringing excellence to substance abuse services in rural and frontier America: 1996 Award for Excellence papers.* CSAT Technical Assistance Publication Series No. 20. Rockville, Md.: Center for Substance Abuse Treatment, pp. 129–34.

Wiscott, Richard, Karen Kopera-Frye, and Ana Begovic. 2002. Later life: Comparing young-old and old-old social drinkers. *Psychology of Addictive Behaviors* 16(3): 252–55.

Wolin, Steven, and Sybil Wolin. 1994. *The resilient self: How survivors of troubled families rise above adversity.* New York: Villard Books.

Change, Motivation, and Intervention for Substance-Abuse Problems

Objectives

1. Define and describe the continuum of change.
2. Identify and explain the key elements to sudden change.
3. Describe the common defenses to change.
4. Identify and describe the stages of change in motivational interviewing.
5. Identify and describe the eight motivational strategies.
6. Identify and describe the active ingredients (i.e., the mnemonic FRAMES) of effective brief counseling.
7. Define intervention, and describe interventions at various stages of recovery.
8. Classify some common dos and don'ts for interventions.
9. Identify and describe the tasks of the four stages of a formal intervention.
10. Outline the differences between a formal (traditional) intervention and a systemic intervention.

✷ Introduction

This chapter explores the interrelated issues of change, motivation, and intervention and how each relates to alcoholism and drug addiction.

It is important to understand the kinds of change that can occur, the determinants of change, and the stages of change and what influences them. Motivation and drive as well as relapse prevention strategies are necessary to stop drinking and/or drugging. Interventions can be made at various levels, from simple concern to taking action through formal intervention.

These issues are worth our focus, and I believe they will be studied even more in the future, to better understand and treat individuals with substance abuse disorders.

✷ Change

The whole subject of change is fascinating and complicated. People change for very personal and individual reasons. Many people can go for years, even a lifetime, wanting to change, intending to change, even verbalizing a desire to change, without taking the action necessary to change.

Why will any given person stop drinking or taking drugs, eat healthier, exercise regularly, commit to a task, pursue a passion, or get out of an imbalanced situation or relationship? The answer is different for each person. Some people will put up with a lot before being forced to make a change. Others will make difficult changes, despite tremendous obstacles, risks, and personal sacrifice, because they feel or know it is what they have to do. In the alcohol/drug recovery field, we often refer to the experience of "hitting bottom," reaching the point where the consequences of drinking or taking drugs are so bad that the individual decides to do something about their drug/alcohol use. The consequences of their addictive behavior have become so demeaning, so shaming, and so foreign to their perception of themselves that users are motivated to take action to do whatever it takes to stop using alcohol or other drugs.

Some people stop using because the negative cycle and negative consequences have gone on for too long. They decide that they are "sick and tired of being sick and tired."

Change can sometimes occur when others influence, directly or indirectly, the motivation to change. Friends, teachers, family members, mentors, or significant others can help the individual to see the need for change and help support change. Certainly, counselors play a pivotal role in helping these individuals explore their perception of their alcohol/drug use, and the need for change. For some users, hearing the same thing from different people, in a timely manner, causes them to consider making a change. What motivates one individual to change, might be quite different for another. Others might make a change because their job is in jeopardy, or because they have been touched in a heartfelt way by someone they love. The counselor is challenged to push the right "button" for each individual.

Change may be gradual, or it can seem sudden and abrupt. William Miller, lead author of *Motivational Interviewing* (Miller and Rollnick, 1991), describes this process of collaboration and gradual influence to motivate the client to explore healthy change. In *Quantum Change* (2001), Miller and coauthor Janet C' de Baca, describe a more sudden and immediate kind of change. A quantum change is a personal transformation that has some key elements:

- *Vivid*—identifiable, distinctive experiences during which the transformation occurred, or at least began
- *Surprising*—not comprehensible as ordinary responses to life events
- *Benevolent*—involves loving kindness
- *Enduring*—it is a permanent transformation
- *Involves conflict*—a rupture in the knowing context

Miller and C' de Baca (2001) quote Bill Wilson, the co-founder of Alcoholics Anonymous, as he describes his quantum change:

> Slowly the ecstasy subsided. I lay on the bed, but now for a time I was in another world, a new world of consciousness. All about me and through me there was a wonderful feeling of Presence. A great peace stole over me and I thought, "No matter how wrong things seem to be, they are all right."

Whether change occurs gradually or suddenly, the outcome is the same—personal transformation.

Resistance is a natural part of the change cycle. Whether it is an adolescent who resists cleaning up his or her room or an adult who delays paying his or her taxes, resistance is embedded in our nature. For some, it is laziness or procrastination, probably related to family-of-origin issues. But most people resist doing something that may bring discomfort or dysphoria or that is just downright uninteresting. Resistance comes out in the various defense mechanisms used by people to avoid taking action on a problem behavior (e.g., substance abuse).

Common Defense Components of Resistance to Change

1. *Denial*—most common
    Counselor tip: Look for the usefulness of the defense to person, what he or she is avoiding and why; wait to point out denial—premature disclosure can "turn off" the client (i.e., you are judging them).
2. *Minimization*—used to maintain self-esteem (e.g., "My drinking/drugging never had an impact on my children, since I drank outside of the house") Counselor tip: Suggest client get feedback from valued and reliable other sources, rather than getting into a tireless debate with client.
3. *Projection*—has important protective function, may cover deeper disturbance Counselor tip: Be sensitive to self-blame and guilt, and the client feeling shamed by any suggestion of criticism; preface feedback with "some people might think."
4. *Rationalization*—clever answers used to avoid responsibility and maintain frozen feelings
    Counselor tip: Avoid your own frustration and anger in trying to get through to a highly intellectualizing client.
5. *Compliance*—hidden form of resistance, may cover up magical expectations Counselor tip: Recognize the potential of provoking rebellion at some point.
6. *Conflict avoidance*—problems handling feelings of anger and disappointment, need to be liked and approved
    Counselor tip: Provoking client to deal with conflict too much may be a hazard.
7. *Obsessive focusing*—all-or-none thinking, may be overly self-critical or overly critical of others, may be perfectionistic
    Counselor tip: Understand the person's situation while suggesting that he or she "lighten up."
8. *Acting out*—lacks awareness of feelings, impulses communicated by behavior, most provocative of defenses
    Counselor tip: Direct to needed change, stay out of harm's way (i.e., be careful not to put self in jeopardy).

Denial

Earlier in this book "denial" was jokingly referred to as a river in Egypt (de-Nile). D-E-N-I-A-L is also described as standing for "I **d**on't **e**ven k**n**ow **I** **a**m **l**ying." It is impossible to make a change if you are in denial. You don't really want to know there is a need for change.

> The essence of bravery is being without self-deception.
> (Pema Chodron, author of *When Things Fall Apart*)

Change is also described as "mindful surrender." Sometimes it is only when we truly let go that things can change. Admitting that you have a problem is the first step toward change.

> Buddhism recognizes that the central issue of our lives, from falling in love to facing death, requires an ability to surrender that often eludes us.
> (Mark Epstein, *Going to Peaces Without Falling Apart* 1998).

The serenity prayer of Alcoholics Anonymous is a good way to remind yourself that you are not in control.

Serenity Prayer
God grant me the serenity
To accept the things I cannot change,
The courage to change the things I can,
And the wisdom to know the difference.

Buddhist teachings (dharma) describe denial and self-delusion as "ignorance" and not a path of "mindfulness."

Procrastination

Procrastination is another obstacle to healthy change. People will gladly put off dealing with difficult issues and problems that block healthy change. In my new book *Awakening to Mindfulness, 10 Steps for Positive Change* (Health Communications 2008), I describe procrastination as the number one reason why people do not implement change.

∝ Motivational Interviewing

William Miller and Stephen Rollnick (1991) developed a form of intervention known as motivational interviewing. They recognized that formal and informal interventions are effective for many individuals who are in denial of having a problem with alcohol or drugs, but for some individuals the traditional form of intervention doesn't work. Despite the intervention, the individual is not motivated to seek abstinence or recovery from alcohol/drugs.

The same holds true for many individuals who, once in alcohol/drug treatment, either terminated treatment early against medical advice or didn't respond when confronted by counselors about their denial. Miller and Rollnick espouse a different approach with individuals who are resistant to traditional intervention methods. Some individuals respond negatively to interventions.

Motivational interviewing draws its strategies from a number of disciplines, including client-centered counseling, cognitive therapy, systems theory, and the social psychology of persuasion. The work of motivational interviewing comes from Miller and Rollnick's contention that there is no one kind of alcoholic or addict or, for that matter, an addictive personality. "This idea of a common alcoholic or addictive personality is supported neither in the original writings of Alcoholics Anonymous, nor by five decades of psychological research" (Miller and Rollnick 1991). It therefore

---

C H A R T   9 . 1

6 Styles of Procrastination

1.   The Perfectionist Procrastinator
     The Perfectionist Procrastinator waits and waits for the perfect time and situation to take action, and misses out on the opportunities for growth.

2.   The Dreamer Procrastinator
     The Dreamer Procrastinator (The Talker) has unrealistic expectations. They talk about what they are going to do, but take little action toward those dreams (i.e., "One day I am going to . . .").

3.   The Worrier Procrastinator
     The Worrier Procrastinator comes up with fearful reasons for not taking action.

4.   The Defier Procrastinator
     The Defier Procrastinator doesn't follow good advice, rejects help, and continues to have the same problems.

5.   The Crisis-Maker Procrastinator
     The Crisis-Maker Procrastinator creates crises to distract from taking "right action." They are "drama" prone. They are so busy putting out fires that they avoid working on the real issues.

6.   The Overdoer Procrastinator
     The Overdoer Procrastinator will focus on one part of the problem, at the expense of ignoring and not taking up the priority issues.

(Adapted from *It's About Time: The 6 Styles of Procrastination and How to Overcome Them* by Sapadin and McGuire).

---

makes sense that alcoholics/addicts need a variety of approaches to engage them into recovery. Perhaps a different approach might reach those alcoholics/addicts who resist traditional confrontive interventions. Motivational interviewing was therefore designed to help clients build commitment and reach a decision to change.

Miller and Rollnick described motivation as a state of readiness or eagerness to change, and they recognized that motivation may fluctuate over time, situation, and circumstance. They described the basic stages of change and the influences a therapist can make in influencing motivation to change. (See Figure 9.1.)

Their approach uses brief, individual counseling, which helps the clients explore and resolve their "ambivalence" about change. Ambivalence is defined as feeling two ways about something, being in conflict between the pros and cons of the status quo (or the pros and cons of changing). Ambivalence is a good description for the conflict many people have about changing, whether it is recovery from alcohol/drugs, unhealthy and self-destructive behaviors (e.g., smoking, overeating), a dysfunctional relationship, a bad work situation, or illegal activities. At the precontemplative stage of change, they are not considering change and may not see or admit problems with the self-destructive behavior (addiction). In the contemplative stage, they are considering change but are ambivalent about it. These are the individuals who waver from day to day and seem easily influenced to go in either direction. When it comes to alcohol/drug abuse and addiction, the alcoholic/addict wants to continue to use alcohol/drugs yet may recognize the risks and negative consequences of use. At the

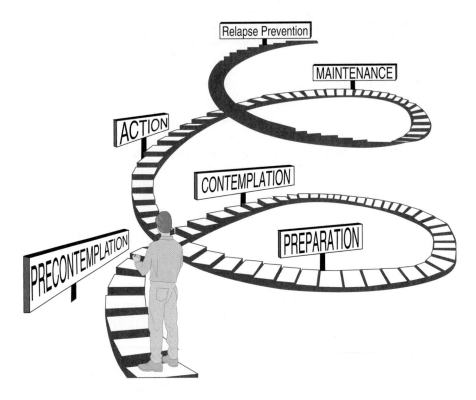

FIGURE 9.1   *The Spiral of Change*
SOURCE: Adapted from J. O. Prochaska, J. C. Norcross, and C. C. DiClemente, *Changing for Good,* Avon Books, New York, 1994 (First Avon Books Printing, Sept., 1995).

determination stage the individual decides to do something. The action stage is when there has been a recent change or an implemented plan of change. The maintenance stage involves a commitment to a long-term change, where the change has become habit, or part of the person's lifestyle. The relapse prevention stage explores strategies to not return to earlier stages. (See Table 9.1 for more information.)

Table 9.2 outlines an approach to a nondirective part of motivational interviewing.

Client-Centered Motivational Interviewing

Motivational interviewing is "client centered," which means that it focuses on eliciting and understanding the client's view.

The motivational interviewing technique is quite different from the intervention model. It is controversial because the active alcoholic/addict wants to continue to drink and will often delay taking action despite significant negative consequences. Many counselors believe that not confronting denial, and giving control back to the alcoholic/addict, will only result in continued destructive, maybe even life-threatening, patterns of alcohol consumption. However, the motivational interviewing approach

TABLE 9.1	
Stages of Change and Therapist Tasks	
Client Stage	**Therapist's Motivational Tasks**
Precontemplative	Raise doubt—increase the client's perception of risks and problems with current behavior. Decrease desirability to status quo, build rapport so you can later provide information about the negative consequences or risks of maintaining the status quo, get to know the client well enough to find out what's important to him or her (what he or she values most). Find something the client did well (maybe it was only being open-minded enough to listen to the counselor's views) and affirm that. Make sure client comes back in the future.
Contemplative	Tip the balance—evoke reasons to change, risks of not changing. Strengthen the client's self-efficacy for change of current behavior. Raise awareness of ambivalence by eliciting and reflecting both sides of the client's ambivalence: the pros and cons of animating the status quo (or the pros and cons of changing, if client prefers to discuss that). Then explore which of these pros and cons mean the most to the client. Try to point out how that status quo is in conflict with the client's deeply held values and how changing might bring the client more in line with those important values.
Determination	Help the client determine the best source of action to take in seeking change.
Action	Help the client take steps toward change. Focus on the plan, what the client is going to do. What is the client willing to do, not willing to do, and ambivalent about doing? People in action still suffer from ambivalence and fear of the unknown, and that ambivalence must be dealt with as you go along. Emphasis on action is on removing barriers to change and problem solving each of these barriers.
Maintenance	Help the client identify and use strategies to prevent relapse
Relapse	Help the client renew the processes of contemplation, determination, and action without becoming stuck or demoralized because of relapse.

has the perspective that people follow through better and are more committed to recovery if they voluntarily make the decision to choose treatment for themselves. Another controversial aspect of motivational interviewing is the counselor eliciting the client's doubts about recovery, as well as the positive aspects. This helps the counselor reflect back to the client the positive and negative aspects of the decision. Case Study 9.1 presents an example of client-centered motivational interviewing.

Effective Motivational Strategies

There are eight general motivational strategies.

1. Giving *advice.* Well-timed and tempered advice to change can make a difference. Advice should (a) clearly identify the problem or risk area, (b) explain why change is important, and (c) advocate specific change.
2. *Removing barriers.* Address blocks to change, such as resistance to go to AA meetings.

T A B L E   9 . 2

The "Nondirective" Part of Motivational Interviewing (MI): OARS* (Tools for Rowing Along with Your Clients)

Open-Ended Questions

Can't be answered with "yes" or "no"

Keep resistance down

Build trust rapidly

Encourage client to talk about what's important to him or her

Reveal what's "delicious" to clients

Help therapist find the "carrot" for change

Affirmations

Very hard to use genuinely; requires much practice

Build self-esteem

Show respect

Reduce treatment dropout rates

Get a "winning streak" going for clients (clients who succeed come back for more
    success)

Reflecting

Takes practice; sounds phony at first

Is like throwing "empathy darts" while client holds up the target

Client will always let you know if you're accurate or not.

Very satisfying for both to be accurate

More than just paraphrasing the client's message content; also reflects underlying
    feelings

Happens after every few sentences spoken by clients

About three of every four statements by MI therapist is a reflection (how do you get
    anything done?)

Summarizing

Gathers together what client said, so it can be heard again (especially the positive
    change talk)

Shows client what's been accomplished during the session

Can help therapist close one topic and move on to another

Can help end sessions on good terms

---

*"OARS" symbolizes the way motivational interviewing therapists act during a session. Whenever you are stuck,
you can fall back on this style of being with your client, until you figure out what your directive strategy is
going to be. Without adding the directive motivational interviewing techniques, OARS will only help you row
about in circles (but at least you're not sinking . . .).

3. Providing *choice.* Few people like to be told what to do. Intrinsic motivation is
    enhanced by the perception that one has freely chosen.
4. Decreasing *desirability.* Weigh the benefits and costs of change against the
    merits of continuing as before.
5. Practicing *empathy.* This kind of empathy is not an ability to identify with
    a person's experiences. Rather, it is a specifiable and learnable skill for

Case Study 9.1

Contemplative and Action Stages

Don

Don knew he had a problem with alcohol/drugs. He took some action by attending AA meetings, yet he still didn't want to stop drinking. He would maintain abstinence for limited periods of time (30–100 days) but then would lapse into drinking. Despite negative consequences at home and at work, and having gone through two inpatient programs, he still was not committed to recovery. He tried to convince himself that he wasn't really an alcoholic, yet he soon found himself in alcoholic binges. Each time he relapsed, he seemed motivated to get sober and work at a program of recovery, yet, despite attending AA, attending outpatient counseling, even working with a sponsor, he was ambivalent about recovery. At the suggestion of his sponsor, he attended several different AA meetings. After attending an AA meeting at a local mission for the homeless, he wondered if he had to "hit bottom" by losing his job, family, and home to stop drinking. The very next day, he talked to an old-timer at another AA meeting who told him, "Maybe things have to get really bad before you get better." He was then convinced that he had to continue to drink until things got worse, before he would stop. In his ambivalence, he called his sponsor with this new idea and was told, "You'll come up with any excuse to continue drinking." His resolve to seek recovery was so ambivalent and such a struggle that he could easily be influenced to go either way—recovery or self-destruction.

Don talked to his outpatient counselor about this conflict during a one-on-one session, and the counselor effectively used motivational interviewing techniques to help Don resolve this ambivalence, so he could move closer to action. The counselor focused more on Don's ambivalence about committing to AA, rather than the global issue of ambivalence about recovery in general.

Counselor:	It's good to see you again, Don. Tell me how have you been doing for the past few weeks, so I can get caught up? [open question]
Don:	Not great, if you really want to know. I haven't drunk or used in over four weeks now. In fact, I'll be thirty days sober tomorrow. But, big deal, I'm more screwed up than ever. I don't mean to sound sorry for myself, but I just feel lousy. And I know I've got to do something, but I don't know which end is up.
Counselor:	Congratulations on making it to one month! You've been working hard and it hasn't been a picnic for you. [affirmation acknowledging client's progress and empathic statement]
Don:	[silent]
Counselor:	But things are tough, and you aren't getting the rewards of feeling better yet. [accurate reflection] Tell me what you mean when you say you're more screwed up now than ever? [open question]
Don:	I was talking with my sponsor yesterday, and he told me he's worried about me. He thinks I'm gonna go out and drink again. He says I'm subconsciously planning a relapse.
Counselor:	What do you think he means? [open question]

(continued on next page)

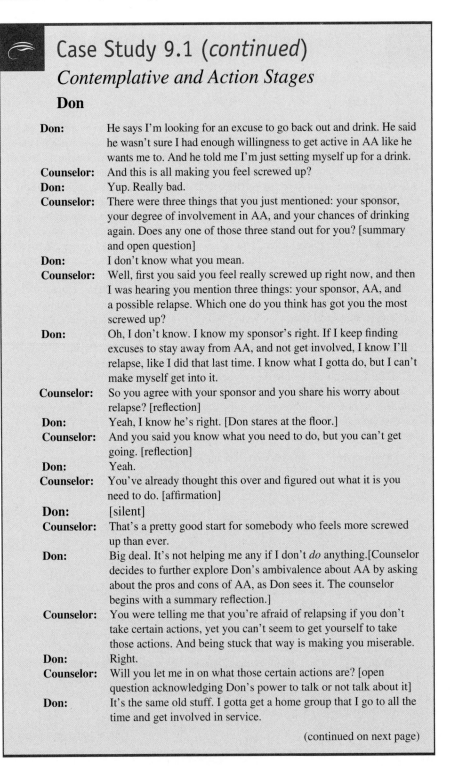

Case Study 9.1 (*continued*)
Contemplative and Action Stages
Don

Don:	He says I'm looking for an excuse to go back out and drink. He said he wasn't sure I had enough willingness to get active in AA like he wants me to. And he told me I'm just setting myself up for a drink.
Counselor:	And this is all making you feel screwed up?
Don:	Yup. Really bad.
Counselor:	There were three things that you just mentioned: your sponsor, your degree of involvement in AA, and your chances of drinking again. Does any one of those three stand out for you? [summary and open question]
Don:	I don't know what you mean.
Counselor:	Well, first you said you feel really screwed up right now, and then I was hearing you mention three things: your sponsor, AA, and a possible relapse. Which one do you think has got you the most screwed up?
Don:	Oh, I don't know. I know my sponsor's right. If I keep finding excuses to stay away from AA, and not get involved, I know I'll relapse, like I did that last time. I know what I gotta do, but I can't make myself get into it.
Counselor:	So you agree with your sponsor and you share his worry about relapse? [reflection]
Don:	Yeah, I know he's right. [Don stares at the floor.]
Counselor:	And you said you know what you need to do, but you can't get going. [reflection]
Don:	Yeah.
Counselor:	You've already thought this over and figured out what it is you need to do. [affirmation]
Don:	[silent]
Counselor:	That's a pretty good start for somebody who feels more screwed up than ever.
Don:	Big deal. It's not helping me any if I don't *do* anything. [Counselor decides to further explore Don's ambivalence about AA by asking about the pros and cons of AA, as Don sees it. The counselor begins with a summary reflection.]
Counselor:	You were telling me that you're afraid of relapsing if you don't take certain actions, yet you can't seem to get yourself to take those actions. And being stuck that way is making you miserable.
Don:	Right.
Counselor:	Will you let me in on what those certain actions are? [open question acknowledging Don's power to talk or not talk about it]
Don:	It's the same old stuff. I gotta get a home group that I go to all the time and get involved in service.

(continued on next page)

Case Study 9.1 (*continued*)
Contemplative and Action Stages

Don

Counselor:	And you feel two ways about choosing a home group. First of all, what are some of your objections to getting one?
Don:	I don't like joining groups because it's corny or something.
Counselor:	Okay. What else?
Don:	I don't want to have to go to the same group every week because I get tired of the people there.
Counselor:	Okay, some groups seem corny to you and you get tired of some people. What else?
Don:	I don't know; that's all I guess.
Counselor:	O.K., what about the other side of the coin? What are the most positive things you might get from choosing a home group?
Don:	Well, it might help me stay sober.
Counselor:	How?
Don:	Just by staying close to a group. They get to know you and, if you start to drop off meetings, somebody might ask you if you're okay.
Counselor:	So people get to know you and care enough to say something to you to help you get back on track, and you might not mind hearing it because you know them, right?
Don:	[Yes.]
Counselor:	So people can help you stay on track. What else might be positive for you if you decided to get a home group?
Don:	Well, they say people get to know your story and you get to know everybody there pretty good, because you hear their stories as well
Counselor:	So if you spend more time with your home group you could get to know them better than the people in other groups if you just "shop around" from group to group.
Don:	Right.
Counselor:	Almost as if each person in your home group were a separate TV show that you tune into each week to see how things are going with them. Kind of entertaining.
Don:	Yeah, I never thought of it that way before
Counselor:	[summarizing] On one hand, you're not much of a joiner and you might get tired of seeing some people every week. But, on the other hand, you could get to know those people better and actually get some support, even enjoyment from being around them each week. Maybe even get so you look forward to going each week?
Don:	I suppose so, although I don't think I'd ever feel really comfortable there. The way it is now, I just go to whatever meeting I feel like. But I never look forward to meetings, because I know I'm just gonna bolt right after it is over.

(continued on next page)

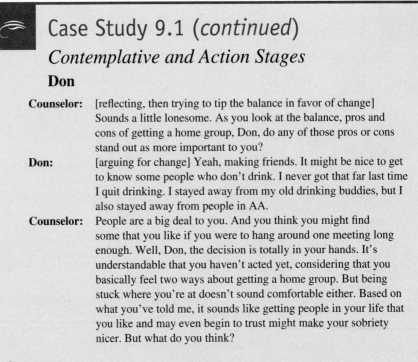

Case Study 9.1 (*continued*)

Contemplative and Action Stages

Don

Counselor:	[reflecting, then trying to tip the balance in favor of change] Sounds a little lonesome. As you look at the balance, pros and cons of getting a home group, Don, do any of those pros or cons stand out as more important to you?
Don:	[arguing for change] Yeah, making friends. It might be nice to get to know some people who don't drink. I never got that far last time I quit drinking. I stayed away from my old drinking buddies, but I also stayed away from people in AA.
Counselor:	People are a big deal to you. And you think you might find some that you like if you were to hang around one meeting long enough. Well, Don, the decision is totally in your hands. It's understandable that you haven't acted yet, considering that you basically feel two ways about getting a home group. But being stuck where you're at doesn't sound comfortable either. Based on what you've told me, it sounds like getting people in your life that you like and may even begin to trust might make your sobriety nicer. But what do you think?

Summary

Counselor tried to move client from contemplation into preparation and action, regarding the specific behavioral issue of getting a home AA group.

[Counselor turns over the responsibility for the decision to Don and then asks if he's ready for action—that is, getting a home group. If the answer is no, the counselor affirms the work that Don did in acknowledging both sides of the painful issue and lets the issue rest for now, closing the topic on good terms, to be returned to later. If the answer is yes, they proceed with discussing an action plan for getting a home group and removing barriers to doing so.]

---

understanding another's meaning through the use of reflective listening, whether or not you have had a similar experience yourself.

6. Providing *feedback*.
7. Clarifying *goals*. Help the client to restate the goal in realistic or attainable terms.
8. Helping *active*. Express actively and affirmatively your interest in your client's change process.

Motivational interviewing is a nondirective approach. Miller and Rollnick (1991) use the mnemonic OARS to describe nondirective counseling. You can "row along with your clients" if you O—ask *open-ended questions,* A—provide *affirmations,* R—*reflect* on client verbalizations, and S—*summarize* what the client says. (See Table 9.2.)

Active Ingredients of Effective Brief Counseling

Miller and Rollnick (1991) have developed the mnemonic FRAMES* to remind counselors of the effective ingredients for motivational interviewing and brief counseling: FRAMES—feedback, responsibility, advice, menu (i.e., a list of choices), empathy, self-efficacy (i.e., you can do it). (See Figure 9.2.)

The general principles of motivational interviewing (see Table 9.2) are the following:

1. *Express empathy.* Acceptance facilitates change; skillful reflective listening is fundamental; ambivalence is normal.
2. *Develop discrepancy.* Awareness of consequences is important; a discrepancy between present behavior and important goals will motivate change; the client should present the arguments for change.
3. *Avoid argumentation.* Arguments are counterproductive; defending breeds defensiveness; resistance is a signal to change strategies; labeling is unnecessary.

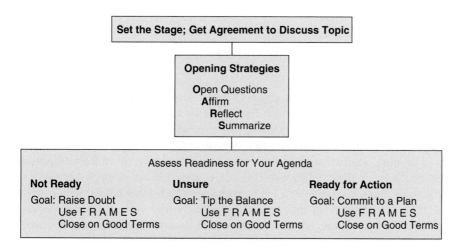

FIGURE 9.2   *One of Many Ways to Do a Brief Intervention*
SOURCE: Miller and Rollnick, *Motivational Interviewing,* 1991.

4. *Roll with resistance.* Momentum can be used to good advantage; perceptions can be shifted; new perspectives are invited but not imposed; the client is a valuable resource in finding solutions to problems.
5. *Support self-efficacy.* Belief in the possibility of change is an important motivator: the client is responsible for choosing and carrying out personal change; there is hope in the range of alternative approaches available.

⋇ Intervention

Everything one does to create awareness of an alcohol/drug problem is an intervention. The slightest suggestion to a friend, colleague, or family member that he or she may be drinking/drugging too much is an intervention. Everyone is different. Those who are at early stages of substance abuse without a family history of alcoholism/addiction may very well pay attention to your observations. If enough people are bringing the drink/drug problem to the person's attention, he or she might decide to do something about it. On the other hand, there are individuals who, if they were hit over the head with a two-by-four, wouldn't recognize their substance-abuse problem.

Interventions at Various Stages of the Alcohol/Drug Use Continuum

Alcohol/drug intervention is any action taken by someone to interrupt the progression of problems with alcohol/drugs. This definition can be expanded to any attempt to help someone from further developing problems with alcohol/drugs. At each stage of alcohol/drug use (i.e., initial contact, experimentation, integrated use, excessive use, addiction), intervention attempts may prevent progression to the next, more damaging stage of alcohol/drug use. This may take the form of an employer expressing concern about an employee's job performance or a teacher talking with parents and letting them know their child is tired and falling asleep in class. There have been a variety of intervention programs in the school system. One such program helps teachers develop core teams (usually involving the school nurse, an administrator, a coach, a dean, etc.), which identify students with behaviors, attitudes, and problems that may indicate alcohol/drug problems. All of these approaches are interventions. Whether it is a conversation expressing concern about alcohol/drug use or a formal intervention, the common goal is to let the individual know that we are concerned about him or her.

In Chapter 4, the various stages of alcohol/drug use are described—nonuse, initial contact, experimentation (situational and circumstantial), integrated use, excessive use (periodic and continuous), and addiction. At each of these stages, there are opportunities for intervention. If one can effectively intervene at earlier stages and interrupt the progression to later stages of alcohol/drug use, the negative consequences may be avoided. Obviously, the later stages of alcohol/drug abuse require more concerted efforts, such as a formal intervention.

The following suggestions illustrate various interventions for children at each stage of the alcohol/drug use continuum.

Stage 1—Nonuse Interventions

- Parental, peer, and other support to maintain nonuse
- Emotional support during difficult times, conflicts, developmental tasks, and emotionally charged events that may make the at-risk individual try alcohol/drugs
- Affirmation and support in activities that promote a good sense of self and alternative activities to alcohol/drug use
- Focus on refusal skills and dealing with peer pressure
- Education and implementation of effective parenting, communication skills, and other alcohol/drug prevention skills

Stage 2—Initial Contact Interventions

Two common problems at this stage are overreaction and underreaction. As a parent, you don't want to be an alarmist and overact in rigid, shaming, and blaming ways to a child's initial contact with alcohol/drugs. You also don't want to ignore the use, disregard the significance, and minimize the impact on the child. As a result,

- Become more aware of the child's behavior and signs of alcohol/drug use.
- Talk with other parents about the child's behavior in their homes.
- Once aware of initial contact, talk with child (i.e., break the no-talk rule); don't ignore the fact that your child used or avoided the opportunity to discuss his or her use of alcohol/drugs.
- If your child has used, let him or her describe the situation, without being judgmental, blaming, or negative.
- Express concerns about safety (e.g., Was your child with friends that he or she could trust? Was it a safe place if problems occurred? Was your child in physical or psychological danger?).
- Without being negative and an alarmist, or lecturing, let the child describe his or her own perception of safety.
- Discuss at-risk factors of alcohol/drug dependence and addiction (especially if there is a family history of alcoholism and/or drug dependence).
- This may be an opportunity to reevaluate other aspects of the child's life (e.g., school, friends, activities).
- This may be an opportune time to explore other family problems and seek an assessment from a counselor who specializes in alcohol/drug recovery and family systems.

Stage 3—Experimentation Interventions

- Focusing on communication and exploration of values, attitudes, and feelings about alcohol/drugs
- Teaching and modeling skills in decision making, conflict resolution, goal setting, and so on

- Teaching and modeling skills in coping with conflicts, dealing with authority figures, and controlling destructive impulses
- Providing information about chemical dependency and addiction
- Providing information about at-risk factors if there is a family history of chemical dependency (e.g., if one parent has or had problems with alcohol/drugs, the child has a four times higher risk of developing problems with alcohol/drugs; if both parents have or had a problem, there is an eight times higher risk for the child to develop problems with alcohol/drugs)
- Identifying, assessing, and perhaps counseling for problems in the family, at school, and so on
- Educating about alcohol/drug prevention and family systems

Stage 4—Interventions at the Integrated Stage

- Identification and communication of concerns and negative consequences as a result of integrated alcohol/drug use
- Expression of concern—in a caring, nonjudgmental way—regarding the well-being of the individual using alcohol/drugs
- Pointing out the individual's denial of an alcohol/drug problem
- Assessment by a trained chemical dependency family counselor to assess alcohol/drug use and family dynamics
- If problems are identified, work on these issues in counseling (i.e., family members attend Al-Anon; take educational classes on chemical dependency, parenting, and family systems; and attend regular counseling).

Stages 5 and 6—Interventions at the Excessive Use and Addiction Stages

All of the previous strategies are appropriate at both the excessive and addictive stages. However, the longer and more pervasive the problems with alcohol/drugs, the more difficult and intense the level of intervention.

- Alcohol/drug assessment, including regular urinanalysis for drugs and blood alcohol tests
- Intensive outpatient counseling for chemical dependency and family issues
- Strong boundary setting and consequences for violation of family rules and alcohol/drug use
- Formal alcohol/drug intervention
- Inpatient/residential treatment for chemical dependency
- Involvement in AA and other self-help meetings, including active involvement in 12-step work with a sponsor

Table 9.3 describes the dos and don'ts of dealing with someone who has an alcohol/drug problem.

TABLE 9.3

Dos and Don'ts of Dealing with Someone Who Has an Alcohol/Drug Problem

1. Deal with your emotions.

If possible, try to be calm, balanced, and caring. This may be difficult; however, remember that if you lose control, you lose.

Do Not

Try to talk with someone while he or she is under the influence of alcohol/drugs; if your child or spouse comes home late at night under the influence of alcohol/drugs, wait until the morning to discuss it.

Threaten to make ultimatums unless you have had time to think them through (e.g., Is it realistic? Can you follow through? What is the impact of the ultimatum on other family members?). Threats said in anger can be unrealistic, inflexible, and abusive. Idle threats or constant threats that are not followed through are meaningless in changing behavior. Threats only set up a lack of consistency, poor trust, and lack of credibility.

Lose your temper, rant and rave, or lose control. It might temporarily make you feel good to let out your frustration and anger, but it does not help the child or adult in addressing the alcohol/drug problem.

Do

Express a willingness to get help and resolve the problem. This is usually in the form of counseling.

Communicate your concern and feelings (e.g., fear, worry, love) without trying to control or lecture the alcohol/drug user.

Set boundaries that are reasonable (to promote appropriate behavior and consistent family rules).

Follow through with consequences for boundaries that were violated.

2. Communicate with behavior-specific examples, rather than generalizations and secondhand or speculative information.

Do Not

Ask why the person is using alcohol/drugs. "Why" questions are often blaming questions, as if asking, "How could you do this to your mother and me?"

Use words such as *drunk, loaded, wasted.* Instead, describe specific behaviors you observe (e.g., slurred speech, staggered gait, etc.).

Generalize about alcohol/drug use. Be specific about alcohol/drug use, if possible (e.g., "I saw you drink five glasses of wine and snort two lines of cocaine").

Use sarcasm, ridicule, and other behaviors that may shame or embarrass the alcohol/drug user. This only perpetuates resentments and often results in later passive-aggressive behavior.

Do

Seek professional counseling to help with family communication about alcohol/drug problems. Seek out a counselor experienced in alcohol/drug treatment and family systems.

3. Trust what you see (behaviors), not what the addict/alcoholic or problem user says.

Do Not

Expect that things will get better on their own. Often, the problem alcohol/drug user will decrease his or her use when he or she suspects that you may do something. Alcoholism and drug addiction are progressive diseases that only get worse over time unless the individual is motivated to change.

Expect that the problem alcohol/drug user will recognize his or her use as a problem. Denial is often the case.

Assume that the alcoholic/addict will be rational and logical. Instead, he or she may exhibit self-deception and delay getting help..

(continued on next page)

TABLE 9.3 (continued)

Dos and Don'ts of Dealing with Someone Who Has an Alcohol/Drug Problem

4. Avoid being distracted from the real issue—the individual's abuse of alcohol/drugs.

Do Not

Spend time or physical and emotional energy on distracting wild goose chases (e.g., finding out who gave the person alcohol/drugs or blaming the school system or other parents). These are all secondary issues. The primary issue is that your child or family member may have an alcohol/drug problem.

Compare the alcohol/drug problems of others that are more involved in alcohol/drug use. This is a form of rationalizing away the problem. Expressions such as "kids will be kids," "he or she will outgrow this," and "most people drink/drug this way" tend to discount the real dimensions of alcohol/drug dependence.

Get distracted by excuses for alcohol/drug abuse (e.g., "I'm experiencing a great deal of pressure right now" or "It's because my girlfriend just broke up with me"). The fact is the person has a problem with alcohol/drugs and is vulnerable to relapse when normal, stressful events happen again.

Take responsibility for the total problem. Avoid self-blaming statements (e.g., "I'm an awful parent" or "I should have_____ ; then he or she wouldn't have an alcohol/drug problem"). Self-blame serves only to distract from the issue at hand—the fact that your child or family member has an alcohol/drug problem and needs help. You cannot go back and change the past; you can only work on the future.

Do

Seek treatment for the addicted person and the entire family. The sooner you do this, the better is the prognosis.

5. Seek professional help for alcohol/drug assessment, education, prevention, intervention, and treatment.

Do Not

Isolate from others and hide the family alcohol/drug problem. The longer you hide the problem from others to avoid feelings of shame and embarrassment, the more damage occurs to your family system.

Get advice from people who may have an alcohol/drug problem themselves or individuals who deny the problem. This only reinforces denial.

Attempt to counsel the family member who has the alcohol/drug problem yourself. This will inadvertently end up being another form of enabling behavior.

Do

Attend Al-Anon, Codependency Anonymous, and other self-help meetings and develop a relationship with a sponsor. This will help you develop a support system necessary to make changes.

Attend educational presentations, classes, and conferences that focus on parenting, family systems, prevention, alcohol/drug recovery, intervention, codependency, and other personal growth issues.

Find a counselor who specializes in alcohol/drug treatment, family systems, and codependency. For more information on choosing a counselor, see Chapter 11.

Take care of yourself and continue with your own recovery, regardless of whether the family member who has the alcohol/drug problem gets help.

Obstacles to Interventions

There are many obstacles that prevent families from getting help for alcohol/drug problems. Getting the family member with the alcohol/drug problem into treatment may not be realistic unless these obstacles are first addressed. Some common obstacles to families getting help are listed in Table 9.4.

Intervention Services

The concept of alcohol/drug intervention began in the 1960s, when Vernon Johnson—at that time a pastor—felt frustrated when he was unable to help spouses of alcoholics. Deciding to abandon the traditional approach of waiting until the alcoholic/addict hit bottom, he tried a strategy that he later called intervention (Johnson 1986).

Merriam-Webster's Collegiate Dictionary, Eleventh Edition, defines *intervene* this way: "to occur, fall, or come between points of time or events." Alcohol/drug intervention is a process that prevents, alters, or interrupts the progression of the disease. The intervention is a process of getting involved or stepping into a situation in an attempt to interrupt the disease and to get the individual into alcohol/drug treatment. Persons who intervene choose to talk about the issue of alcohol/drug dependence that is destructive to the individuals, their families, and friends. Due to the alcoholic/addict's strong denial system, a trained interventionist with an expertise in chemical dependency treatment must lead or facilitate the intervention.

TABLE 9.4

Obstacles to Reaching Parents and Families

- Denial of family dysfunction/imbalance and alcohol/drug problems
- Skepticism about alcohol/drug messages that don't fit parents' own experience
- Assumption by parents that children's alcohol/drug use will be O.K.
- Distorted, depressed view of life by dysfunctional families
- Fear of being stigmatized or labeled as dysfunctional
- Fear of loss of confidentiality
- Narcissism of parents
- Lack of insurance resources for parenting/counseling services
- Lack of energy/time by parents
- Distrust of the system
- Lack of credible message sources for cultural/racial minority groups
- Lack of concern/respect for experts' opinions about alcohol/drugs
- Lack of awareness of community resources, discomfort with middle-class settings
- Overwhelming need for services for basic survival
- Cultural mores

SOURCE: Office for Substance Abuse Prevention 1990.

Intervention services are offered by most chemical dependency inpatient and residential treatment centers. Trained chemical dependency counselors also specialize in conducting interventions. The choice of the interventionist is a critical element in determining the success of an intervention. Local, state, and national alcohol/drug help lines are excellent referral sources for finding trained and experienced interventionists.

Intervention Approaches

There are a variety of approaches to the alcohol/drug intervention, including formal and informal chemical dependency interventions, in which each interventionist has his or her own style of conducting the intervention. The principles described in this chapter form a basic framework within which most interventionists work.

Professional Intervention Assistance

Whatever the format or style, conducting an intervention without professional guidance is often doomed to failure, no matter how powerful the individual. Untrained, grandstanding individuals who coerce someone into chemical dependency treatment often cause further resistance by the individual needing help. Do not use this information to try to conduct an intervention on your own; consult a professional interventionist for help.

Intervention as a Caring Response

The most important aspect of an intervention is that it is a caring effort designed to interrupt the disease of alcoholism and drug addiction. Individuals involved in an intervention can be effective only if they maintain a caring, behavior-specific approach and support each other within the basic guidelines of their intervention group.

Goals of Intervention

The primary goal in developing an intervention is to get the addicted person to recognize that he or she has an alcohol/drug problem and to get that person into appropriate chemical dependency treatment. Treatment is usually a minimum 21- to 28-day inpatient or residential program.

Secondary goals of the intervention are to

1. Provide an opportunity for those who care about the alcoholic/addict to express concern about the impact the alcoholic/addict's dysfunctional behavior has had on them.
2. Provide information on alcohol/drug addiction and family patterns of interaction, such as enabling behavior, to the significant others (parents, spouses, family members, employers, and peers).
3. Promote the development of a healthy family system and provide resource information for family members to continue working on their issues.

Family Interventions

Interventions are 100 percent effective in that, regardless of whether the alcoholic/addict decides to get help and go to treatment, family members go on with their recovery. The family has begun a process of change. The growth that the family members experience in developing an intervention can empower them to continue to be true to their feelings and to their own individual recovery, whether or not the alcoholic/addict decides to seek treatment. Via the intervention process, the family members learn about the disease of alcohol/drug addiction. They recognize their own enabling behavior and the role they play in the dynamics of the disease. The intervention may be the first time in a long time that the family members have interacted by functionally discussing their feelings. It may be the first time they have candidly discussed the impact that the alcoholic/addict's alcohol or drug use has had on each of them.

Candidates for Intervention

Using a formal intervention process on adolescents, or young adults who are developmentally still at the adolescent stage, is usually ineffective. Adolescents often feel violated by the process of intervention. Because they are still exploring their own issues of identity and boundaries, they feel that it is unfair for family members to be planning an intervention without their knowledge. Adolescents fail to recognize or acknowledge that all previous direct efforts have not been effective in getting them to listen and understand the true dimensions of their problems.

Interventions are far more effective in getting individuals into treatment, when addicts recognize that their behavior has been a problem. The addict who still values and respects members of the intervention group is the best candidate. In some situations, addicts have alienated so many people that only job-related people are left. This relationship with an employer or business associates might be the integral element that makes some addicts good candidates for intervention.

Stages of Formal Intervention

The four basic stages of a formal intervention are assessment, preintervention, intervention, and postintervention. The rest of this chapter describes these stages with many examples and a case study.

Assessment

Families consider an alcohol/drug intervention because a family member recognizes that the family needs to do something about the person with the alcohol/drug problem. Likely, people have approached the addict about getting help on numerous occasions. Despite their efforts, the addict still chooses not to recognize the problem or get help. The alcoholic/addict's goal is to continue drinking or drugging.

A family member begins the intervention process by contacting a professional who conducts interventions. The interventionist schedules an appointment with family members to assess the alcohol/drug problem and to determine if an intervention is appropriate.

An experienced interventionist is trained to assess alcohol/drug problems. In the initial assessment sessions, several family members, friends, colleagues, and even the employer describe what they know about the alcohol/drug use of the person being assessed for the intervention. Individuals seeking to intervene on a family member with an alcohol/drug problem are often at a late stage of frustration with the alcoholic/addict's dysfunctional and destructive behavior. Many look at the intervention as a last-ditch alternative. Despite the family's urgency to conduct an intervention, the interventionist conducts a proper assessment to determine if the person really does have an alcohol/drug problem.

The key element of the assessment is eliciting *behavior-specific information* and avoiding hearsay and generalized information. The interventionist needs specific times, dates, and firsthand knowledge of the actual level of consumption of alcohol and drugs. Some assessment questions are "What makes you think the individual has a problem with alcohol/drugs?" "What have been the consequences of this individual's alcohol/drug use?" The interventionist asks family members to explain or clarify the

Frequency of use, amounts used (dose and routes of administration), and set and setting of use
Patterns of use—binges, periods of nonuse, and cycle of use
History of negative consequences—overdoses, medical complications, and physical and emotional harm
Periods of abstinence, if any, and methods used
Any medical conditions that affect alcohol/drug use
Use of coffee, cigarettes, and medications and other addictions
Difficulties with the criminal-justice system
Financial problems and interpersonal problems

Family members at the assessment sessions are asked to describe specifically what they know about the addict's use of alcohol and drugs and resulting dysfunctional and destructive behavior. The assessment clarifies the dimensions of the problem with alcohol/drugs. The family, and others present, usually recognize, confirm, and validate their own worst fears—the individual has an alcohol/drug problem.

Another extremely important aspect of the assessment is to determine whether the person you are going to intervene on is able to listen and understand. Someone who is going to physically attack, verbally explode, or rage at others at the intervention is not appropriate for an intervention. During the assessment stage, interventionists often ask the family members and others present, "How does the person you are planning to intervene on deal with anger?" "What do you think his or her reaction is going to be to the intervention?" These questions should elicit responses that determine if the individual is violent and if there have been some physical violations in the past. Sometimes individuals can be paranoid and/or delusional, especially if they have been using cocaine, crack, or freebase. Obviously, you do not want to do an intervention if there is a high risk that the individual will be violent or unable to listen and understand. One alternative is to videotape the intervention and give it to the addict.

Some people have a negative reaction to the concept of an alcohol/drug intervention. They believe that it is an invasion, or a violation, of the individual and his or her right to use alcohol/drugs. For the intervention to be effective, it must be planned without the knowledge of the person being intervened on. Some individuals have difficulty with this behind-the-scenes aspect. Once the interventionist has assessed that an intervention is warranted, members of the intervention group must decide whether they are comfortable proceeding with the intervention.

Case Study 9.2 illustrates the perils of initiating an intervention without first doing a proper assessment.

Preintervention

The preintervention stage consists of all the sessions necessary to prepare for the actual intervention to take place. The ingredients essential for a successful intervention include (1) the commitment and participation of meaningful and significant others (family members, friends, relatives, peers, and children); (2) a proper assessment by the interventionist; and (3) specific, nonjudgmental information about the individual's alcohol and drug behavior.

In preparation for the intervention, preintervention sessions develop a cohesive group of significant others—a group that has the goal of getting the alcoholic/addict into appropriate treatment.

The interventionist begins developing this group by educating the members, giving them information about the dynamics of chemical dependency. The education emphasizes the progressive nature of the disease of alcoholism/drug addiction, which affects the entire family.

The group members then develop their scripts and role-play the intervention. Role-playing allows the group to anticipate the reactions of the person they are going

Case Study 9.2
Intervention Without Proper Assessment
J. R

J. R., an aspiring vice president in a developing company, contacted an interventionist and requested an intervention for another vice president in the same company. The family members of the person with the supposed alcohol problem believed that Roger had been drinking regularly but were not sure that he had an alcohol problem. Insisting that his co-worker's drinking was a problem, J. R. was unable to come up with any behavior-specific examples of increased alcohol use. Despite the limited information and secondhand generalizations, the interventionist decided to go ahead with the intervention. The result was disastrous. Roger did not have an alcohol problem and quickly identified sabotage by his colleague, who desired his sales territory. Needless to say, Roger was justified in proceeding with litigation against the interventionist for not conducting a proper assessment.

to intervene on. The group members can then redevelop their intervention to make it more effective.

The alcoholic/addict is a master in distracting the intervention group from the goals of the intervention. When each family member communicates generalizations and judgments, the alcoholic/addict picks at their statements and distracts the group, thus weakening their ability to get the alcoholic/addict to commit to treatment. Therefore, the members of the intervention group must develop and communicate behavior-specific examples of the alcoholic/addict's dysfunctional and self-destructive behavior.

The following examples illustrate generalized statements, followed by the alcoholic/addict's distracting statements. The appropriate behavior-specific statement follows each set of generalized and distracting responses.

Example 1

Generalized and blaming statements: "Boy, you were really wasted at the party picnic and got violent. You were drunk and loaded on cocaine."

Alcoholic/addict distracting statements: "What do you mean wasted? You were drinking just as much as I was. Weren't you? Boy, are you hypocritical. You use cocaine."

Behavior-specific statements: "John, I'm here because I care about you. On Saturday, July 4, 1991, at the company picnic, I saw you drink five beers from 1 to 3 p.m., then snort six lines of cocaine, which was followed by two more beers. You sat down in the outfield during the softball game and fell asleep. When I went over to wake you up, you threw a punch at me, right in front of the head of our company. You left the field. I found you a half hour later, with a six-pack in the back of your car. Two of the cans of beer were already empty. I am worried about you. I'm afraid you are going to lose your job. You've been like a brother to me. I pray that you will get help. I know it's the alcohol and drugs."

Example 2

Generalized and blaming statements: "You are an awful husband and father. You are always using drugs and drinking too much. Last night you were drinking and snorting cocaine all night. You scared the kids to death that night by yelling so loud at them, like a madman."

Alcoholic/addict distracting statements: "You think you are such a great mother? I remember the time you. . . ."

Behavior-specific statements: "John, I'm your wife and I'm here because I care about you. On Friday night, November 3, I went to the church meeting. When I came home at 10:15 p.m., I smelled alcohol on your breath and clothes. There was an empty gram bottle of cocaine on the kitchen table and three lines of cocaine still on the mirror. There were 12 empty beer cans on the living room floor and the kids were hiding in their closet upstairs. When I went into their room, they ran to me, shaking and out of control. That night I had to sleep with them because they were so frightened. The next day, they told me you threw beer cans at them and told them you would kill them if they didn't stop bothering you. I love you, John; I know it's the alcohol and drugs. I would like all of us to get help."

Each person involved in the intervention uses the following script format to avoid generalized, blaming statements:

"I'm here because I care about you. You are my _____. I *care* about you."
"I saw _____" (describe the behavior-specific incidents that occurred)
"I feel _____" (embarrassed, hurt, frightened, worried, ashamed, etc.)
"I know it's the drugs." (or the alcohol or cocaine)
"I want you [us] to get help."

Script Example

> "John, I'm here because *I care* about you. We've been friends a very long time. During Christmas, *I saw* you snort half a gram of cocaine. In the next hour, you drank four beers. *I felt embarrassed* when you were trying to kiss your niece. *I felt ashamed. I saw* the hurt on your wife's face. *I know it's the cocaine. I know it's the alcohol. I want you to get help.*"

Some interventionists prefer the words "I want you to get help." Others prefer "I want us to get help" because everyone in the family is going to get help to stop enabling the alcoholic/addict's use of alcohol/drugs.

During the preintervention, the intervention group members determine

1. When the intervention will take place
2. Where the intervention will take place—usually a neutral setting such as the interventionist's office is best
3. Who will bring the person to the intervention
4. Their scripts, role-play the intervention, and determine the most effective way of communicating their message
5. In which order each member will talk during the intervention
6. Who is going to ask for a commitment to listen from the person being intervened on
7. That arrangements have been made with the alcohol/drug treatment program; insurance and other details have been completed; and a bed is reserved at the treatment center starting on the day of the intervention
8. All contingencies, so that the individual can go directly to the treatment program; bags have been packed and are in the car; and a family member drives the addict directly to the treatment program.

Every detail is planned, even the seating arrangement. The actual intervention session will start and flow as planned. The family members will be prepared to continue their own recovery, regardless of the addict's decision. The session will not escalate into an uncontrollable situation. The family will approach the intervention as a process, rather than a static event. Bear in mind that if the preintervention sessions have gone well, the interventionist is available to help the family members during the intervention, but most often he or she plays a minimal, facilitating role.

Intervention

Each intervention is unique. However, they all have the same common ingredients for success, such as a nonjudgmental tone and behavior-specific caring responses by family and friends. The following is an example of an intervention.

Audrey is an attractive, energetic 33-year-old. She owns a very successful travel agency. She is the single parent of two children: Andy is 12 years old and Bridget is 7 years old. Audrey is dynamic, aggressive, and—the most critical feature—an alcoholic.

Audrey's sister, Mary, 39, is concerned enough to seek intervention for her sister. Both sisters grew up in an alcoholic family system. Their father died of alcoholism when Mary was 16 and Audrey was 9 years old. Those involved with the intervention are the following:

Mary—Audrey's older sister

Ann—Audrey and Mary's mother, a very successful businesswoman

Roger—Mary's son, Audrey's nephew, a 20-year-old student at the University of
    Washington

Andy—Audrey's 12-year-old son

Mary has taken Audrey to the interventionist's office under the pretense that they have been having some family counseling sessions for her son Roger. She said they wanted Audrey to participate in one session. All the family members are present at the office, waiting for Audrey and Mary to arrive.

Mary:	Audrey, this is Dr. Fields. [Shakes hands.] Just sit right here. Audrey, we are all here because we care about you. We are concerned about you and the children. We would like to be able to talk to you about our concerns. We would each like to say some things. We need your commitment to listen to us and not to respond until we are finished. You will have an opportunity to respond then. Will you promise to first listen to us and not talk until we are finished?
Audrey:	But, I thought we were here for Roger.
Mary:	We are here for you, Roger, and all the family members.
Audrey:	Yeah, but you didn't let me know what this was about.
Mary:	Audrey, we wanted you to come. Will you just hear us out? Then you can have your chance.
Audrey:	I, I . . . don't . . . yeah, I guess so. O.K., I'll listen to what you have to say. [Establishing ground rules allows each family member to talk without being distracted by the addict's ambiguous arguments. Having the addict agree to listen and not talk back is an essential ingredient for the intervention to be successful. Even though Audrey has been deceived in getting her to the intervention, she knows or suspects what the meeting is about. She is curious and is even challenging the group to try to affect her.]
Roger:	Thank you. You've been like a big sister to me, even though you are my aunt. You have provided a lot of opportunities to me. You've taken me on vacations and introduced me to all sorts of people, activities, and even jobs that I never would have had access to. I care

about you a great deal. You've been a tremendous influence and I am very proud of you. I am here because I love you.

Lately, however, I find that I'm not so proud of you anymore. I'm worried about you. I'm worried about Andy. I'm worried about Bridget. At your birthday party on January 7, you came home smelling of alcohol. You had three margaritas within an hour. I saw you in the kitchen, downing two doubles, as if they were water. You stumbled out of the kitchen and fell and cut your lip.

Audrey: That was my birthday party. Don't you understand?

Roger: You promised you would listen. After you cut yourself, when Andy, Bridget, and I came into the kitchen to help, you screamed and yelled at us to get away. Andy was so frightened he hid in his room and Bridget couldn't stop crying. They said they were so frightened that you were going to hit them again.

This isn't the first time this has happened. The same thing happened when we went down to Mexico. You had four drinks at the airport bar and four drinks on the flight. I was so embarrassed when you were flirting with the man next to you. The kids were embarrassed when you were kissing him and when you yelled at me for interfering. When we got to our hotel, the first thing you did was to order more booze.

In February, I was at the travel agency and you went into the bathroom. You invited me in and you had some lines of cocaine that you offered me. I saw you do ten lines of cocaine and then come out and act as if everything was O.K. You made six trips to the bathroom in the hour that I was there.

Audrey: I didn't do that much. As if you are so innocent!

Roger: You promised that you would listen and not interrupt. I was with you the night you got arrested for driving under the influence of alcohol. The kids were frightened sitting in the back seat. Despite my arguing with you, you insisted on driving. I was so frightened that we all would be killed. I went along because I felt guilty that you would kill yourself and the kids. I tried to take the keys away from you, but you wouldn't let me. I was so angry with your boyfriend, Al, for insisting that you were O.K., when you couldn't even walk straight. I was so angry with you when the police arrested you in front of your children. But I was more upset with myself for allowing myself to get drawn into the whole situation.

Audrey, despite all of this I love you and the children and I want you to get help.

Audrey: What kind of help?

Roger: [No response, head tilted down to ground, feeling emotionally spent.]

Ann: Audrey, you were a beautiful child; I gave birth to you. I love you a great deal. You were always so fun loving, energetic, and interested in so many things. We went shopping the other day, last Wednesday, and you had four beers at lunch, after you said you would cut back. You told me that you were just wired. You were agitated, nervous, jittery. Audrey, I'm frightened for you. When we came home from the travel agency last Friday, you smelled of alcohol. You were driving erratically. I was afraid we would get pulled over and you'd be arrested again. When I told you that you were in no condition to drive, you yelled at me to stop nagging.

Audrey: You, you're always telling me what to do. You're always bothering me. You're always involved in my life, telling me how to parent my kids.

Ann: That day, I saw you drink three beers before we left the agency.

Audrey: You guys are in this together. I don't even know why I'm here.

Roger: You said you'd listen.

Audrey: How can I listen to you if you keep on getting together? How could you guys get together behind my back to do this?

Ann: We're here because we care about you. We love you. I know it's the drugs. I know it's the alcohol. I want us to get some help.

Mary: We've grown up together. We've always been close. I love you. I care about you. Last week, we went out to Morgan's restaurant. You drank five margaritas within an hour and a half. You were snorting cocaine in the bathroom. You left the restaurant with two men whom you didn't know. I am really frightened for you. The next day you called me and told me you had a problem with alcohol and wanted help. Two days later, on Sunday, when I asked you about getting help, you said that you were doing much better and were getting your act together.

It was only a week later, that Friday night, when you were back at Morgan's. I saw you drink three doubles in an hour. You insisted that I stay. It was too hard to stay and watch you order another drink. I'm afraid that you are hurting yourself. I worry about you. I want my younger sister back. I want you to get help.

Andy: [Tears rolling from his eyes] Mommy, I am afraid when you drink and use drugs that you will hurt me. I am afraid that you will hurt Bridget. I want you to go get help. Will you?

Audrey: [Hugs Andy] Yes, I'll get help. I love you and don't want you to be frightened.

Mary: We have reserved a bed at the treatment center and Roger will drive you there.

Audrey: You mean you want me to go right now?

Mary: Yes.

Audrey: But what about the appointments at the agency?

Mary: I've arranged for Natalie to come in and manage the agency while you are gone.

Audrey: But what about the meeting with the accountant on Thursday?

Ann: I can cover the meeting, since I know all about the new book-keeping system.

Audrey: What about clothes?

Mary:	I packed some of your things in a suitcase. Anything else you want I can get to you tomorrow.
Audrey:	Can the children come and visit?
Mary:	After the first week, there are regular family visits and a family counseling program. We chose this program because it specializes in providing counseling for young children.
Audrey:	I guess you thought of everything.
	[In reality, the family did think of everything. Any potential form of denial was anticipated, so that Audrey and her family could get the help they needed.]

In the event that Audrey did not agree to go into treatment, the family had prepared another bottom-line script. The purpose of the bottom-line script is to let the addict know that if she refuses to go into treatment, the family is not going to continue to enable her alcohol/drug use, as they have in the past. In implementing the bottom-line script, family members have to be willing to follow through with their bottom lines. Otherwise, there is no point in stating them. For example, if Audrey had refused to go into treatment, the bottom-line stage of the intervention would have followed:

Roger:	Audrey, I care about you. You've been a person that I greatly admire. I love you a great deal. I'm frightened about the alcohol and drugs. I'm fearful that you'll hurt yourself or the kids. If you don't go into treatment, I can no longer come over to the house. I won't see you until you get help. It's too difficult for me to see you killing yourself.
Ann:	Audrey, I love you. You are a wonderful, caring mother. I see you teaching the kids to read and doing wonderful, creative things with them. You'll always be my daughter. If you don't get help I'm going to have my lawyer start the process of declaring you unfit. It hurts me to do this, but I can't allow the children to be abused the way they are. I know it's the alcohol and drugs, and I want us to get help. [Ann cries.]
Mary:	We've been more than sisters. We've been best friends. If you don't get help, I'll help Mom get the children in a safe environment and away from the alcohol and drugs. I'm afraid for the children and their future. Please get help.

The bottom-line script is implemented only if the individual refuses to get treatment. If the individual still refuses treatment after the bottom line, the intervention is over, and the family members implement the bottom line.

Postintervention

The trauma and emotion of the intervention affects all of the family members and friends involved in the intervention. Immediately after a successful intervention, families are often relieved and hopeful. However, the road to family recovery has just begun. The family should get together with the interventionist within a month, prior to the end of the 30-day inpatient program attended by the person who was intervened on. This gives the family members an opportunity both to reflect on their original commitment to the intervention and on their own enabling behavior and to reiterate their commitment to recovery.

⚔ In Review

- According to Miller and C' de Baca (2001) a quantum change (i.e., epiphany) has the following common elements:

    Vivid
    Surprising
    Benevolent
    Enduring
    Involves conflict

- Common defense components of resistance to change (Choppel) are

    Denial
    Minimization
    Projection
    Rationalization
    Compliance
    Conflict avoidance
    Obsessive focusing
    Acting out

- Any attempt to create awareness in others that they might have a problem with alcohol or other drugs is an intervention.
- Intervention is defined as an action taken by someone to interrupt the progression of problems related to alcohol/drugs.
- Motivational interviewing is a client-centered approach that uses cognitive therapy, systems theory, and social psychology.
- The stages of motivational interviewing are

    Precontemplative
    Contemplative
    Determination
    Action
    Maintenance
    Relapse prevention

- There are eight general motivational strategies:

    - Giving advice
    - Removing barriers
    - Providing choice
    - Decreasing desirability
    - Practicing empathy
    - Providing feedback
    - Clarifying goals
    - Helping active

- The general principles of motivational interviewing are
  - Express empathy
  - Develop discrepancy
  - Avoid argumentation
  - Roll with resistance
  - Support self-efficiency
- Stages of a formal intervention:
  - Assessment
  - Preintervention
  - Intervention
  - Postintervention

⚹ Discussion Questions

1. Discuss a change you are considering and/or have made, and outline your beliefs, thinking, and actions for each of the stages of change as they apply:

   Precontemplative
   Contemplative
   Determination
   Action
   Maintenance
   Relapse prevention

2. Discuss your opinion and concerns about a formal intervention. Organize a debate on the topic.
3. Plan a role-play of a formal intervention, assign a counselor, family roles, and the person you are going to intervene on, and go through the stages from assessment, preintervention, intervention, and postintervention.
4. Discuss any interventions, informal or formal, in which you have been involved.

⚹ References

Alcoholics Anonymous. 1976. *The history of how many thousands of men and women have recovered from alcoholism,* 3d ed. World Services.

Brazier, David. 1997. *The feeling Buddha.* New York: Fromm International.

Chodron, Pema. 2000. *When things fall apart, heart advice for difficult times.* Boston: Shambhala.

Epstein, Mark. 1998. *Going to pieces without falling apart, lessons from meditation and psychotherapy.* New Jersey: Broadway Books.

Johnson, Vernon E. 1986. *How to help someone who doesn't want help.* Minneapolis: Johnson Institute Books.

Miller, William, and Janet C'de Baca. 2001. *Quantum change: When epiphanies and sudden insights transform ordinary lives.* New York: Guilford Press.

Miller, William, and Stephen Rollnick. 1991. *Motivational interviewing: Preparing people to change addictive behavior.* New York: Guilford Press.

Sapadin, L., and J. Maguire. 1997. *It's about time: The 6 styles of procrastination and how to overcome them.* New York: Penguin.

Disorders Co-occurring with Substance Abuse

Objectives

1. Define co-occurring disorders.
2. Identify the number of people who suffer from serious mental illness (SMI) and SMI and substance abuse-disorders.
3. Explain the differences between a depressive mood and an affective disorder.
4. Assess the depth of depression disorders using the criteria of severity, frequency, duration, and precipitating factors.
5. Describe in diagnostic criteria the differences between the following affective disorders:
   - Major depression
   - Dysthmia
   - Atypical depression
   - Bipolar disorder
   - Cyclothymic disorder
6. Describe and identify common characteristics of the manic phase of bipolar disorder.
7. Explain the difference between a personality trait and a personality disorder.
8. Explain the relationship between personality disorders and substance-abuse disorders.
9. Identify diagnostic criteria and assessment questions you might ask in identifying antisocial personality disorder.
10. Identify the characteristics of borderline personality disorder and describe how alcohol/drugs complicate(s) the disorder.
11. List some assessment questions you might ask to help identify abandonment issues and abandonment depression.
12. Define narcissistic personality disorder and describe how alcohol/drug use complicates the disorder.
13. Explain the role of trauma in co-occurring disorders.
14. List the American Psychiatric Association's ten questions for the treatment of psychiatric disorders.

∗ Introduction

A number of psychiatric disorders are prevalent with substance-abuse disorders. We commonly call these "dual disorders" or disorders co-occurring with substance abuse. They include both affective (feeling) disorders and personality disorders.

Affective disorders that often co-occur with substance abuse are depression and bipolar disorder; personality disorders are most frequently narcissistic disorder and borderline personality disorder.

This chapter explores the dimensions of these co-occurring disorders and how they interact with substance abuse.

⋇ Definition of a Co-occurring Disorder

The terms *dual disorders, comorbid disorders,* and *co-occurring disorders* have been used interchangeably to describe the condition of having both a psychiatric diagnosis and a chemical dependency diagnosis. The symptoms produced by psychiatric disorders and chemical dependency can overlap. The concept reminds us of this overlap in symptoms and highlights the need to make an accurate diagnosis, so that appropriate treatment can be provided.

Until recently, counselors in the mental health and chemical dependency fields took a somewhat provincial outlook. Each has accused the other of minimizing the importance of his or her own perspective. In many ways, the situation has become like the story of the blind men asked to describe an elephant. Each described it according to the body part he could touch but without regard to the remaining, unseen portions of the beast. Recent years have witnessed the emergence of a greater understanding and acceptance of the dual disorders or co-occurring disorder concept. Increasingly, members of both fields are educating themselves about each other's areas of specialty.

Clinically, we think of patients as existing on a continuum between purely psychiatric disorders at one end and purely chemical dependency problems on the other. Most patients lie somewhere between the extremes. An evaluation would take into account the relative position on the continuum. Today, it is rare to find a patient who has purely one condition, either psychiatric or chemical dependency. Many psychiatric patients are affected by alcohol/drugs, and many patients with alcohol/drug problems have psychiatric symptoms.

It is common to see prevalence rates of substance abuse ranging between 40 and 60 percent of any psychiatric population. A report of a commission of mental health providers in New York State estimated that, of the 75,000 individuals hospitalized in New York each year for psychiatric conditions, close to 40,000 admissions "involve persons with dual disabilities or a serious psychiatric illness and an alcohol and/or drug abuse condition" (Bauer 1987).

A more recent, community-based survey of 20,291 people found that 53 percent of the surveyed drug abusers and 39 percent of the alcohol abusers had at least one mental illness, and 29 percent of the mentally ill in the survey abused either alcohol or drugs (Regier et al. 1990). National surveys report co-occurring disorders (COD) as common in the adult population. The National Survey on Drug Use and Health (NSDUH) estimated that in 2002, 4 million adults met the criteria for both serious mental illness (SMI) and substance dependence and abuse. According to the survey, among adults with SMI, 23.2 percent were dependent on or abused alcohol or illicit drugs, while the rate among adults without SMI was only 8.2 percent (Sacks and Ries 2004).

The evolution of the co-occurring disorders concept has paralleled our expanded understanding of the biological nature of both alcoholism and certain mental disorders.

The 1990s was labeled the "decade of the brain," as we learned more about brain functions and their relation to affect. Research suggests that the causes of mental illness such as schizophrenia, depression, anxiety disorders, and affective disorders are substantially, if not primarily, biological. Genetic research of families with a history of alcoholism has supported the biological nature of alcoholism. There is a higher rate of alcoholism and other drug abuse in the families of patients with affect and mood disorders and vice versa. Quite possibly the genetic traits that predispose one to depression or other mental illness may be the same or similar genetic traits for chemical dependency.

The two major co-occurring disorders covered in this chapter are (1) affective (feeling) disorders and chemical dependency and (2) personality disorders and chemical dependency.

⚹ Serious Mental Illness (SMI) and Substance Abuse

The number of people who have serious mental illness seems astounding in our American culture, considering our high standard of living. In 2002, there were 33.2 million adults aged 18 or older with SMI (SAMHSA June 2004) (see Figure 10.1).

Of the adults who had SMI, 13.4 million had only SMI, and 4 million had SMI and a substance-abuse disorder. SMI and a substance-abuse disorder is a co-occurring disorder that has gained much needed attention over the last few years. The substance abuse tends to complicate an already complicated situation for the severely mentally ill person. These patients are very challenging and require a more organized effort to stabilize (see Figure 10.2).

Of those, 12.2 percent, or 4 million, had a co-occurring disorder of both serious mental illness and a substance-use disorder. Only 12 percent of this population received treatment for both mental health and substance-abuse disorders, indicating

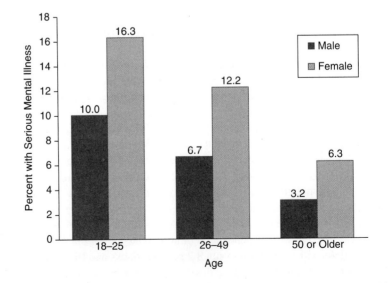

FIGURE 10.1   *Serious Mental Illness among Adults Aged 18 or Older, by Age and Gender: 2002*

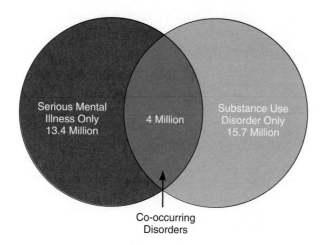

FIGURE 10.2   *Co-occurrence of Serious Mental Illness and Substance Use Disorders among Adults Aged 18 or Older: 2002*
Note: Circles are not drawn to scale.
SOURCE: SAMHSA, Office of Applied Studies. National Survey on Drug Use and Health, 2002.

the limited extent of adequate assessment and treatment approaches. Many of these co-occurring disorder patients (52%) received no treatment at all, or treatment for only one disorder (34% for mental disorder; only 2% for substance-abuse disorder) (SAMHSA Sept/Oct 2004) (see Table 10.1 for further discussion).

TABLE 10.1

Facts about Serious Mental Illness (SMI)

- In 2002, there were 17.5 million adults aged 18 or older with SMI during the 12 months prior to being interviewed. This represents 8.3 percent of all adults in the United States. On average, adults with SMI were younger, less educated, and more likely to be female than adults without SMI.

- Adults with SMI were more likely to be either unemployed or not in the labor force (36.4 percent) than were persons without SMI (31.2 percent).

- Of the three age groups considered in this report, *adults aged 18 to 25 had the highest rate of SMI (13.2 percent), followed by adults aged 26 to 49 (9.5 percent) and adults aged 50 or older (4.9 percent).*

- Overall, the rate of SMI was almost twice as high among females (10.5 percent) as it was among males (6.0 percent).

- The two racial/ethnic groups with the highest prevalence of SMI were those reporting more than one race (13.6 percent) and American Indians and Alaska Natives (12.5 percent).

- In 2002, there were 5 million adults aged 18 or older who had SMI and used an illicit drug in the past year. This represented 28.9 percent of all persons with SMI.

SOURCE: SAMHSA 2004.

⊀ Affective (Feeling) Disorders and Substance-Use Disorders

The Difference Between a Depressive Mood and a Depressive Disorder

It is common to feel down, sad, or even depressed after experiencing disappointment, frustration (blocked goal), setback, or trauma. Feelings of sadness, melancholia, grief, and loss are normal aspects of life. Working through the grief or loss is an essential feature of growth. However, when these depressive feelings persist beyond the common period of time to work through them, an affective disorder may be developing.

It is also normal to feel bad or low in early recovery from abusing alcohol and other drugs. Some of this is due to withdrawal from the chemicals, but problems in mood may persist even after withdrawal. Chemical dependency causes financial, civil, criminal, interpersonal, and family problems in the lives of many alcoholics/addicts—all of which can cause lasting pain. However, what is going on if the depression continues beyond normal alcohol/drug recovery?

Everyone experiences symptoms of depression from time to time. When symptoms become severe and persistent, however, diagnosis of an affective (feeling) disorder could be warranted. As researchers and clinicians have used various systems of classifying depression over the years, they have increasingly recognized the different types and subtypes of depression. What differentiates various types from one another is their **severity, frequency, duration,** and **precipitating factors.**

Affective disorders are different from the normal emotions of feeling down or sad. The following questions may help distinguish common depressive feelings from an affective disorder:

Severity: How deep is your depression? How low do you feel? Are you suicidal or self-destructive?

Frequency: How often do you feel depressed?

Duration: How long does the depression last? Are there periods when you are not depressed?

Precipitating factors: What triggers your depression? Do you know what is causing your depression?

Regardless of what causes depression initially, once it has been present for long enough it locks in and takes on a life of its own. This is another way of saying that the brain changes physiologically in response to internal or external events that have persisted for a sufficient time. After the physiological changes have taken place, a number of biological, or physical, signs of depression emerge. These *vegetative signs* include disturbances in the basic biological functions that the brain regulates. Vegetative signs of depression include the following:

- Disrupted sleep patterns
- Difficulty with appetite and weight regulation

- Decreased cognitive functioning (including problems with concentration, memory, and problem solving)
- Decreased libido, or sex drive
- Lack of motivation, decreased energy (anergia)
- Difficulty experiencing pleasure (anhedonia)

Denial and Depression

The psychological aspects of depression bring with it feelings of shame, as outlined in Chapter 6. Many individuals are extremely frightened to be labeled depressed, labeled manic-depressive (with bipolar disorder), or labeled with other affective and mood-cycling disorders. The denial of these feeling disorders is often self-medicated with the use of alcohol/drugs in an attempt to avoid the shame. Despite the fact that a vast majority (99 percent) of individuals suffering from affective disorders can be helped, only one in three depressed individuals seeks help. It is estimated that over 10 million people suffer from depressive illness, and 2 million people suffer from bipolar disorder. Serious depressions are "whole body" disorders affecting body, feelings, thoughts, and behaviors (U.S. Department of Health and Human Services 1987). "Substance use disorders and mood and anxiety disorders that develop independently of intoxication and withdrawal are among the most prevalent psychiatric disorders in the United States" (Grant et al. 2004).

Most people view themselves as weak and inferior in not having the will power to overcome depressive illness. This is much like the denial of the disease of alcoholism and drug addiction. In fact, depressive disorder is a disease much like alcohol/drug addiction in that it has a known etiology, gets progressively worse over time, and has significant negative consequences if untreated. Case Study 10.1 presents an example of an individual who suffers from both depression and substance addiction.

Categories of Mood Disorders

Common affective disorders include the following:

- Major depression
- Dysthymic disorder (a low-grade depression)
- Atypical depression (depression related to sudden loss)
- Organic depression
- Bipolar disorder, formerly referred to as manic-depressive illness (severe mood swings)
- Cyclothymic (mood-cycling) disorder (a less severe form of mood swings)

Case studies in this section give you an understanding of the dynamics of the affective disorder and chemical dependency. In some case studies, chemical dependency is the primary diagnosis. Other case studies demonstrate that, even after sobriety, the underlying affective disorder still persists and requires treatment.

Many mood disorders are treated with antidepressant medications.

Case Study 10.1
Major Depression and Addiction
Elaine

Elaine is a 53-year-old divorced woman with two previous psychiatric hospitalizations for severe depression. These were treated successfully with antidepressant medication. She returned to her psychiatrist after a 10-year absence due to progressively worsening depression for 2 months. Further questioning revealed that she had experienced anxiety symptoms last year and her gynecologist had prescribed diazepam (Valium). She took the medication in low doses as prescribed until sustaining a neck injury in an automobile accident 5 months ago. At that time, the doctor prescribed narcotic pain medication. Initially, she took the pain medication as prescribed but later took the medication in increasing doses. She found that her pain and anxiety symptoms were manageable with the higher doses and she simultaneously increased her daily dose of Valium, taking a moderate to heavy dose at night to help her overcome her physical discomfort and to improve sleep. Her escalating use of the medication surprises her, since she had never used similar drugs in the past and had avoided alcohol and street drugs because of religious beliefs. She is troubled by a growing preoccupation with suicide and fears that she may commit suicide, as her mother and maternal grandmother did. A physical exam by her internist later in the day revealed slightly elevated blood pressure, sweaty palms, and slightly dilated pupils.

Discussion Questions

What are the signs of depression?
What role do you think age played in this case?
Can you describe a case that is similar to this and identify signs?
Give some examples of maladaptive behaviors as a result of depression.

Major Depression

This depressive syndrome may occur as a single episode or as repeated episodes over the years. This diagnosis generally connotes a severe depressive episode with fairly clear onset and accompanying vegetative signs. Individuals suffering from major depression exhibit difficulty in the most basic of tasks (e.g., getting out of bed, brushing their teeth).

Episodes of major depression typically last from 6 to 12 months and then clear sometimes even without treatment. However, an episode can last significantly longer. Episodes of depression that are longer in duration require adequate and careful attentiveness and sensitivity to potential suicide attempts. (See Table 10.2.)

Case Study 10.2 takes a look at a familiar storybook character who suffers from depression.

T A B L E   1 0 . 2

Diagnostic Criteria of Major Depressive Disorder

A. At least five of the following symptoms have been present during the same
two-week period and represent a change from previous functioning; at least
one of the symptoms is either (1) depressed mood or (2) loss of interest or
pleasure. (Do not include symptoms that are clearly due to a physical condition,
mood-incongruent delusions or hallucinations, incoherence, or marked loosening
of associations.)

1. Depressed mood (or can be irritable mood in children and adolescents) most
of the day, nearly every day, as indicated either by subjective account or
observation by others

2. Markedly diminished interest or pleasure in all, or almost all, activities most
of the day, nearly every day (as indicated either by subjective account or
observation by others of apathy most of the time)

3. Significant weight loss or weight gain when not dieting (e.g., more than
5% of body weight in a month), or decrease or increase in appetite nearly
every day (in children, consider failure to make expected weight gains)

4. Insomnia or hypersomnia nearly every day

5. Psychomotor agitation or retardation nearly every day (observable by others,
not merely subjective feelings of restlessness or being slowed down)

6. Fatigue or loss of energy nearly every day

7. Feelings of worthlessness or excessive or inappropriate guilt (which may
be delusional) nearly every day (not merely self-reproach or guilt about
being sick)

8. Diminished ability to think or concentrate, or indecisiveness, nearly every
day (either by subjective account or as observed by others)

9. Recurrent thoughts of death (not just fear of dying), recurrent suicidal
ideation without a specific plan, or a suicide attempt or a specific plan for
committing suicide

B. 1. It cannot be established that an organic factor initiated and maintained the
disturbance.

2. The disturbance is not a normal reaction to the death of a loved one
(uncomplicated bereavement). *Note:* Morbid preoccupation with
worthlessness, suicidal ideation, marked functional impairment or
psychomotor retardation, or prolonged duration suggest bereavement
complicated by major depression.

C. At no time during the disturbance have there been delusions or hallucinations for
as long as two weeks in the absence of prominent mood symptoms (i.e., before
the mood symptoms developed or after they have remitted).

D. Not superimposed on schizophrenia, schizophreniform disorder, delusional
disorder, or psychotic disorder.

SOURCE: American Psychiatric Association, *Diagnostic and Statistical Manual of Mental Disorders,* Fourth Edition,
Revised, Washington, D.C., American Psychiatric Association, 1994.

Case Study 10.2
Eeyore Syndrome

The donkey, Eeyore, in the children's story *Winnie-the-Pooh,* could be clinically described as suffering from major depression or dysthymic disorder.

When Eeyore is asked by Pooh and other characters in the story, "Would you like to go swimming today?" Eeyore answers, in his low, depressed voice in a number of negative statements, "No, I'm so tired today and it's too far to walk to the swimming hole," or "I might get sun burned on a sunny day like today," or "It's too hot and I might get overheated."

Eeyore worries about everything. Instead of enjoying being with his friends, he isolates himself. Instead of enjoying the activity (swimming) and a beautiful summer day, he can't see anything positive. He is constantly in the black cloud of depression, even though it is a bright, sunny day.

Discussion

Remember, two major signs of depression demonstrated by "Eeyore" are

- anergia (a lack of energy for activities that one would normally be motivated to do—e.g., swimming on a sunny summer day)
- anhedonia (an inability to gain pleasure from something that normally would be pleasurable—e.g., playing/swimming with friends)

Dysthymic Disorder

Dysthymic disorder is a mood disorder of longer term than major depression but is a lower-grade depression. Patients with dysthymic disorder frequently comment that they have never felt completely happy, or that if they do achieve a period of feeling well, it is relatively short-lived. Anxiety symptoms, headaches, and muscle tension are frequent, in addition to symptoms of depression. (See Table 10.3.) Patients with dysthymic disorder come to assume that their own baseline mood is normal; they are frequently surprised that they actually do experience improvement with treatment. Only 25 percent of patients with major depression receive adequate diagnosis and treatment; it is very likely that the percentage is even lower for dysthymic disorder, given the less intense and less notable degree of symptoms. Case Study 10.3 presents an example of dysthymic disorder.

Atypical Depression

Atypical depression is not a common condition, as the symptoms and duration of symptoms are different from those of major depression or dysthymic disorder.

Atypical depression is frequently the diagnosis for many adult children of alcoholics. Usually, a patient with atypical depression experiences intense and sudden

---

T A B L E   1 0 . 3

Diagnostic Criteria for Dysthymic Disorder

A. Depressed mood (or can be irritable mood in children and adolescents) most of the day, more days than not, as indicated either by subjective account or observation by others, for at least two years (one year for children and adolescents)

B. Presence, while depressed, of at least two of the following:
   1. Poor appetite or overeating
   2. Insomnia or hypersomnia
   3. Low energy or fatigue
   4. Low self-esteem
   5. Poor concentration or difficulty making decisions
   6. Feelings of hopelessness

C. During a two-year period (one year for children and adolescents) of the disturbance, never without the symptoms in A for more than two months at a time

D. No evidence of an unequivocal major depressive episode during the first two years (one year for children and adolescents) of the disturbance. *Note:* There may have been a previous major depressive episode, provided there was a full remission (no significant signs or symptoms for six months) before development of the dysthymia. In addition, after these two years (one year in children or adolescents) of dysthymia, there may be superimposed episodes of major depression, in which case both diagnoses are given.

E. Has never had a manic episode or an unequivocal hypomanic episode

F. Not superimposed on a chronic psychotic disorder, such as schizophrenia or delusional disorder

G. It cannot be established that an organic factor initiated and maintained the disturbance—e.g., prolonged administration of an antihypertensive medication.

SOURCE: American Psychiatric Association, *Diagnostic and Statistical Manual of Mental Disorders,* Third Edition, Revised, Washington, D.C., American Psychiatric Association, 1987.

---

depressions in response to interpersonal loss or threatened interpersonal loss. We may, in fact, be talking about a condition similar to that described by James Masterson (1976) as abandonment depression.

This condition is common in patients who may also have severe personality disturbances, such as borderline personality disorder. Psychodynamically, a sudden severe depression in response to feelings of loss, rejection, and/or abandonment may be related to a childhood loss so traumatic that it triggers this depression when feelings of loss are activated in present-day situations.

Atypical depression is also different because these patients may not report a loss of appetite and insomnia but, instead, experience an increase in appetite and sleep. Perhaps this is also indicative of the frequent problems in body image, binge patterns of eating, and other eating disorders that these clients exhibit. Patients with atypical depression may increase alcohol/drug use in a similar manner.

Case Study 10.4 presents an example of atypical depression.

Case Study 10.3
Dysthymic Disorder
Duane

Duane is a 39-year-old married male who completed inpatient treatment for alcoholism and cocaine dependence nearly 3 years ago. Since then he has maintained sobriety while regularly attending his aftercare counseling sessions and cocaine and Alcoholics Anonymous meetings. He has also been involved in individual and group counseling to deal with the effects of growing up in an alcoholic and emotionally abusive family system. Despite these efforts, he continues to experience symptoms of low energy, periods of irritability, and an inability to have fun without a great deal of effort. His therapist has referred him for a psychiatric evaluation.

Most notable in Duane's history is that earlier he was abstinent from alcohol and drugs for approximately 4 to 5 months. During that time, he experienced the same depressive symptoms. Besides alcoholism, his family history includes several relatives with depression. A recent physical exam was unremarkable.

Discussion

Explain why his relapses might occur after 4 to 5 months.
As his counselor, what would you recommend to cope with the depression?
What kinds of physical, emotional, and interpersonal activities might help this client?
What kind of cognitive-behavioral approaches might be taken?

Organic Depression

Depression may also occur as a result of organic factors, such as brain tumors, head injuries, nutritional deficiencies, physical illness, or alcohol/drug use. Many chemically dependent patients have nutritional deficiencies as a result of decreased intake, malabsorption, and poor eating habits. Alcohol is especially high in calories with poor nutritional value. Other drugs disrupt the appetite (e.g., cocaine reduces appetite) and create problems in nutrition. After initial recovery from alcohol/drug use, depression may continue for a while due to nutritional causes. However, once a normal diet and vitamin therapy have been reimplemented, organic (nutritional) depression should improve.

Head injuries are fairly common, especially in end stage alcoholics, and may contribute to cognitive deficits as well as mood disturbances. Pancreatic cancer is also more common in the alcoholic population and can look identical to major depression clinically.

Prolonged use of opiates, benzodiazepines, alcohol, sedative hypnotics, and especially stimulant drugs can produce depression. Users of cocaine and amphetamines typically experience a crash at the end of a binge pattern of cocaine use. This occurs because of the depletion of the neurotransmitter that the stimulant drug causes to be released in greater than normal quantities.

Case Study 10.4

Atypical Depression

Gail

Gail is 28 years old, single, and an accountant. She is extremely shy and often feels uncomfortable in social situations. She is 7 years sober and attends AA meetings regularly. Gail cries easily whenever she is involved in conflict. She suffered a number of losses in her childhood, including the loss of her father, who was reported missing in action in the Vietnam War. Around the same time, Gail's maternal grandmother, to whom Gail was extremely close, died while sleeping in the same bed with Gail. Gail has also had to deal with the issue of having been sexually abused at 12 years of age.

After Gail began counseling, her self-confidence improved. But she still felt sad, so she got an evaluation from a psychiatrist experienced in alcohol and drug recovery. The psychiatrist recommended an antidepressant. After 2 weeks, Gail felt tremendous relief and realized that she had been struggling with depression for quite some time.

Discussion Questions

Can you describe the stages of grief (DABDA)?
How does grief get complicated by an "atypical" depression?
What would you recommend for Gail's shyness?

Bipolar Disorder

Bipolar disorder is the highest affective (feeling) disorder associated with co-occurring disorders. In other words, of all the affective disorders (e.g., major depression, dysthymia, etc.), bipolar disorder is found more often with co-occuring substance-abuse disorders. Some common themes found with clients who have bipolar disorder and substance abuse are

- A strong emphasis on depression, as opposed to mania
- Predominance of hopelessness
- Specific pattern of medication noncompliance
- Patients labeling of their substance abuse as self-medication (Weiss 2004)

The first bipolar disorder described and understood was the classic manic-depressive illness. Manic-depressive illness consists of repeated depressive episodes over the years; these episodes are typically briefer than those in a major depression. In addition, a manic-depressive has less frequent but equally intense highs, or manic episodes. Characteristics of the manic phase of the disorder include the following:

- Euphoria
- Irritability
- Racing thoughts
- Decreased need for sleep

Case Study 10.5

Bipolar Disorder

Gustav

Gustav is a 45-year-old salesman with a history of binge drinking and erratic job performance. He goes on 2- to 3-week binges every spring and uses alcohol only socially at other times. He feels remorseful about these binges. In the weeks preceding a binge, he typically is quite productive, energetic, and successful in making sales. Gustav comments that his springtime burst in earnings helps compensate for his lackluster winter performance, when he typically feels lethargic and moody. In the past, he has used cocaine intermittently during the winter months to help brighten his mood. His finances have not allowed him to do cocaine in recent years. His occupational history is notable for multiple sales jobs across the country. He has made a number of impulsive springtime moves to pursue hot job possibilities. He does not find this unusual because his father, uncle, and brother all have similar histories. Closer questioning reveals that during the springtime bursts of increased sales activity, he has less need for sleep, a feeling of euphoria, and an increased philosophical preoccupation. Co-workers have commented on his high energy level and rapid speech. He has no history of previous psychiatric treatment.

Gustav's history reveals a patient with a bipolar disorder who binge drinks when he is high. There is a seasonal component to his mood swings, as he experiences manic symptoms in the springtime and symptoms of depression in the winter. Notably, he has a family history of similar mood swings and a personal history of minimal alcohol or drug use when he is not high. He is a good candidate for treatment with a mood-cycling agent, such as lithium, and would benefit from counseling on how to manage his impulses to drink. He should use available resources for support, such as AA.

Discussion Questions

Why is this client/patient so difficult to treat?
What would you recommend for treatment?
How would you "engage" this client in counseling?
Would you get permission and talk to family members for counseling with Gustav?
What problems and sabotaging do you anticipate in counseling Gustav?

- Excessive spending
- Grandiosity
- Pressured speech
- An increased preoccupation with sexuality, religious, and/or philosophical themes

A manic episode may also include delusional beliefs and disorganization of thinking. Highs may not always involve euphoria; many patients simply become much more irritable, bizarre, and erratic in their behavior. Case Study 10.5 presents an example of bipolar disorder.

Descriptions offered by people with bipolar disorder give valuable insights into the various mood states associated with the illness (NIMH 2001):

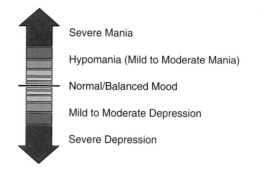

Severe Mania

Hypomania (Mild to Moderate Mania)

Normal/Balanced Mood

Mild to Moderate Depression

Severe Depression

Depression: I doubt completely my ability to do anything well. It seems as though my mind has slowed down and burned out to the point of being virtually useless. . . . (I am) haunt(ed) . . . with the total, the desperate hopelessness of it all. . . . Others say, "It's only temporary, it will pass, you will get over it," but of course they haven't any idea of how I feel, although they are certain they do. If I can't feel, move, think or care, then what on earth is the point?

Hypomania: At first when I'm high, it's tremendous . . . ideas are fast . . . like shooting stars you follow until brighter ones appear. . . . All shyness disappears, the right words and gestures are suddenly there . . . uninteresting people, things become intensely interesting. Sensuality is pervasive, the desire to seduce and be seduced is irresistible. Your marrow is infused with unbelievable feelings of ease, power, well-being, omnipotence, euphoria . . . you can do anything . . . but somewhere this changes.

Mania: The fast ideas become too fast and there are far too many . . . overwhelming confusion replaces clarity . . . you stop keeping up with it—memory goes. Infectious humor ceases to amuse. Your friends become frightened . . . everything is now against the grain . . . you are irritable, angry, frightened, uncontrollable, and trapped.

A variety of bipolar disorders have somewhat different patterns. Some patients experience recurrent depressive episodes with smaller and less intense manic episodes (hypomania) in between. During a hypomanic episode, a patient might typically experience all of the preceding symptoms except for the psychotic symptoms, such as disorganization of thinking, delusional material, and bizarre behavior.

Patients with bipolar disorder are typically plagued by mood instability; they may experience mood swings as frequently as daily. Patients who have significant mood swings, more than four times per year, are said to have a rapid cycling bipolar disorder. A growing accumulation of evidence suggests that some of these rapid cycling bipolar disorders may actually be a variation of epilepsy. Some of these patients may respond favorably to the medication that had previously been used only for epilepsy.

Mood-Cycling Disorder

The frequency of the cycling and the amplitude of the highs and lows are aggravated by alcohol/drug use. A relatively low-grade mood-cycling pattern may become much more aggravated with the use of alcohol/drugs, and the symptoms may become more clinically apparent.

Patients who otherwise have no psychotic symptoms, such as delusions, hallucinations, or disorganization of thinking, and have a mood-cycling disorder may develop psychotic symptoms, given the extra push from alcohol/drug use. (This is especially apparent with cocaine, amphetamines, hallucinogens, and even marijuana use.) Again, this stresses the importance of taking a thorough alcohol/drug history with each patient.

⋇ Affective Disorders and Suicide

One can clearly understand why depressive disorders may lead to suicidal ideation and suicide. The combination of depression and alcohol/drug use places patients at an even higher risk for suicide. Self-destructive acts that otherwise might be contemplated and dismissed are frequently acted on impulsively by those who are intoxicated and disinhibited. In earlier chapters, we discussed alcoholism and drug addiction as a kind of death wish. Disaster might also occur when a depressed, forgetful patient is drinking and inadvertently takes an overdose of antidepressant medication. The antidepressants, especially the tricyclic antidepressants, are lethal when mixed with alcohol.

The vicious psychological pattern of affect (feelings) plus shame can also contribute to suicidal ideation and actions—for example,

depressive feelings + shame = feelings of despair

Shame is exemplified as "I shouldn't feel depressed; I'm weak to have these feelings. I feel unable to control my feelings and there must be something inferior about me."

This cycle continues to the next stage of

feelings of despair + shame = suicidal ideation

The shame takes the form of thoughts such as "I'm not worthy. There is no hope; things won't change; I don't have any choices. Things are so painful and never change; they only get worse. There is nothing to get any pleasure or joy from life."

The next and often fatal stage is

suicidal ideation + shame = suicide

It is no wonder that initial or normal feelings of sadness, or melancholia from unresolved trauma from childhood, is avoided and not grieved. The individual suffering from depressive illness is fearful that any negative experience will start in motion this cycle of depression to self-destruction. As a result, feelings of sadness and emotional pain are often self-medicated with alcohol/drugs. One can see the importance of supportive counseling for depressed patients in addition to the appropriate use of antidepressant medication.

❧ Personality Disorders and Substance-Use Disorders

Personality Traits versus Personality Disorder

In describing people's personalities, we may think of traits that describe the way people behave, experience life, and interact in relationships. Personality is an important dimension that defines who we are. "Each of us is known not only by his or her physical features, occupation, and family background, but especially by what is called personality" (Nace 1990).

The American Psychiatric Association (APA) defines personality as "the ingrained pattern of behavior that each person evolves, both consciously and unconsciously, as the style of life or way of being in adapting to the environment" (APA 1984).

Most personality traits have both adaptive and maladaptive qualities or features. For example, being logical and organized are valuable traits in a computer programmer. But always being ruled by logic and being compulsively organized can also be maladaptive, since these traits may limit one's capacity to be emotionally expressive. On the other hand, a creative and artistic person might not be as suited to a situation or an occupation that requires logical, politically correct, and decisive action. We all have a mix of personality traits, which define us as individuals. When personality traits are persistently maladaptive and lead to chronic difficulty in interpersonal, occupational, and social functioning, there is a personality disorder.

The fourth edition of the *Diagnostic and Statistical Manual of Mental Disorders* (APA 1994), known as the *DSM-IV*, recognizes eleven personality disorders and divides them into three clusters, or groups (see Table 10.4):

Cluster A is characterized by odd and eccentric traits and may lead to psychiatric conditions, such as delusional disorder or schizophrenia.

TABLE 10.4

Personality Disorders

To qualify for a personality disorder diagnosis, an individual's traits and behaviors must be longstanding and must cause significant impairment in social or occupational functioning or subjective distress. The following are the eleven DSM III-R personality disorders.

Cluster A	Cluster B	Cluster C
Paranoid	Antisocial	Avoidant
Schizoid	Borderline	Dependent
Schizotypal	Histrionic	Obsessive-Compulsive
	Narcissistic	Passive-Aggressive

SOURCE: American Psychiatric Association, *Diagnostic and Statistical Manual of Mental Disorders*, Fourth Edition, Revised, Washington, D.C., American Psychiatric Association, 1987.

Cluster B is characterized by behavior that is erratic, emotional, or dramatic. This cluster has the strongest association with substance abuse, particularly antisocial and borderline personality disorder.

Cluster C is characterized by feelings of fear and anxiety. Substance abuse occurs in this group, but not as frequently as in Cluster B.

Personality Disorder and Chemical Dependency Disorder

The difficulties in differentiating between a personality disorder and an alcohol/drug disorder are often confounded by a common overlap in behaviors associated with each disorder. "Some behaviors that are symptomatic of particular Axis II disorders (manipulativeness, exploitativeness, dishonesty) may be integral or sometimes even adaptive aspects of addicted behavior, particularly among individuals who use illicit drugs" (Weiss 1996).

Personality-disordered individuals may be attracted to alcohol/drugs to self-medicate feelings of discomfort, anxiety, depression, anger, grief, and even shyness. V. M. Hesselbrook and associates (1983) reported that 52 percent of a sample of male alcoholics had a current or lifetime diagnosis of antisocial personality disorder.

Kleinman and colleagues (1990) found that, of 76 lower-social-class cocaine abusers, 71 percent had at least one personality disorder and 40 percent had two or more. The four most common personality disorders identified were

- Antisocial personality disorder—21 percent
- Passive-aggressive personality disorder—21 percent
- Borderline personality disorder—18 percent
- Self-defeating personality disorder—18 percent

Weiss and Mirin (1986), in their study of an upper-middle-class addict population, found borderline personality disorder and narcissistic personality disorder to be the most common diagnoses.

Craig (1988) used the very sensitive Millon Clinical Multiaxial Inventory and found that, of 121 opiate addicts from the Chicago area, all of them (100 percent) had at least one personality disorder and 27 percent had more than one. The most common diagnoses were

- Antisocial personality disorder—22 percent
- Narcissistic personality disorder—18 percent
- Borderline personality disorder—16 percent
- Dependent personality disorder—16 percent

This surprising result brings up the question of whether drug abuse and addiction lead to behaviors that are characteristic of personality disorders. Edward Kaufman, author of *Psychotherapy of Addicted Persons* (1995), points out that the characteristics inherent in substance abusers—such as unstable and intense interpersonal relationships; inappropriate, intense, out-of-control anger; affective instability; and physically self-damaging acts—can all meet the diagnostic criteria for borderline personality disorder and other personality disorders. Widiger et al. (1986) state that there is good evidence that many substance abusers who are diagnosed as having borderline personality disorder are really "pseudoborderline."

It is clear from the research that personality traits and personality disorders play a major role in substance abuse. The extent and depth of the role personality plays in substance abuse is confounded by the old "chicken or egg" question. Did the personality disorder cause substance abuse, or did substance abuse lead to behaviors that resemble the criteria for a diagnosis of a personality disorder? Case Study 10.6 presents an example of an individual who suffers from depression when withdrawing from an addictive substance. Case Study 10.7 describes personality problems for an individual who is addicted to alcohol.

Antisocial Personality Disorder
Antisocial Personality Disorder and Chemical Dependency

Antisocial personality disorder (ASPD) is estimated to be found in 2 to 3 percent of the male population. Of all the personality disorders, the strongest relationship with

Case Study 10.6
Depression and Withdrawal Symptoms
Evan

Evan is a 27-year-old male who is receiving inpatient treatment for his cocaine dependency. He was referred for a psychiatric evaluation because of his current severe depression symptoms. He had been freebasing cocaine for 2 to 3 months prior to admission to the treatment unit 3 days ago. Now he is feeling severely depressed and experiencing cocaine cravings.

Evan has no history of depression and no family history of psychiatric disorders. During childhood, he experienced hyperactivity and had mild learning disabilities. He notes that since beginning drug use in his midteens, he has preferred stimulant drugs ("they calm me down"). He has received inpatient treatment for cocaine dependence once previously and had 2 years of complete abstinence before relapsing several months ago. During his clean time, he experienced no mood difficulties but continued to feel somewhat hyper.

Evan is a patient who experiences severe depression as part of cocaine withdrawal. There is no reason to suspect an underlying problem with depression, given his personal and family history. He would benefit from a short course of treatment with desipramine, an antidepressant that is particularly effective for treating acute depression and cocaine cravings during cocaine withdrawal. Such treatment typically lasts for 2 to 4 weeks.

Discussion Questions

What relapse prevention strategies might you suggest for Evan? (See Chapter 11 for relapse-prone behaviors.)
Could Evan be diagnosed with ADHD? What symptoms indicate this?
What do you think Evan's prognosis is for recovery?
What would he need to do to increase the probability that he would sustain recovery and sobriety?

Case Study 10.7
Alcoholism

Charlie

Charlie is a 53-year-old married engineer at a local aerospace company. He has a long-standing, but progressively worsening, history of irritability, nervousness, and difficulty sleeping. Charlie is under the care of Dr. Greenhorn, a physician just out of his internal medicine residency. Dr. Greenhorn assumed the practice of Charlie's previous physician and golfing buddy, Dr. Barleycorn.

Dr. Greenhorn reviews the previous medical record and notes difficulties with stomach irritation and ulcers, elevated triglyceride and cholesterol levels, and persistent complaints of decreased libido, or sex drive. Charlie requests some of the sleeping pills that Dr. Barleycorn had prescribed. Further questioning reveals a history of regular heavy drinking, which began when Charlie and Dr. Barleycorn were fraternity brothers. This heavy drinking behavior persisted over the years. Charlie typically drinks three or four mixed drinks or glasses of beer per weeknight and six or seven drinks per night on the weekends. He can recall going 2 to 3 days without alcohol during a church retreat several years ago. At that time, he felt very shaky and irritable. Physical examination reveals a moderately enlarged liver, and laboratory studies reveal elevated liver enzyme levels and mild anemia.

Discussion Questions

Do you think his personal relationship with his previous physician has been a
  problem? If so, explain why.
Why do you think Charlie has sleeping problems?
What would you recommend?

---

substance abuse is with antisocial personality disorder. ASPD has been found in 15 percent of alcoholic men, as compared with a 4 percent lifetime prevalence in nonalcoholic men (Helzer and Pryzbeck 1988). Hesselbrook, Meyer, and Kenner (1985) found ASPD to be the most common additional diagnosis in a hospitalized sample of more than 200 male alcoholics—49 percent met the diagnostic criteria for ASPD. The diagnosis is predominately attributed to men, whereas borderline personality disorder is primarily found in women. The ratio of men to women with antisocial personality is approximately 8 to 1. In contrast, the ratio of women to men is 8 to 1 for borderline personality disorder.

Childhood Precursors of Antisocial Personality Disorder

Conduct disorders and attention-deficit hyperactive disorder (ADHD) in children are precursors of both substance abuse and antisocial personality disorder. Early assessment, intervention, and counseling with these young people and their families are recommended to address current problems and to prevent future problems.

Denial, Alcohol/Drugs, and Antisocial Personality Disorder

The shame attached to identifying one's personality traits as causing problems in life and in relationships often results in denial. It is easier to blame others for conflicts, problems, and personality issues than to take responsibility. A major feature of a personality disorder is that the individual may not consider the personality trait that is causing conflict as undesirable. The individual might attribute others' complaints about them as the fault of others—"The hell with them if they can't take a joke."

The traditional denial defense mechanisms of rationalization and minimization are used to deny the true dimensions of a personality disorder. Integrity, honesty, and responsibility are discounted in the self-centered behavior of the ASPD.

Difficulty *regulating behaviors* (poor impulse control, recklessness, and a failure to anticipate consequences) and *affect intolerance* (the inability to recognize, regulate, and tolerate emotions) lead to substance abuse (Khantzian 1981).

Nace and associates (1983) described alcohol/drugs as providing immediate gratification followed by regressive behaviors. These regressive behaviors include the following:

- *Impulsivity*—cannot delay gratification; has stimulus-bound decreased frustration tolerance; is impatient; overreacts to situations; is inconsistent
- *Self-centeredness*—is stubborn and defiant; lacks empathy; exhibits grandiosity; either overvalues or undervalues self; sees things in either/or, rather than shades of gray; can't compromise; exhibits perfectionism, sees self as unique
- *Passivity*—is withdrawn; is isolated; feels helpless; is "mentally lazy"; avoids self-revelation
- *Affect intolerance*—has difficulty in recognizing feelings; fears feelings; has decreased ability to endure or regulate painful emotional states

Some questions that may identify antisocial personality traits are the following:

- Do you exaggerate your achievements and talents?
- Are you preoccupied with thoughts of great success, power, brilliance, beauty, achievement, or idealized love?
- Do you often want a great deal of attention and admiration?
- Do you have a tendency to dominate conversations and activities (perhaps "showing off")?
- Do you expect special favors but feel you don't have to return them?
- Do you sometimes feel surprised and angry that people do not do what you want them to?
- Do you ever take advantage of others so that you can get what you want?
- Do you sometimes disregard the rights or personal boundaries of others?
- Do you alternate between thinking too much and too little of a person?
- Do you sometimes feel you don't care enough about other people's pain and feelings?
- Do you change jobs frequently? Have you changed jobs three or more times in the past 5 years, but not because of the kind of job or because of economic or seasonal fluctuations?

- Have you been unemployed for 6 months or more during a period of 5 years, when you might have been able to work?
- Have you walked off jobs at various times without having another job already lined up?
- If you have children, do you feel you adequately provide food, safety, and shelter for them?
- Have you spent money on drugs, alcohol, or personal items that probably should have been spent on *necessities?*
- Have you committed repeated thefts or engaged in illegal occupations (fencing, selling drugs, prostitution, pimping, etc.)?
- Have you had multiple arrests or been convicted of a felony?

Extreme difficulties in relationships with your spouse or partner could also indicate antisocial personality traits. The following are some further questions to consider.

- Have you been separated (whether legally married or not) or divorced several times?
- Have you had ten or more sexual partners in one year?
- Do you sometimes feel that you are overly irritable and aggressive?
- Have you frequently been involved in physical fights or assaults?
- Have you ever physically abused your spouse or children?
- Have you failed to plan ahead for the future or have you been extremely impulsive?
- Have you lied repeatedly, used aliases, or "conned" others to get what you wanted?
- Have you frequently driven while drunk?

The *DSM-IV* diagnostic criteria for ASPD are shown in Table 10.5. Case Study 10.8 presents an example of the problems an individual with ASPD can create for himself and others.

Borderline Personality Disorder and Chemical Dependency

The second most common personality disorder that has a high incidence of substance abuse is borderline personality disorder. A number of studies have reported co-occurring substance abuse and borderline personality disorder—43 percent (Koenigsberg et al. 1985), 28 percent (Johnson and Connelly 1981), and 13 percent (Nace, Saxon, and Shore 1983).

In Chapter 6, we described abandonment depression as the common factor in borderline personality disorder. As previously mentioned, the term *abandonment depression* was coined by James Masterson to describe a personality disorder that has six key elements: (1) feelings of emptiness and void; (2) hopelessness and helplessness; (3) panic; (4) guilt; (5) suicidal depression; and (6) homicidal rage.

Someone suffering from abandonment depression probably had a highly stressful separation from parent(s) or a primary caregiver early in life (18 months to 2 years

TABLE 10.5

Diagnostic Criteria for Antisocial Personality Disorder

A. There is a pervasive pattern of disregard for and violation of the rights of others occurring since age 15, as indicated by three (or more) of the following:

1. Failure to conform to social norms with respect to lawful behaviors as indicated by repeatedly performing acts that are grounds for arrest

2. Deceitfulness, as indicated by repeated lying, use of aliases, or conning others for personal profit or pleasure

3. Impulsivity or failure to plan ahead

4. Irritability and aggressiveness, as indicated by repeated physical fights or assaults

5. Reckless disregard for safety of self or others

6. Consistent irresponsibility, as indicated by repeated failure to sustain consistent work behavior or honor financial obligations

7. Lack of remorse, as indicated by being indifferent to or rationalizing having hurt, mistreated, or stolen from another

B. The individual is at least 18 years.

C. There is evidence of conduct disorder with onset before age 15 years.

D. The occurrence of antisocial behavior is not exclusively during the course of schizophrenia or a manic episode.

SOURCE: American Psychiatric Association, *Diagnostic and Statistical Manual of Mental Disorders,* Fourth Edition, Washington, D.C., American Psychiatric Association, 1994.

of age). The separation could have been caused by natural events (death, separation, divorce, health, etc.), or the parent(s) might not have been emotionally available.

Some common questions that may help identify abandonment follow. Did you have parents or guardians who

- Were not open or available to you physically and emotionally?
- Attacked you verbally or physically or blamed you for many of their problems?
- Gave mixed messages, called *double binds,* saying one thing but meaning something else?
- Had unreasonably high expectations or standards for you or had ambiguous expectations of how you should behave, what you should do, and how you should feel?
- Did not show you warmth or sensitivity, did not make you feel secure or safe, or did not pay much attention to your feelings, concerns, and conflicts?
- Discounted your sense of self or violated your physical and psychological boundaries, such as by committing physical, emotional, or sexual violations?
- Disparaged, blamed, or rejected you if you had any difficulty with developmental tasks?

Case Study 10.8
Antisocial Personality Traits

Tony

Tony is a 24-year-old construction worker. He says he began working after leaving high school at the age of 15. As a child, he was hyperactive, and his behavior problems caused him to perform poorly in school. Thus, school was frustrating for Tony and his teachers.

Tony told lies, stole, and fought with other children. His family took him to a counselor (a behavioral specialist) after Tony repeatedly set fires. During one school year, Tony was treated with Ritalin, a medication that helps children calm down and stay focused, and he did better in school. But during summer vacation he stopped taking the medication and refused to resume taking it the next fall.

Since dropping out of high school, Tony has held a number of jobs. Usually he gets fired because he fights with his co-workers or doesn't show up for work; this irritates Tony, who feels victimized. Although his employment—or lack of it—has caused financial problems, Tony admits that he has lied and not paid his bills. He tells friends, creditors, and bill collectors, "The check is in the mail," or "I'll send the payment as soon as. . . ." Although he has a relationship with a woman, he has also had several one-night stands with other women he has met at bars. He has snorted and smoked cocaine, often squandering his money while partying with friends and women he picks up. His parents have bailed him out financially several times. Tony's attitude was "They have the money, so they should be able to help me out."

After two DUIs, Tony was referred to a chemical dependency program as part of a deferred prosecution. He is now slowly working on both his chemical dependency and his personality problems.

Discussion Questions

What is your prediction for Tony's sobriety?
What would help Tony stay sober?
Do you think Tony could be "rigorously honest"?

- Disregarded, ridiculed, blamed, or teased you?
- Jokingly or seriously threatened to abandon or leave you?
- Made you feel that your fears were unwarranted or inappropriate?
- Did not understand you or were insensitive to your needs and desires?

Patients with borderline personality disorder have a marked instability of mood and often form intense interpersonal attachments. They typically feel abandoned and rejected during instances of real or perceived interpersonal loss. Many borderline patients engage in repeated self-destructive or suicidal acts during episodes of intense depression and despair. Theoretical explanations of the origin of this personality disorder range from developmental to biochemical explanations. In all probability, the condition is a result of both nature and nurture (i.e., inadequate bonding and parenting during early years and a genetic predisposition). Most clinicians agree that borderline patients have a great deal of difficulty regulating their degree of attachment to others. They want the closeness and trust that intimacy brings but fear the dependency, vulnerability, and possible rejection that may occur. Not surprisingly, these patients have a high incidence of chemical dependency as they attempt to blunt the intensity of their emotions by using alcohol/drugs. They are especially prone to becoming dependent on addicting prescription drugs, such as benzodiazepines. Their impulsivity, frequent thoughts of suicide, and substance abuse make them especially at risk when prescribed psychiatric medication. Many psychiatric medications are lethal when taken in amounts only 5 to 10 times the usual dosage, especially if the individual is already toxic with alcohol or drugs.

Abstinence from alcohol/drugs is essential in treating borderline patients, as their already fragile mood stability is quite sensitive to alcohol/drugs. Such patients generally need psychotherapy. When medication management is indicated, doctors commonly prescribe antidepressant or mood-cycling agents. Which medication the patient receives depends on the clinical symptoms that are most troublesome (more on treatment of dual disorders appears in Chapter 11).

Do you have a pattern of unstable and intense personal relationships? For instance, does your attitude about your relationships keep changing? Do you idealize or romanticize your friends? Do you put them down, manipulate them, or often use them to meet your own needs? Do you find yourself treating some friends very well and some very poorly? Do you have intense anger that is not really justified? Or do you lack control of your anger? Are you concerned about your self-image, your gender identity, your long-term goals or career choice, your friendship patterns, your values, or your loyalties? (If you are concerned, you might have thoughts like these: "*Who am I?*" or "*I feel just like my sister when I'm good.*") Do you have deep mood swings? Are you depressed when alone? Do you try very hard to avoid being alone? Do you feel empty or bored most of the time?

Table 10.6 lists the *DSM-IV* diagnostic criteria for borderline personality disorder. Case Study 10.9 illustrates the dual disorder of borderline personality disorder and substance addiction.

Narcissistic Personality Disorder

The *DSM-IV* definition of narcissistic personality disorder is "a pervasive pattern of grandiosity, need for admiration, and lack of empathy" (see Table 10.7). The narcissist can have several of the following qualities:

- A grandiose sense of self-importance
- A preoccupation with fantasies of unlimited success, power, brilliance, beauty, or ideal love
- Trouble in interpersonal relationships
- Requires excessive admiration
- Unreasonable expectations of others
- Interpersonally exploitive of others
- Lacks empathy

TABLE 10.6

Diagnostic Criteria for Borderline Personality Disorder

A pervasive pattern of instability of interpersonal relationships, self-image and affects, and marked impulsivity beginning by early adulthood and present in a variety of contexts, as indicated by five (or more) of the following:

1. Frantic efforts to avoid real or imagined abandonment
2. A pattern of unstable and intense interpersonal relationships characterized by alternating between extremes of idealization and devaluation
3. Identity disturbance: marked and persistently unstable self-image or sense of self
4. Impulsivity in at least two areas that are potentially self-damaging (e.g., spending, sex, substance abuse, reckless driving, binge eating)
5. Recurrent suicidal behavior, gestures, or threats or self-mutilating behavior
6. Affective instability due to a marked reactivity of mood (e.g., intense episodic dysphoria, irritability, or anxiety usually lasting a few hours and only rarely more than a few days)
7. Chronic feelings of emptiness
8. Inappropriate, intense anger or difficulty controlling anger (e.g., frequent displays of temper, constant anger, recurrent physical fights)
9. Transient, stress-related paranoid ideation or severe dissociative symptoms

SOURCE: American Psychiatric Association, *Diagnostic and Statistical Manual of Mental Disorders,* Fourth Edition, Washington, D.C., American Psychiatric Association, 1994.

- Envious of others
- Arrogant attitude

Combine these qualities with the abuse of alcohol and/or other drugs, such as cocaine, and you have the potential for real problems. (See Case Study 10.10.)

Trauma and Substance Abuse Disorder (SUD) in Adolescents

It is interesting to consider the diverse and multiple pathways that explain the high incidence of trauma and substance abuse disorders (SUD) in adolescents.

These possible pathways are

1. Substance-abuse disorders preceding trauma because substance abuse by the adolescent increased the likelihood for the adolescent to engage in risky behaviors that cause trauma.
2. Substance-abuse disorders interfere with the adolescent's ability to cope effectively with the trauma.
3. Substance-abuse disorders occur when adolescents try to self-medicate the stress symptoms of trauma. (Giaconia et al. 2003)

Case Study 10.9
Borderline Personality Disorder
Francine

Francine is 26 years old and single. Her alcoholic parents divorced when she was 3 years old. She lived with her mother, who drank heavily and had a series of live-in boy-friends. Her mother was physically and emotionally unavailable and spent a great deal of time at bars. Her mother's boyfriends physically and sexually abused Francine. To try to cope, Francine began using alcohol in midadolescence. She was also sexually promiscuous. She was involved in shoplifting and occasionally went on eating binges. Today, she acknowledges that she drinks to blunt emotional pain.

As an adult, she has had intense relationships with men. When a relationship breaks up, her rage and anger have been equally intense. Francine cannot cope with rejection in relationships and says she feels "empty inside" when she thinks she has been abandoned. Her sudden shifts in mood and her occasional threats of suicide have alienated boyfriends and other friends.

Although she drinks alcohol to lessen the intensity of her feelings, it ultimately causes deeper depression and leads to impulsive, self-destructive behavior. Several times, when her relationships have broken up, Francine has taken overdoses and cut her wrists.

Francine ended a previous therapy after three or four sessions—she said the therapist was getting "too close" and she felt too vulnerable. But she is once again in counseling and is making progress in dealing with her addiction and the personality traits that have caused problems.

Discussion Questions

What is the prognosis for Francine?
What would help her to maintain recovery and sobriety?
Do you think her problems in relationships are important? Explain.
Do you think she would benefit from all-women AA meetings and/or a women's
    therapy group? Why? Explain.

⚹ Treatment of Disorders Co-occurring with Substance Abuse

Treatment of co-occurring disorders means addressing both the mental illness and the substance abuse. Treating one and ignoring the other will only result in relapse. American Psychiatric Association (1994) Practice Guidelines for the Treatment of Psychiatric Disorders include these:

1. Establish and maintain a therapeutic alliance with the client.
2. Manage the client's psychiatric (or substance use) symptoms and monitor the status of these over time.

TABLE 10.7

Narcissistic Personality Disorder

A pervasive pattern of grandiosity (in fantasy or behavior), need for admiration, and lack of empathy, beginning by early adulthood and present in a variety of contexts, as indicated by five (or more) of the following:

1. Has a grandiose sense of self-importance (e.g., exaggerates achievements and talents, expects to be recognized as superior without commensurate achievements)
2. Is preoccupied with fantasies of unlimited success, power, brilliance, beauty, or ideal love
3. Believes that he or she is "special" and unique and can only be understood by, or should associate with, other special or high-status people (or institutions)
4. Requires excessive admiration
5. Has a sense of entitlement, i.e., unreasonable expectations of especially favorable treatment or automatic compliance with his or her expectations
6. Is interpersonally exploitative, i.e., takes advantage of others to achieve his or her own ends
7. Lacks empathy: is unwilling to recognize or identify with the feelings and needs of others
8. Is often envious of others or believes that others are envious of him or her
9. Shows arrogant, haughty behaviors or attitudes

SOURCE: American Psychiatric Association, *Diagnostic and Statistical Manual of Mental Disorders*, Fourth Edition, Washington, D.C., American Psychiatric Association, 1994.

---

3. Provide education regarding the disorder(s) and treatment.
4. Determine the need for medications and other specific treatments.
5. Develop an overall treatment plan.
6. Enhance adherence to the treatment plan.
7. Help the client and family adapt to the psychosocial effects of the disorder(s).
8. Promote early recognition of new episodes and help identify factors that precipitate or perpetuate these episodes.
9. Initiate efforts to relieve and improve family functioning.
10. Facilitate access to services and coordinate resources among different service providers.

Working with co-occurring disorders requires a strong team approach and good communication among mental health caregivers (case counselor, psychologist, psychiatrist, group counselor, etc.) so that the client doesn't "fall between the service gaps." This supportive team approach also can counter recurrent sabotaging by client and family members, treatment and medication noncompliance, and inconsistency in care and messages to the client and his or her family (i.e., it avoids triangulation).

For more information on the treatment of co-occurring disorders and difficult clients, see Chapter 11.

Case Study 10.10
Narcissism and Cocaine

Aaron

Aaron is 38 years old and a partner in a marketing and advertising firm. He is the tall, handsome, dark, and not-so-silent type. He epitomizes the singer Carly Simon's line "You're so vain, you probably think this song is about you." He is good looking and well educated, but his self-centeredness pervades his conversation. The first half-hour of the therapy session he talked about his success, his six-figure income, and his "trophy" wife. He then began to describe some business problems and his anxiety about some unethical and illegal business he was doing and the possibility of legal and criminal action. As he went on, he soon talked about a conflict with the Internal Revenue Service over some deductions he took and the unpaid and overdue interest on those deductions. This threatened his financial situation, which was already compromised by his cocaine binges. Upon further discussion, he revealed that his partners were upset with him because his cocaine use was interfering with business. His partners had become aware of Aaron forging their signatures, without their approval, in order to withdraw funds from the company. Aaron admitted he did this because he needed the money to repay a cocaine debt.

He was in his second marriage. He had one child by the first marriage and two young children by the second marriage. His current wife had filed for divorce and moved with the two children back east to her family.

In subsequent sessions Aaron was able to realize that his own behavior and personality had caused his downfall. The more successful he got, the more entitled he felt. The more demanding he got, the more angry and disrespectful were his interactions with others. He blamed others and held them responsible for his unhappiness. This vicious cycle continued in a self-sabotaging criticism and contempt of others that led to even more dissatisfaction, shame, and isolation. The cocaine binges would then further the downward cycle. Aaron's inability to modulate his own emotions (especially anger), combined with his cocaine binges, led to further distrust of others and, eventually, to paranoia. His periods of abstinence with cocaine (a few months at a time) became shorter and shorter, as his world became more and more chaotic.

His arrogance caused him to reject AA and other self-help methods, and he still maintained resentment about his 30-day stay in a residential drug treatment program that he had completed a year ago. He was obsessed with childhood incidents related to his parents, describing a narcissistic mother and distant father, and his constant feelings "that no matter whatever I did, it was not good enough."

Aaron tried to stay sober, but he refused to go to any self-help meetings. He tried to reestablish his relationship with his partners, but they were done with him. He went on one last cocaine binge, borrowing some money from an old friend who also used cocaine. With his business relationships destroyed, the IRS after him, and his marriage coming to an end, he had nowhere to turn. He considered suicide as an option, but ironically he was so self-absorbed that he really didn't see that as a way out. He considered a "geographical relocation" and then flew back east to try to reunite with his wife and children. That was short-lived, as he relapsed while on the East Coast, getting drunk and then using cocaine.

(continued on next page)

Case Study 10.10 (*continued*)
Narcissism and Cocaine

Aaron

Tired and depressed, emotionally bankrupt, he surrendered and entered a 90-day residential treatment program. It took him a few years to stabilize. He is currently sober for 2 years, participating in AA and a recovery therapy group, has reached an agreement with the IRS, is working in the counseling field, sees his children when he can, and is a lot more humble. Fortunately, Aaron has achieved a relatively "happy ending." Many others have been less fortunate, suffering worse outcomes, and some have died.

⋇ In Review

- The term *co-occurring disorder* refers to the condition of having both a psychiatric diagnosis and a chemical dependency diagnosis.
- Four million adults in the United States had serious mental illness (SMI) co-occurring with substance-abuse disorder. Only 12 percent of this population received treatment for both disorders.
- This chapter describes the problems related to mood disorders and chemical dependency, with specific emphasis on major depression, dysthymia, atypical depression, bipolar disorder, and mood-cycling disorder.
- What differentiates these various types of affective (feeling) disorders are their severity, duration, frequency, and precipitating factors. Common vegetative signs of a mood disorder are disrupted sleep, difficulty with appetite and weight regulation, decreased cognitive functioning (including problems with concentration, memory, and problem solving), decreased libido or sex drive, lack of motivation, decreased energy (anergia), and difficulty experiencing pleasure (anhedonia).
- Bipolar disorder is the highest affective (feeling) disorder associated with co-occurring disorders.
- Some common themes found with clients who have bipolar disorder and substance abuse are
  - A strong emphasis on depression, as opposed to mania
  - Predominance of hopelessness
  - Specific pattern of medication noncompliance
  - Patients labeling of their substance abuse as self-medication (Weiss 2004)
- This chapter also explores the co-occurring disorder of personality disorders and chemical dependency. Most personality traits have both adaptive and maladaptive qualities or features. When personality traits are persistently maladaptive and lead to chronic difficulty in interpersonal, occupational,

and social functioning, there is a personality disorder. The major personality disorders most frequently associated with chemical dependency are antisocial personality disorder, borderline personality disorder, and narcissistic personality disorder.

- There is a high incidence of trauma and substance-abuse disorders in adolescents.
- The possible pathways of trauma are
    - Substance-abuse disorders preceding trauma because the substance abuse by adolescents increased the likelihood for the adolescent to engage in risky behaviors that cause trauma.
    - Substance-abuse disorders interfere with the adolescent's ability to cope effectively with the trauma.
    - Substance-abuse disorders occur when adolescents try to self-medicate the stress symptoms of trauma. (Giaconia et al. 2003)

Discussion Questions

1. Which do you think occurs more often—depression and then substance abuse, or substance abuse and then depression? State your reasons for your position.
2. Discuss the differences and give examples of the differences between major depression, dysthymia, atypical depression, bipolar disorder, and cyclothymic disorder.
3. Explain and describe the differences between a personality disorder and a personality trait.
4. Describe treatment approaches to co-occurring disorders. Illustrate each approach with case examples.

References

American Psychiatric Association [APA]. 1984. *Psychiatric glossary.* Washington, D.C.: American Psychiatric Press.

American Psychiatric Association [APA]. 1994. *Diagnostic and statistical manual of mental disorders.* 4th ed. Washington, D.C.: Author.

Bauer, Anne. 1987. Dual diagnosis patients: The state of the problem. *Information Exchange (TIEUNES)* 9(3, July): 1–4, 8.

Craig, R. J. 1988. A psychometric study of the prevalence of DSM-III personality disorders among treated opiate addicts. *International Journal of the Addictions* 23(2): 115–24.

Daley, Dennis C., and Howard B. Moss. 2002. *Dual disorders: Counseling clients with chemical dependency and mental illness.* 3d ed. Center City, Minn.: Hazeldon Foundation.

Fields, Richard, and Russell Vandenbelt. 1992a. *Understanding mood disorders and addictions* [pamphlet]. Center City, Minn.: Hazeldon Educational Materials.

Fields, Richard, and Russell Vandenbelt. 1992b. *Understanding personality problems and addiction* [pamphlet]. Center City, Minn.: Hazeldon Educational Materials.

Giaconia, Rose M., et al. 2003. Comorbidity of substance use disorders and posttraumatic stress disorder in adolescents. In *Trauma and substance abuse: Causes, consequences, and treatment of comorbid disorders,* edited by Paige Ouimette and Pamela J. Brown. Washington, D.C.: American Psychological Association, pp. 227–42.

Grant, Bridget F., et al. 2004. Prevalence and co-occurrence of substance use disorders and independent mood and anxiety disorders: Results from the National Epidemiologic Survey on Alcohol and Related Conditions. *Archives of General Psychiatry* 61: 807–16.

Helzer, J. E., and T. R. Pryzbeck. 1988. The co-occurrence of alcoholism with other psychiatric disorders in the general population and its impact on treatment. *Journal of Studies on Alcohol* 49: 219–24.

Hesselbrook, M. N., R. E. Meyer, and J. J. Kenner. 1985. Psychopathology in hospitalized alcoholics. *Archives of General Psychiatry* 42: 1050–55.

Hesselbrook, V. M., E. G. Shaskan, and R. E. Meyer. 1983. Summary of bio/genetic factors in alcoholism. *NIAAA Research Monograph Series* 9: 159–66.

Johnson, R. P., and J. C. Connelly. 1981. Addicted physicians take a closer look. *Journal of the American Medical Association* 245: 253–57.

Kaufman, Edward. 1995. *Psychotherapy of addicted persons.* New York: Guilford Press.

Khantzian, E. J. 1981. Some treatment implications of the ego and self-disturbance in alcoholism. In *Dynamic approaches to the understanding and treatment of alcoholism,* edited by M. H. Bean and N. E. Zinberg. New York: Free Press.

Kleinman, P. H., A. B. Miller, and R. B. Millman. 1990. Psychopathology among cocaine abusers entering treatment. *Journal of Nervous and Mental Disease* 178: 442–47.

Koenigsberg, H. E., et al. 1985. The relationship between syndrome and personality disorder in DSM-III: Experience with 2,462 patients. *American Journal of Psychiatry* 142(2): 207–12.

Masterson, James. 1976. *Psychotherapy of the borderline adult: A developmental approach.* New York: Brunner/Mazel.

Nace, E. P. 1990. Substance abuse and personality disorder. In *Managing the dually diagnosed patients: Current issues and clinical approaches,* edited by D. F. O'Connell [Special issue]. *Journal of Chemical Dependency Treatment* 3(2): 183–98.

Nace, E. P., J. J. Saxon, and N. A. Shore. 1983. A comparison of borderline and nonborderline alcoholic patients. *Archives of General Psychiatry* 40: 54–56.

National Institute of Mental Health [NIMH]. 2001. *Bipolar disorder.* NIMH Publication No. 01-3679, Washington, D.C.: Dept. of Health and Human Services.

Regier, Darrel A., et al. 1990. Comorbidity of mental disorders and alcohol and other drug abuse: Results from the Epidemiologic Catchment Area (ECA) Study. *Journal of the American Medical Association* 19: 2511–18.

Sacks, Stanley, and Richard K. Ries. 2004. Substance abuse treatment for persons with co-occurring disorders. A Treatment Improvement Protocol 42. Rockville, Md.: U.S. Dept. of Health and Human Services, SAMHSA/CSAT.

SAMHSA. June 2004. Serious mental illness and its co-occurrence with substance use disorders, 2002. Analytic Series A-24. Rockville, Md.: U.S. Dept. of Health and Human Services.

SAMHSA. Sept./Oct. 2004. 4 Million have co-occurring serious mental illness, substance abuse. *SAMHSA News* 12(5): 15–18.

U.S. Department of Health and Human Services. 1987. *Helpful facts about depressive illnesses* [DART pamphlet]. Rockville, Md.: National Institute of Mental Health.

Weiss, R. D., and S. M. Mirin. 1986. Subtypes of cocaine abusers. *Psychiatric Clinics of North America* 9: 491–501.

Weiss, Roger. 1996. Personality parallels. *Professional Counselor Magazine,* January/February, pp. 15–16, 40–41.

Weiss, Roger. 2004. Treating patients with bipolar disorder and substance dependence: Lessons learned. *Journal of Substance Abuse Treatment* 27: 307–12.

Widiger, T., et al. 1986. Diagnostic criteria for the borderline and schizotypal personality disorders. *Journal of Abnormal Psychology* 95: 43–51.

Alcohol/Drug Recovery Treatment and Relapse Prevention

Objectives

1. Describe the four major treatment programs that were available from 1960 to 1980: therapeutic communities, outpatient methadone clinics, outpatient drug-free programs, university-affiliated clinical research centers.
2. Describe the impact that cocaine use in the 1980s had on treatment approaches and facilities.
3. Classify the elements of most drug/alcohol treatment programs operating today.
4. Describe the advantages of Alcoholics Anonymous as a recovery model.
5. Identify some of the reasons given for resisting Alcoholics Anonymous.
6. Describe the differences between Rational Recovery and Alcohlics Anonymous.
7. Identify and describe the stages of recovery from withdrawal to resolution and when they occur (i.e., at how many days of sobriety).
8. Describe the behavioral, cognitive, and emotional symptoms of each stage of recovery and the impact on relationships at each stage.
9. Describe the early phase of recovery as it relates to safety and stabilization.
10. List and give examples of some common denial defenses.
11. Describe the differences between the public, private, blind, and discovery self.
12. Identify and describe the eleven curative factors in group psychotherapy as they relate to alcohol/drug recovery.
13. Identify the five major family modalities for alcohol/drug treatment and some of the goals of family treatment.
14. Explain the difference between a full-blown relapse and a lapse.
15. Describe the differences between relapse-prone behaviors and recovery-prone behaviors and why we say "most relapses are planned."
16. List the many causes for relapse as outlined by Marlatt and Gordon.
17. Classify some triggers for relapse based on the categories of time, place, things, and people.
18. Explain the meaning of the Alcoholics Anonymous serenity prayer:
    God grant me the serenity
    To accept the things I cannot change,
    The courage to change the things I can,
    And wisdom to know the difference.
19. Explain the dimensions of the controlled drinking controversy.
20. Describe the special treatment needs for clients with co-occurring disorders.
21. Describe the boundaries and treatment guidelines for
    - Dependent clingers
    - Demanders

- Manipulative help-rejectors
- Self-destructive deniers

22. Describe the relationship of alcohol/drug abuse to suicide, and list some warning signs of suicidal intentions.
23. Define and describe the applications of mindfulness in alcohol/drug recovery.

⋈ Introduction

Approximately 1 million people in the United States currently receive treatment for drug or alcohol addiction. This final chapter gives an overview of alcohol/drug treatment and relapse prevention. Sobriety from alcohol/drugs is an ongoing process. Recovery is a lifelong process involving not only the recovering addict/alcoholic but also his or her entire family system.

This chapter highlights treatment issues and approaches for specific alcohol/drug and co-occurring disorders. You are encouraged to explore referenced material, take counseling courses specific to alcohol/drugs, and pursue supervised internships for more in-depth counseling skill development.

⋈ History of Alcohol/Drug Treatment

Drug Addiction Treatment, 1960–80

The four basic kinds of treatment that had federal, state, and local government support in the 1960s were

1. Therapeutic communities
2. Outpatient methadone clinics
3. Outpatient drug-free programs
4. University-affiliated clinical research centers

Therapeutic Communities

In 1958, Synanon was established as a model for most therapeutic communities, and the approach was expanded to other programs, including Day Top Village, Phoenix House, and Odyssey House in New York, and Delancey Street and The Family in California.

By 1978, a national organization, Therapeutic Communities of America, was organizing and unifying the goals of more than 300 therapeutic communities.

These communities were essentially residential programs, where alcoholics/addicts lived together in a family atmosphere, which promoted

- Addicts helping addicts to recovery in a structured lifestyle
- Confrontational and group therapies
- Adherence to the principles of AA and the 12 steps
- Honesty, drug abstinence, self-reliance, and personal responsibility through example

Methadone Treatment

The monumental methadone treatment work of Dole and Nyswander (1965) became a treatment model that spread throughout the United States. In 1980, forty-eight out of fifty states had methadone treatment programs.

Dole and Nyswander believed that heroin addiction is a metabolic disease and that a single administration of a narcotic can change a person's metabolism. Therefore, multiple administrations of the narcotic has even more potency in changing the person's nervous system. Dole and Nyswander searched for a medication to replace the metabolic need and craving for opiates (heroin). They found methadone, a long-acting, orally administered drug that eliminates the craving for heroin and other opioids. By successfully reducing the need for heroin, methadone reduces the antisocial, crime-related behavior of many addicts.

Methadone treatment involves detoxification and maintenance. *Detoxification* helps patients gradually reduce their dependence on opiates by giving them decreasing doses of methadone over 21 days. After detoxification, the individual is then drug free.

Maintenance essentially helps addicts develop a productive nondrug-using life-style. In effect, methadone replaces the devastating addiction to heroin and other opiates. Methadone does not affect the pleasure centers as do opiates, and addicts do not experience highs. The craving for heroin is stopped with the rather benign dependence on methadone. There is still some controversy with methadone maintenance because addicts are still dependent on another drug—methadone.

The treatment methods in both methadone detoxification and methadone maintenance include individual and group education, counseling sessions, self-help 12-step recovery, and rehabilitative services.

Outpatient Programs

A variety of outpatient treatment clinics existed in the 1970s and 1980s, including medically supervised programs and storefront centers. Medically supervised programs provided crisis-oriented medical services for alcohol/drug detoxification and overdose. At storefront drop-in/crisis counseling centers, treatment was unstructured, often focusing on crisis intervention, legal and criminal-justice counseling, medical care and/or health-related services, welfare and social services, employment, and counseling for family and interpersonal problems. The outpatient clinics served as a community-based entry point into the health care system for drug users in low-income communities.

University Research Centers

The drug revolution of the 1960s saw some significant changes. Drug use was no longer confined to inner-city, lower socioeconomic groups. When drugs began affecting the campus population, government spending increased for alcohol/drug research and treatment. During the same period, the government foresaw that large numbers of soldiers returning from Vietnam would need treatment for heroin addiction.

As a result, university-based research treatment centers opened, and many affiliated with the Veterans Administration. These centers tested new pharmacological aids. They evaluated medications, such as naltrexone, propoxyphene, levo-alpha-acetylmethadol (LAAM), and clonidine, for treatment of opiate craving and addiction.

Alcohol Treatment, 1970–80

Private commercial, inpatient, and residential 28- to 30-day treatment programs rapidly expanded during the 1970s. Their tremendous financial success caused these programs to become a major standard of alcohol treatment. The 28- to 30-day length of stay was developed as a standard, not as a result of empirical study but, instead, as the negotiated arrangement between the hospital-based inpatient providers and the insurance companies. These inpatient programs were also successful because they were modeled after AA 12-step principles and integrated AA self-help meetings as part of the program.

When former first lady Betty Ford entered an alcohol treatment facility, public disclosure of her alcoholism did much to bring this kind of treatment into public view and acceptance (Ford 1987). "Her forthright discussion of her alcoholism and addiction and subsequent sponsorship of the Betty Ford Treatment Center provided a turning point in the alcoholism field" (Rawson 1991).

Disinterest in Alcohol/Drug Treatment, 1970s and 1980s

In the late 1970s, public interest in therapeutic communities, methadone treatment, outpatient programs, and university research centers seemed to wane. A variety of factors caused this loss of interest. First, the anticipated epidemic of heroin addicts returning from Vietnam was not realized. Many returning soldiers withdrew from heroin on the long boat and plane ride back home. For many of these young men, heroin use was inconsistent with their lifestyles back home. Others did not have the connections at home to maintain their addiction to heroin. Most discontinued opiate use without significant involvement in the treatment system.

Second, a dramatic reduction took place in the use of hallucinogens, sedative-hypnotics, and amphetamines. The primary nonopiate drugs used by the white population shifted primarily to marijuana and cocaine. At the time, the treatment community and general public thought marijuana and cocaine had a low risk for dependency. Most experts were still referring to marijuana and cocaine as psychologically dependency-producing rather than addicting. That mistake caused one of the major drug problems of the 1980s.

Third, the confrontive strategies of some therapeutic communities got out of control. Many therapeutic communities were exposed as dysfunctional systems much like the alcoholics/addicts' dysfunctional families of origin. Fourth, there was also opposition and public disenchantment with methadone maintenance on the principle that, rather than recovering, heroin addicts were addicted to a new drug—methadone.

Fifth, the efficacy and success of drop-in counseling centers was questioned. The criminal-justice system was often in conflict with these centers because clients were protected from criminal prosecution. Funding misappropriation and failure to adequately document client charts created tremendous conflict between centers and various government funding sources.

Due to these developments, public interest in drug addiction problems had decreased by the late 1970s. Although a treatment network had been established and some promising new treatments were in development, there appeared to be a societal loss of interest in drug addiction treatment. The one drug problem that obviously was going to persist was heroin. However, heroin was predominately a lower-income, inner-city, minority problem. Since middle-class Americans did not appear to be significantly at risk from heroin problems, there was to be a loss of commitment to continued funding for new treatments. Funding levels in many of the programs dropped, resulting in a reduction in treatment slots and a reduction in ancillary services for the remaining slots. Research funding decreased, and many of the clinical strategies developed during the 1970s were put on the back burner. As the 1980s began, the drug treatment system appeared to have lost momentum (Rawson 1991).

Changes in the 1980s
Cocaine Epidemic

The explosive emergence of cocaine addiction in the 1980s challenged the alcohol/drug treatment system to develop new treatment strategies. In 1984, Mark Gold and Arnold Herman described cocaine as a major public health concern. What experts thought was a rather benign, psychologically dependency-producing drug became known as the most addicting drug to date.

Animal studies, human studies, and clinical human reports all validate cocaine as the most highly addicting drug. Thus, warnings not to try it even once are not scare tactics but frightening reality. Sidney Cohen, the most prolific writer in the drug field, predicted in the early 1980s that "if cocaine were readily available and inexpensive, this would create the biggest drug epidemic we had ever known." His prediction has come true with crack cocaine.

In the early 1980s, there were no treatment programs for cocaine addiction. This new addict population, however, soon found treatment at inpatient alcohol treatment facilities. Facility directors responded to the need by developing cocaine treatment programs. Financial reward motivated these inpatient facilities, which saw a tremendous treatment population developing. Their television commercials added taglines stating, "We treat cocaine addiction, too." The constant flow of sports figures, celebrities, and other public figures further created an attractive notoriety for these treatment programs.

The cocaine epidemic was even further catapulted into the public consciousness with the development of freebase cocaine. In the mid-1980s, crack cocaine use made cocaine available to all socioeconomic levels. Crack cocaine was marketed to new populations: those who could not afford cocaine in the inner city and young people. "Smokable cocaine, preprocessed in ready-to-smoke dosage units flooded major American cities from 1985 to today. Use of the drug in this form produced addiction very rapidly, and the availability of the drug in lower-cost dosage units made cocaine available to lower-income users. This combination produced a fire storm of addiction among lower income, minority, inner-city residents" (Rawson 1991).

Risk of AIDS

Exacerbating our crack cocaine epidemic is the AIDS crisis. The fact that the HIV virus can be spread by high-risk sexual practices and the sharing of needles used to inject drugs has identified intravenous drug users as being at high risk for the spread of the virus.

Treatment in the Twenty-First Century
Extended Length of Stay for Residential Programs

The traditional 30-day residential or inpatient alcohol/drug treatment program is the current mainstay of treatment in the first decade of the twenty-first century. However, there is the recognition that treatment for some individuals may need to be longer. Many programs extend treatment for 90 or more days. Most programs provide, after the initial 30-day program, an extended care program of from 30 to 180 additional days (usually at a less expensive residential setting). Treatment for adolescent alcohol/drug problems is even more difficult. Many adolescent programs extend lengths of stay as well. For example, a therapeutic school for substance abuse requires a minimum of 9 months. Many of these programs also offer more experiential components to break through the denial. These adolescent programs often involve wilderness experiences, equine therapy, experiential group therapies, and other experiential modalities.

The following are some of the modalities that most alcohol/drug programs now include in treatment:

- Treatment for co-occurring disorders
- Specialized treatment for trauma
- Adjunct tracks for eating disorders
- Specialized treatment for sexual addictions and sexual disorders
- Cognitive-behavioral therapies
- EMDR and other techniques for trauma
- Dialectical behavior therapy (DBT) for borderline personality disorder
- More emphasis on family members and family systems (e.g., family week at the residential program)
- Medications to reduce craving and for affective disorders
- Outpatient treatment as an alternative to inpatient/residential treatment when appropriate
- Specialized tracks for gambling addiction

❧ Need for Support
Self-Help Meetings/Alcoholics Anonymous

The most widely used approach for recovery from alcoholism and drug addiction is self-help groups. Alcoholics Anonymous (AA) was founded in the early 1930s by Bill W., a stockbroker, and Bob S., a surgeon. Both of these men found that willpower alone was not enough to keep them from using alcohol. After admitting to each other their common disease and shared frustration with alcohol recovery, they discovered that they could help each other remain sober through mutual support. They soon discovered that others had the same experiences in struggling with recovery from alcoholism, and the movement was begun. Small groups of alcoholics met on a regular basis to share their experience, strength, hope, and support for one another. In 1938, the basic principles of AA were first outlined as the now famous Twelve Steps. (See Table 2.1.)

Alcoholics Anonymous has been the most successful program of recovery to date. There are AA meetings every day in almost every city and town in the United States. Throughout other parts of the world, more than ninety countries have AA meetings. The fellowship crosses all religious and racial barriers; the only requirement for membership is a desire to stop drinking.

"There are no dues or fees for AA membership; they are self-supporting through their own contributions. AA is not allied with any sect, denomination, politics, organization, or institution; does not wish to engage in any controversy; neither endorses nor opposes any causes. Our primary purpose is to stay sober and help other alcoholics to achieve sobriety" (Alcoholics Anonymous 1978).

Advantages of AA as a Recovery Model

Lawson, Peterson, and Lawson (1983) identified the following key factors that contribute to the success of AA as a recovery model:

1. Mutual sharing by members, which provides solutions to alcohol-related problems and helps alleviate guilt by showing members that others have acted irrationally also
2. Provision of a regular support group of individuals working toward the goal of abstinence
3. Frequent and regular meetings to help members structure their time
4. Availability of AA as an adjunct to other treatments, such as counseling and psychotherapy
5. Absence of membership fees and nondiscrimination by race, sex, or socioeconomic status
6. Establishment of comprehensive goals covering the emotional, behavioral, and spiritual life of the members

A number of studies have found favorable treatment outcomes from participation in AA (e.g., Armor, Polich, and Stambul 1978; Bateman and Peterson 1971; Browne-Mayers, Seeley, and Brown 1973; Kish and Herman 1971). In 1965, a study by Robson, Paulus, and Clark found that 71 percent of regular AA attendees improved and 57 percent improved from attending no more than ten meetings.

Despite these figures, treatment programs that are exclusively AA-oriented without the incorporation of other treatment methods and modalities have been less effective. Costello (1975) found that the effectiveness of intermediate care was doubled (18 to 36 percent) when the unit converted from an exclusively AA-oriented model to a program with many treatment methods, AA being one of them.

Resistance to Attending AA and Other Self-Help Groups

For a variety of reasons, individuals in early alcohol/drug recovery often resist attending self-help meetings. Some of the reasons they give are the following:

1. Difficulty with the concept of a higher power, or references to God
2. Lack of tolerance by self-help members, at times, to

      a.   Use medication for affective or feeling disorders and other psychological conditions

      b.   Help understand that there are different types of alcoholism

      c.   Reject treatment (therapy and other treatment modalities)

3.   People are uncomfortable in group settings and are concerned with the group's maintaining strict confidentiality

4.   The disruptive influence of people (especially court-referred) who don't have a true desire to be sober

Despite these drawbacks, which can be overcome, AA and other self-help meetings have been a positive and extremely beneficial source of inspiration and hope for millions of recovering alcoholics/addicts.

Application of Self-Help to Other Problems

Other standard self-help meetings that have adapted the AA 12-step model for a variety of problems, include the following:

NA—Narcotics Anonymous
CA—Cocaine Anonymous
MA—Marijuana Anonymous
Al-Anon—for family members of alcoholics
Narcanon—for family members of drug addicts
Alateen and Alatot—for teenagers and youngsters of alcoholics
ACA—for Adult Children of Alcoholics
FA—Families Anonymous
OA—Overeaters Anonymous
CODA—Co-Dependents Anonymous

There are self-help meetings for survivors of incest and sexual abuse; meetings for those addicted to gambling or compulsive sexuality; and meetings to help those having problems with spending and those grieving the loss of a child. There are even self-help groups for people suffering from similar physical, psychological, and emotional conditions. In California, while working in a community mental health center, I ran across a group for people suffering from bipolar disorders. The group appropriately called itself the "Ups and Downs Group." Whatever the condition, the self-help model is being applied as a successful treatment modality, especially when it is integrated with a variety of other treatment modalities. Alcohol/drug self-help meetings are the most widely used modality for recovery from alcoholism and drug addiction.

Rational Recovery

Rational Recovery (RR) was started by Jack Trimpey in 1986 as an alternative to Alcoholics Anonymous and other self-help meetings. The principles of RR are based on the rational-emotive approach developed by Albert Ellis, Ph.D. The major focus of rational recovery is on changing the way people think and feel about themselves and their use of alcohol/drugs. "In RR, we learn to take control of our emotions so that we are not compelled to reach for an anesthetic when we are feeling bad" (Trimpey 1996). Trimpey, a clinical social worker in California, wrote *The Small Book* (1985), which attacked the principles of the AA *Big Book*. Unfortunately Trimpey's book is too intent on bashing AA, rather than outlining another alternative for people who have problems with AA meetings or principles.

In 1990, Trimpey set up a for-profit organization, Rational Recovery Systems, Inc. Many people had problems with the incongruity of a self-help meeting that had a for-profit motive. In 1993, a new organization, RRSN (Rational Recovery Self-Help Network), was developed as a nonprofit organization, with new bylaws and elected officers. Trimpey also developed Addictive Voice Recognition Training (AVRT) in 1993–94. Many psychologists who were involved in the original Rational Recovery groups developed a new organization, called SMART Recovery. SMART Recovery is based on rational-emotive behavioral therapy and cognitive-behavioral approaches.

F. Michler Bishop's article "Rational-Emotive Behavior Therapy and Two Self-Help Alternatives to the 12-Step Model" (1995) outlines in more detail the history and dimensions of these approaches. The article describes some of the common tenets of these approaches as the following:

1. People are largely responsible for their behaviors, including addictive behaviors.
2. A person can recover; that is, a person can gain control over his or her addictive behaviors.
3. Lifetime membership is not required; many people can recover in a year or two.
4. Labeling of all kinds is discouraged; a person does not have to call himself or herself an alcoholic to begin to recover.
5. Alcoholism may or may not be a disease; however, a person has to find a way to cope and take responsibility for his or her life in any case.
6. The value of a person is not linked to his or her behavior, addictive or otherwise. A person will not be a better person if he or she gives up alcohol or some other addictive behavior; he or she may be a happier person, a person who has better relationships and can keep a job, but behavioral change does not affect the "goodness" of the self.
7. A person is not necessarily, ipso facto, "in denial" if he or she does not accept the basic AA tenets.
8. A person is not doomed to a life of alcoholism if he or she does not accept help from AA, a rehabilitation clinic, a hospital, and so on. People can recover on their own with or without the help of professionals and/or self-help groups.

Regardless of your own viewpoint about Alcoholics Anonymous, the Rational Recovery movement poses another alternative that may help a specific population. However, the approach may also cause others to continue to deny their alcoholism and drug addiction and continue to suffer the negative consequences of their alcohol/drug use.

⋊ Stages of Alcohol/Drug Recovery

Richard Rawson and associates (1988) outlined five basic stages of cocaine recovery, which also apply to alcohol/drug recovery. (See Table 11.1.) The time periods for each stage vary from individual to individual and are based on the kinds of drugs used. The stages are

    0–15 days—withdrawal
    15–45 days—honeymoon
    45–120 days—the wall
    120–180 days—adjustment
    180–360 days—resolution
    1 year—after resolution and beyond

Withdrawal Stage

Most of the physical aspects of withdrawal clear up after 3 to 7 days. Emotional feelings of anxiety, fatigue, pain, and depression persist throughout the first 15 days. Patients require education and direction during the withdrawal phase. Once patients go through the initial physical withdrawal, they want to leave treatment to avoid the emotional issues. (See Table 11.2.)

Honeymoon Stage

The honeymoon stage is the opposite of the withdrawal stage. (See Table 11.3.) The neophyte to recovery has gone through the difficult withdrawal stage and now feels energetic, confident, and optimistic. Cravings for alcohol/drugs are usually reduced and moods improve. This may lead clients to believe that recovery is easier than they thought it would be. Unwittingly, they begin to stray from the elements of their recovery program that helped them stay sober. Their behavior becomes more unstructured, inconsistent, and at times frenetic. They may go through a manic cycle,

TABLE 11.1	
Stages of Recovery	
Stage	**Time Course***
Withdrawal	0–15 days
Honeymoon	15–45 days
The Wall	45–120 days
Adjustment	120–180 days
Resolution	180–360 days

*These generalized categories are rough estimates for periods of time when alcohol/drugs are not used. The actual time course for each stage of recovery may be quite different for each individual and alcohol or drug used.

SOURCE: Richard Rawson et al., "Neurobehavioral treatment for cocaine dependency" in *Journal of Psychoactive Drugs* 22 (2): 159–71. Haight-Ashbury Publications, San Francisco, Calif. Reprinted by permission.

TABLE 11.2

Withdrawal Stage (0–15 Days)

Behavioral Symptoms	Cognitive Symptoms	Emotional Symptoms	Relationships
Increased need for sleep	Difficulty concentrating	Depression	Hostility
Behavioral inconsistency	Cravings for alcohol/drugs	Anxiety	Confusion
Impulsive, erratic behavior	Short-term memory	Self-doubt	Maladaptive coping
Anergia (lack of energy)	disruption	Shame	responses
			(inappropriate
			actions and behavior)
			Fear

SOURCE: Richard Rawson et al., "Neurobiological treatment for cocaine dependency," in *Journal of Psychoactive Drugs* 22 (2): 159–71. Haight-Ashbury Publications, San Francisco, Calif. Reprinted by permission.

doing many things and overextending themselves. These behaviors then disrupt their recovery. This is the time when patients are most at risk to return to alcohol use, marijuana use, or other drug use. They may convince themselves that they had a problem with a particular drug, not that they are at risk with all alcohol/drugs.

The Wall Stage

After 45 days of sobriety, the largest percentage of relapses to alcohol/drugs occur, as shown in Table 11.4. Personal and interpersonal issues are emotionally experienced more fully during this stage. Relapse vulnerability increases as patients start feeling these emotional issues and begin to further sort out some of the problems in their lives and in their relationships. Patients often get discouraged and may verbalize that they "feel this will go on indefinitely." Patients may lose hope, strength,

TABLE 11.3

Honeymoon Stage (16–45 Days)

Behavioral Symptoms	Cognitive Symptoms	Emotional Symptoms	Relationships
High energy (perhaps manic)	Inability to prioritize	Optimism	Denial of addiction disorder
Poorly directed behavior	Abbreviated tension span	Overconfidence	Desire for things to return to
Excessive work and/or play	Inability to recognize	Feelings of being cured	normal
Return to alcohol, marijuana,	relapse potential		Conflict between spouse
or other drug use			or partner, family, and
			treatment

SOURCE: Richard Rawson et al., "Neurobiological treatment for cocaine dependency," in *Journal of Psychoactive Drugs* 22 (2): 159–71. Haight-Ashbury Publications, San Francisco, Calif. Reprinted by permission.

TABLE 11.4

The Wall Stage (46–120 Days)

Behavioral Symptoms	Cognitive Symptoms	Emotional Symptoms	Relationships
Sluggishness, anergia (lack of energy) Sexual disinterest/ dysfunction Insomnia Discontinuation of treatment, recreational, exercise, diet, and/or occupationally appropriate behaviors Resumption of alcohol, marijuana, and/or other drug use	Cognitive rehearsal of relapse, thinking, planning, or playing over the idea of relapse Euphoric recall, remembering the feelings and good times of drug/alcohol use Increased frequency of drug/ alcohol thoughts, dreams, and cravings Denial or rationalization of emotional feelings and reactions Difficulty concentrating	Depression Anxiety Fatigue Boredom Anhedonia (inability to feel pleasure with things that normally give pleasure) Irritability	Mutual blaming Irritability Devaluation of progress Threatened separation or expulsion from home

SOURCE: Richard Rawson, et al., "Neurobiological treatment for cocaine dependency," in *Journal of Psychoactive Drugs* 22 (2): 159–71. Haight-Ashbury Publications, San Francisco, Calif. Reprinted by permission.

and motivation to continue in their process of recovery. This is a time when the supportive elements of their recovery program need to be strengthened, even though patients may attempt to alienate those who can help. Group counseling can be especially helpful at this stage. Others in the group who have gone through this difficult stage can share their struggle and ultimate success and lend support.

Adjustment Stage

The achievement of working through the intense feelings of the wall stage gives patients new hope and energy for recovery. Patients begin to accept that this is a life-long struggle. The achievement of being sober for 120 or more days affirms the addicts' ability to be sober for a long time. This is the longest time that most patients have ever been sober. (See Table 11.5.)

Resolution Stage

Completion of an intensive 6-month program signals a shift from learning new skills to monitoring for relapse signs, maintaining a balanced lifestyle, and developing new areas of interest. Some clients may need individual psychotherapy or relationship work. (See Table 11.6.)

Period After the Resolution Stage

After the resolution stage, the individual may need to do more in-depth counseling on family of origin and family systems issues. Issues of underlying affective disorders and other psychiatric disorders may also be more fully explored during this stage.

TABLE 11.5

Adjustment Stage (121–180 Days)

Behavioral Symptoms	Cognitive Symptoms	Emotional Symptoms	Relationships
Return to activities that may have been inappropriate and had relapse potential in early stages Return to normal behavior	Reduced frequency of drug/alcohol thoughts, dreams, and cravings	Reduced depression, anxiety, irritability Continued boredom Loneliness	Emergence of long-term relationship problems Resistance to assistance with relationship problems

SOURCE: Richard Rawson, et al., "Neurobiological treatment for cocaine dependency," in *Journal of Psychoactive Drugs* 22 (2): 159–71. Haight-Ashbury Publications, San Francisco, Calif. Reprinted by permission.

The factor most predictive of alcohol/drug treatment success is the counselor's attitude about treatment. When counselors truly believe that they can help patients, and have the necessary insight and training, treatment tends to be more successful. The same holds true for treatment programs.

"Since the addictive alcoholic patient is fundamentally hostile, his behavior is unconsciously designed to arouse negative feelings and to invite retaliation. Hostility and retaliation must be constantly guarded against by all treatment personnel" (Chafetz, Blane, and Hill 1970). Many mental health counselors are uncomfortable working with alcoholics/addicts because of the hostility and resistance of these patients in complying with treatment. The alcoholic/addict's grandiosity and denial of reality causes him or her to always be just one step away from terminating treatment and to rationalize away the need for change. "The pervasive hopelessness that some clients feel regarding themselves and their lives is apt to be projected into the treatment process and the counseling relationship, so that the client feels, 'This is useless; it isn't going to get me anywhere" (Marks, Daroff, and Granick 1987).

TABLE 11.6

Resolution Stage (181 + Days)

Behavioral Symptoms	Cognitive Symptoms	Emotional Symptoms	Relationships
Emergence of other excessive behavior patterns: gambling, sex, work, eating, alcohol use	Questioning of the need for long-term monitoring and supports	Emergence of psychodynamic material Boredom with abstinence	Conflict between recovery principles and relationship needs

SOURCE: Richard Rawson, et al., "Neurobehavioral treatment for cocaine dependency," in *Journal of Psychoactive Drugs* 22 (2): 159–71. Haight-Ashbury Publications, San Francisco, Calif. Reprinted by permission.

Breaking through denial and the evasive tactics of alcoholics/addicts and their families requires a special kind of counselor. M. Duncan Stanton described that counselor as needing to be energetic to engage clients/patients and their families into treatment.

Addicts and alcoholics are constantly testing counselors' competency by pushing boundaries and testing to see if counselors know what they are talking about. Denial is the defense mechanism of addiction; alcoholics/addicts wonder if counselors are strong enough to break through their denial system. Counselors also need to conduct an accurate assessment of both alcohol/drug problems and affective and personality problems (see Figure 11.1).

Due to shameful feelings about self, alcoholics/addicts naturally seek or provoke rejection, hostility, anger, frustration, and even rage. Alcoholics/addicts test the counselor, as they do everyone in their own family systems. If counselors become provoked, alcoholics/addicts can play familiar "bad child at odds with authority" roles.

To effectively engage alcoholics/addicts and their families in treatment, counselors must exhibit a combination of both patience and boundary setting. Counselors need to be powerful yet sensitive, while recognizing both the need for limit setting and the inner vulnerability and sensitivities of the patients. Counselors must establish control of the therapeutic process, while being flexible to the patients' weak ego-strength and sensitivity to shame.

Group counseling is an effective treatment modality because alcoholics/addicts can be confronted in a caring way by other alcoholics/addicts. Each person in the group observes other group members struggling with similar issues and modeling growth and success in that struggle to maintain abstinence and sobriety.

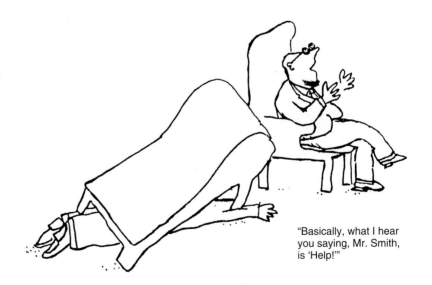

"Basically, what I hear you saying, Mr. Smith, is 'Help!'"

FIGURE 11.1   *The Need for a Good Assessment*

✻ Counseling and Chemical Dependency

Early Phases: Safety and Stabilization

In the early phases of counseling with substance abusers, the therapist must be concerned with *safety* and *stabilization.*

Safety and stabilization focus on a variety of factors that help the recovering alcoholic/addict maintain sobriety and a basic sense of balance in his or her life. Mistakenly, in their zealousness to uncover traumatic content, therapists may open up wounds without first determining if the individual has the emotional strength, resources, and support network to help him or her heal these wounds. Opening up these wounds may exacerbate already fragile relationships with family members and the spouse or partner. The result inevitably is a relapse to alcohol/drug use.

Not long ago, psychoanalytically trained therapists maintained that they could cure alcoholics/addicts. Psychoanalysts tended to approach alcohol/drug users with the fixed, often rigid perception that all addicts have personality and/or affective disorders, such as narcissism, depression, bipolar disorder, and borderline personality disorder. The psychoanalysts then tried to treat alcoholics/addicts by personality reorganization and lumped all of the disorders together. The psychoanalysts attempted to show the addicts that the etiology of their drinking/drugging was due to personality disorders. "Analysts had unreal expectations of their patients, such as that they could give up their drug use immediately while in therapy, come in at fixed times, fit into the fifty-minute sessions, and adhere to the requirements of therapy" (Brill 1981).

Probing into feelings so early in recovery often caused alcoholics/addicts to re-experience traumatic emotional issues that they were not emotionally ready or able to deal with. As a result, alcoholics/addicts did what they had done before when feeling emotionally vulnerable—go back to using alcohol/drugs.

Unfortunately, this treatment still continues today, as professionals try to validate their theoretical models, without insight into when and how it is appropriate to deal with underlying issues and feelings. These psychoanalytical issues are best dealt with when alcoholics/addicts have maintained a significant period of sobriety (usually 1 to 5 years), have a strong support system, have the ego strength to tolerate the feelings, and have the insight and motivation to work on these issues. This happens during Stage 3 of alcohol/drug treatment, as Table 11.7 shows. The first phase of counseling, therefore, focuses on strengthening both the alcoholic/addict's alcohol/drug recovery support system and the therapeutic alliance.

In the early stages of counseling with alcoholics/addicts the therapist needs to be extremely active, focusing on relapse prevention, helping the client overcome fears of and resistance to AA or other self-help programs, facilitating the development of a sponsor relationship, focusing on stress and anger management, and using other factors that will meet safety and stabilization needs. The need for interventions to stop the drinking and drugging and a solid period of sobriety are prerequisites for successful counseling/psychotherapy (Fox 1958; Tiebout 1962).

TABLE 11.7

Stages of Drug Alcohol Treatment

Stage of Treatment	Patient Status	Treatment
1	"I can't drink." (need for external control)	Alcohol detoxification, directive psychotherapy, AA, Al-Anon, family therapy, Antabuse
2	"I won't drink." (internalized control)	Directive psychotherapy, supportive psychotherapy, AA, consider discontinuing Antabuse
3	"I don't have to drink." (conflict resolution)	Psychoanalytically oriented psychotherapy

SOURCE: S. Zimburg, "Principles of Alcoholism Psychotherapy" in *Practical Approaches to Alcoholism Psychotherapy,* 2d ed, edited by S. Zimberg, J. Wallace, and S. B. Blume, Human Science Press, 1985

Breaking Through Denial

At early stages of recovery there is denial of the extent of the impact of alcoholism/drug addiction. There is denial as to the extent and consequences of the drug use and behaviors on the individual and family members.

Common Denial Defenses

Minimization
Projection
Rationalization
Compliance
Conflict avoidance
Obsessive-compulsive behavior
Acting out

Affect (Feeling), Recognition, and Modulation

Once stabilization and safety needs are addressed, the next stage of counseling may focus on affect, recognition, and modulation. The therapist slowly works with the client in labeling and tolerating feelings. The counseling can then take many forms, exploring a variety of issues relevant to the chemical dependency. Throughout this process, regular review of relapse dynamics and support for a stable and secure recovery from alcohol/drugs are maintained.

Counseling approaches explore both the conscious and the unconscious levels of feelings. The Johari window (Table 11.8) is a training model that describes the domain of counseling. Counseling focuses on all four of these areas of self:

1. *Public self:* The public self includes all the aspects about the individual that are known by the individual and others close to the individual (e.g., age, marital status, hobbies, job, interests, basic personality type).

2. *Private self:* The private self involves information that the individual is aware of but others don't know (e.g., sexual practices, mistakes in the past or present, private feelings or thoughts, family of origin issues).

TABLE 11.8		
Johari Window		
Others		**Self**
	Things You Know About Self	**Things You Don't Know About Self**
Things They Know About You	1. Public	3. Blind
Things They Do Not Know About You	2. Private	4. Discovery

SOURCE: Adapted from *Group Processes: An Introduction to Group Dynamics* by Joseph Luft. Mayfield Publishing Company, Copyright © 1984, 1970, and 1963 by Joseph Luft. Reprinted by permission.

3. *Blind self:* The blind self includes things the individual is not consciously aware of that others are aware of about the individual (e.g., personality characteristics; denial about others' behavior or own behavior; lack of awareness of interpersonal, occupational, social, and marital issues).
4. *Discovery self:* Discovery self is the category of the future. These things are not in the conscious awareness of the individual or of others and will be discovered in the future (e.g., the natural changes that occur in life's unexpected journey).

By placing a major emphasis in counseling on Category 2, the private self, and Category 3, the blind self, individuals can see changes in Category 1, the public self, and Category 4, the discovery self. When individuals are defensive or unwilling to deal with their feelings about their private selves and blind selves, there are limitations to progress and personal change. Clients would do well to follow Louise Hay's (1984) advice: "If you think of the hardest thing for you to do and how much you resist it, then you're looking at your greatest lesson at the moment. Surrendering, giving up the resistance, and allowing yourself to learn what you need to learn, will make the next step easier."

Other techniques that are often included as part of the counseling approach to chemical dependency recovery include relaxation training (e.g., biofeedback), stress reduction, anger management, problem-solving/coping skills, communication skills, exercise, nutrition, life management (i.e., balance in activities), relationships, and work.

The common goals of all counseling approaches are education; the provision of information and resources; catharsis (patients' release of emotion and feelings); connectedness and trust, which facilitates disclosure of feelings and concerns; support for positive growth; awareness and insight; and personality change (reorganization).

Group Therapy

Therapy groups have the same guidelines as individual counseling. Members adhere to strict confidentiality and do not socialize outside of the group. The group's purpose is to provide a safe environment to explore individual and interpersonal issues.

Most therapy groups are led by professional counselors trained in group therapy and experienced in the dynamics of chemical dependency recovery, family systems, and related areas of expertise. Some therapy groups have co-therapists, usually male-female counseling teams that co-lead and clarify issues in the group.

Therapy groups can take many forms. I have found more success leading all-male recovery groups, and female therapists have seen a benefit to all-female therapy groups. This avoids some of the sexual and gender-specific issues that may distract from the focus on alcohol/drug recovery. Most groups have from four to eight members to allow adequate opportunity for interaction by all group members.

As discussed in Chapter 7, Yalom outlined eleven curative factors of group psychotherapy:

1. Instilling hope
2. Sharing universality
3. Imparting information
4. Fostering altruism
5. Recapitulating the primary family group
6. Developing socializing techniques
7. Imitating behavior
8. Sharing interpersonal learning
9. Developing group cohesiveness
10. Sharing catharsis
11. Exploring existential factors

Family Treatment

Peter Steinglass (1979) outlined five major family modalities for alcohol/drug treatment:

1. Pure family therapy is based on a family systems mode, in which all family members are present at the same time in therapy sessions.
2. Individual or group treatment approaches fulfill specific criteria suggested by a family therapy theory of alcoholism, such as the concept of homeostasis.
3. Therapies involving concurrent therapeutic work with both the alcoholic and family members rely on a more traditional, individual, psychodynamic theoretical base.
4. Specific therapies designed for the spouses or partners of alcoholics
5. Supportive treatments assist nonalcoholic family members in dealing with common problems related to having an alcoholic family member.

Following are some of the goals of the family treatment modality:

1. Develop family commitment for recovery.
2. Identify enabling behaviors and counter them.
3. Encourage leveling or open communication.
4. Validate members' reality and feelings regarding the chemical abusing member and the negative consequences of chemical abuse.
5. Educate the family to the family disease concept.
6. Elaborate on concrete rules and consequences.
7. Plan and define family leisure activities.
8. Solidify the parental coalition.

9. Specify attitudinal and behavioral changes for each member.
10. Prepare relapse prevention guidelines and family response.

According to Steinglass (1979), the advantages of a family systems approach are the following:

1. It bridges the disparity between psychodynamic and stress-reduction explanations of drinking.
2. It explains diversity in alcoholic families by redirecting the focus from common etiological characteristics in alcoholic families to the common function of alcohol to maintain imbalanced family systems.
3. It gives therapists an understanding of alcoholism as a total system's behavior.

⚡ Relapse Prevention

Recognizing the Signs of Relapse

One must be trained to recognize the signs and problems that may cause relapse. (See Table 11.9.) The defense mechanisms of denial (rationalization and minimization) may be invoked to avoid looking at the potential for relapse. Many alcoholics/addicts tend to discount the stressful situations and distressful lifestyles and behaviors that contribute to relapse. The alcoholic/addict trained in relapse prevention can recognize these problem areas and avoid being blindsided by high-risk relapse situations. (See Table 11.10 and Figure 11.2.)

Habit

Alan Marlatt and Judith Gordon (1985) described the following stages in changing a habit:

1. Preparation for change, involving commitment, desire, and motivation to change

TABLE 11.9	
Relapse-Prone versus Recovery-Prone	
Denial and Evasion	**Recognition and Problem Solving**
Relapse-Prone	**Recovery-Prone**
Evade or deny the sticking point	Recognize a problem exists
Stress	Accept that it is O.K. to have problems
Compulsive behavior	Detach to gain perspective
Avoid others	Ask for help
Problems	Respond with action when prepared
Evade/deny new problems	

SOURCE: ° Terence T. Gorski, The Cenaps Corporation, Homewood, Ill., 708-799-5000. Published by Herald House Press, Independence, Mo., 1-800-767-8181.

TABLE 11.10

Analysis of Situations for Relapse

Situations	Example	Sample Number	Percent (%)
Frustration/anger	Patient tried to call his wife (they were separated); she hung up on him; he became angry and took a drink.	14	29
Social pressure	Patient went with friends to a bar after work. They put pressure on him to join the crowd, and he was unable to resist.	11	23
Intrapersonal temptation	Patient walked by a bar and just unconsciously walked in for no real reason; could not resist the temptation to take a drink.	10	21
Negative emotional state	Patient living alone, no job, complained of feeling bored and useless; could see no reason he should not take a drink.	5	10
Miscellaneous other situations	Patient reported that everything was going so well for him that he wanted to celebrate by having a drink.	5	10
No situation given or unable to remember		3	7

SOURCE: Data from Alan Marlatt and Judith Gordon, *Relapse Prevention,* Guilford Press, New York, 1985.

2. Implementation of the specific behavioral change (such as to eat healthy, balanced meals or to stop using alcohol/drugs)
3. Maintenance of change in long-term goals

Marlatt and Gordon quote Mark Twain: "Quitting smoking is easy; I've done it hundreds of times." Deciding to change a habit is easy. However, implementing the change is a bit more difficult, and maintaining change is the most difficult stage because it's an ongoing, long-term goal.

For alcoholics/addicts, the beginning step is admitting that they are powerless over alcohol/drugs and have the desire to stop using. Quitting is just the beginning of the journey; implementing the change by working a program of recovery is the next

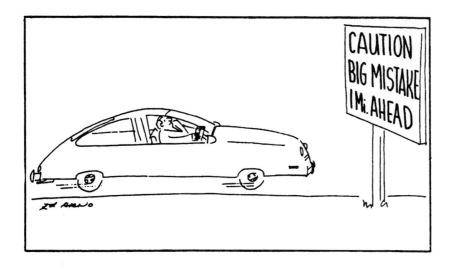

FIGURE 11.2   *Caution: Relapse Ahead*
SOURCE: Drawing by Ed Arno; © 1980 The New Yorker Magazine, Inc. Reprinted with permission.

difficult step. Maintaining that program despite stressful situations and life events is the most difficult, day-at-a-time struggle for recovering alcoholics/addicts.

The first 120 days of chemical dependency recovery are the most difficult because it is a significant period of time to establish a period of maintenance. Even after this primary period of maintenance, there is still no guarantee. Stressful situations, places, times, and interpersonal interactions may still cause a relapse. Even after a year of maintenance, there are pressures, as evidenced by the many alcoholics/addicts who have problems at their 1-year anniversary of sobriety. After 2 to 5 years of sobriety, alcohol/drug use is not a choice for most, even during stressful periods.

Case Study 11.1 describes the difficulties of addiction and recovery when both partners in a couple have substance addictions.

Causes of Relapse

Marlatt and Gordon (1985) identified three major categories that cause recovering alcoholics to be vulnerable to relapse:

1. *Negative emotional states* cause 35 percent of all relapses. In these situations, individuals experience negative emotional states, moods, or feelings, such as frustration, anger, anxiety, depression, or boredom. (See Table 11.11.)
2. *Interpersonal conflict* causes 16 percent of all relapses. These situations involve an ongoing or a relatively recent conflict associated with any interpersonal relationship, such as marriage, friendship, relationships with family members, employer-employee relations. Arguments and interpersonal confrontation occur frequently in this category. (See Table 11.12.)
3. *Social pressure* causes 20 percent of all relapses. In these situations, individuals respond to the influence of another person or group of people exerting pressure on them to engage in the taboo behavior. (See Table 11.13.)

Case Study 11.1

The Ideal Coupling

Alcohol and Cocaine

Alice was 35 and Gary was 29 when they first met. He was struggling to be a movie producer, and she was working as the office manager in an off-Broadway theater. They were opposites in many ways.

Gary grew up in the shadow of his father's accomplishments as a major Hollywood movie producer. His family was Jewish, wealthy, and had no history of problems with drugs/alcohol. Alice grew up on the East Side of New York. Her father was an alcoholic, and her mother was dependent on Valium and pain medication. She grew up in a rigid, abusive family system, with strong Catholic indoctrination.

Gary began smoking marijuana at age 13 and used hallucinogens throughout the early 1970s. Despite his drug use, he was bright enough to graduate high school and was accepted to a college film program that he failed to complete. Gary was talented and bright. His underlying shyness stemmed from a fear of rejection and a fear of failure. He would vacillate between grandiosity and hopelessness.

Alice began drinking alcohol at the age of 10 and had adverse reactions when she tried marijuana. Her drug of choice was alcohol. An extremely rebellious child, Alice had a tough time in Catholic school and barely graduated. Alice was bright, aggressive, and resourceful. Despite their different backgrounds both Gary and Alice had fathers who were emotionally unavailable, and smothering mothers who were enmeshed and needy of their affection.

The differences between Alice and Gary initially made them a good team. Gary was working on a film project in New York City when they first met. She was the perfect partner, someone who could encourage him when he was feeling insecure or down. He was the sensitive partner who represented everything that Alice didn't have when she was growing up. Alice was also able to bridge the relationship with Gary's father, which enabled Gary to get support and contacts for film projects and allowed Alice to access the powerful father figure that she never had growing up. Things were going well as Alice and Gary struggled in New York City. They enjoyed their friends, the lifestyle, and the exposure to the inner workings of the city.

Unfortunately, New York City also represented Alice's shame-based childhood; contact with her mother triggered sad memories. As a result, Alice pressured Gary to move back to Los Angeles where the major studios were and where his father's contacts could move his career faster.

Once in Los Angeles, other things moved faster, but not Gary's career. Alice quickly moved into the fast-lane lifestyle. Her flirtations and attention to others made Gary extremely jealous and angry. Before too long, Alice was again drinking heavily, and Gary's attempts to have her cut back only escalated further conflicts. At the same time, Gary was again smoking marijuana heavily. A short time later, he was snorting cocaine and eventually smoking freebase cocaine. Periodically, they swore off alcohol and cocaine. However, in a few days they would have an argument and return to using. The conflicts between Gary and his family created feelings of shame and rage. Initially, Alice was close with his family but when she began drinking and hanging out, she was

(continued on next page)

> ### Case Study 11.1 (*continued*)
> #### *The Ideal Coupling*
> #### Alcohol and Cocaine
>
> snubbed by them. This brought back her feelings of rejection, shame, and feeling lesser than everyone else. Next, they taught each other about their drugs of choice, and soon they both were using alcohol and cocaine on an addictive level. With her entrepreneurial aggressiveness, Alice began dealing cocaine to support their habit, and Gary scammed his parents for additional money to keep them in cocaine, alcohol, and the fast-lane lifestyle. They continued to abuse cocaine and alcohol; after a 24- to 36-hour cocaine binge, they drank alcohol to counteract the depressive crash of the cocaine. Many times they drank alcohol excessively, which lead to cocaine use. Most of these binges were followed by 2 to 5 days of sleep, excessive food binges, and a generally reclusive existence. Once a partnership of different backgrounds, now their partnership was based on alcohol and cocaine addiction.
>
> My contact with them began when Alice was trying to get sober and struggling to get Gary into treatment. Alice finally got out of this dysfunctional codependent relationship based on alcohol and cocaine. She entered an inpatient drug/alcohol treatment program. Two years later, Alice told me that she was the director of marketing for a drug/alcohol treatment program. She had not been in contact with Gary but suspected that he was doing drugs/alcohol with a new girlfriend and going through the same addictive cycle.
>
> #### *Discussion Questions*
>
> What problems occur when couples try to get sober at the same time?
> Do you think couples should enter the same treatment? Explain.
> Explain the codependency issues in this case.

Sometimes recovering alcoholics/addicts do not develop or maintain all aspects of their recovery program. Table 11.14 lists some of the reasons certain persons are more prone to relapse. These factors may lead people to make impulsive decisions to test their recovery by using alcohol/drugs. In effect, this testing of their willpower to go back to controlled alcohol/drug use frequently leads to relapse.

Cravings and Urges

Thoughts, desires, even dreams about using alcohol/drugs are very common in chemical dependency recovery. A variety of things can trigger this craving for alcohol/drugs, and cravings acted on can lead to relapse. The most effective way of coping with cravings and urges is to detach from the craving. "Instead of identifying with the urge (e.g., I really want a cigarette right now) the client can be trained to monitor the urge or desire from the point of view of a detached observer (I am now experiencing the craving/urge to smoke). By externalizing and labeling the craving/urge and watching it come and go through the eyes of the observer, there will be

TABLE 11.11

Negative Emotional States

Difficulty Managing Negative Emotional States	Difficulty Managing Stress Effectively	Difficulty Dealing with Feelings from Family of Origin	Difficulty with Blocked Goal-Directed Activities	Physical States That Contribute to Negative Emotional States
Feelings of depression, anxiety, rage, and distress exacerbated by feelings of shame and a poor sense of self	Feelings of confusion and overreaction to problems and conflicts	Feelings of emotional pain, loss, grief, separation, abandonment, violation, rejection, and isolation	Feelings of aggressiveness and rage Feelings of being hassled by normal daily living Feelings of boredom, loneliness, isolation, uselessness, helplessness, or hopelessness; lack of purpose in life	Physical health problems, pain, illness, injury, fatigue, specific physical disorders (e.g., chronic or recurrent pain caused by headaches, menstrual cramps, back pain) Physical states associated with prior substance abuse

TABLE 11.12

Interpersonal Conflicts

Conflicts with Partner/Spouse	Conflicts with Family	Other Stressful Interpersonal Conflicts
Once sober, the recovering person begins to see dysfunctional aspects of the relationship. Different stages of recovery: one person is working on her recovery program and the other is not actively working on his issues. New adjustment in relationship due to recovery Fear that the relationship will not be maintained or improve	Recognition of family dysfunction may lead to unresolved feelings of loss, abandonment, violation, and rejection; then these issues are stuffed and not worked out. Family system does not change or adapt to alcoholic/addict's recovery but maintains some dysfunctional patterns of communication and interaction.	Separation; divorce; or continued physical, sexual, or emotional violations Conflicts with employer, employees, friends, and other social situations Pattern of excessive fighting, arguments, and conflicts that go unresolved and are a repetitive cycle Pleasing people, avoiding conflicts, not telling others how one feels, acquiescing, and avoiding anger and other feelings associated with conflict

TABLE 11.13	
Social Pressure	
Peer Group	**Isolating**
Return to old alcohol/ drug–using peer group	Withdrawing from friends who support recovery; nonattendance or passive involvement with support group, such as AA or NA
Hang out with alcohol/drug users	Not maintaining contact with sponsor, counselor, or aftercare program
	Emotionally shutting down, not sharing feelings with others who are trusted and supportive of recovery; AA's motto is "Silence is the enemy of recovery"

TABLE 11.14
Other Risk Factors for Relapse
Miscellaneous Factors
High-stress personality type
Mood swings, temper, rage
Shutting down, withdrawing emotionally
Overseparation and overattachment
Difficulty establishing intimacy and maintaining appropriate boundaries in relationships
Personality disorders: narcissism, bipolar disorder, borderline personality, codependent personality, depression (affective disorder), anxiety disorders, obsessive-compulsive disorders, and others
High-risk lifestyle: constant changes, high-stress job (i.e., always wheeling and dealing), financial and employment roller coaster, partner/spouse relationship changes and/or conflicts, always around others who use alcohol/drugs (entertainment industry, business-related drinking, bars, nightclubs, etc.)
Financial: problems in managing finances, inability to control spending, making inappropriate financial commitments and taking on inappropriate financial obligations
Problems in employment, career change with poor planning
Trouble with back taxes and the Internal Revenue Service or other previous debt
Thinking and Perceptual Factors
Self-defeating or self-sabotaging thoughts
Painful memories and/or euphoric recall of alcohol/drug use
Return of denial and inability to consciously recognize loss of control over alcohol/drugs
Poor judgment and negative or grandiose thinking, which leads to impulsive self-destructive decisions
Overreacting, crisis building, and creating problems when things are beginning to go better
Spiritual Factors
Feeling at a loss, not feeling that life has meaning
Difficulty maintaining sobriety or having a reason for staying sober
Existential despair: not seeing a function of or reason for living

a decreased tendency to identify with the urge and feel overwhelmed by its power" (Marlatt and Gordon 1985).

Recovering alcoholics/addicts can identify triggers leading to cravings for alcohol/drugs and develop an awareness as to why cravings occur. Then the alcoholics/addicts can structure their lives either to avoid these triggers or to desensitize themselves to the trigger.

A trigger is "a stimulus which has been repeatedly associated with the preparation for, anticipation of, or the actual use of alcohol/drugs. These stimuli include people, places, things, times of day, emotional states, and alcohol/drugs" (Rawson 1989). The following lists of time, place, thing, and people triggers show how diverse triggers are.

Time

- Periods of idle or leisure time
- Periods of extended stress
- Payday, holidays, Fridays, and Saturdays
- Birthdays and anniversaries
- Specific times of the day or evening
- Vacation
- Periods of unemployment

Place

- Drug dealers' home, bars, and parties
- Neighborhoods where drugs are dealt
- Clubs, concerts, and social events
- Places where alcohol/drugs have been used before

Things

- Drug dealers' car, telephone number, or name
- Large amounts of cash, $100 bills, and bank machines
- Paraphernalia: pipes, syringe, and rolling papers
- Movies, films, and television shows about alcohol/drugs and alcohol/drug lifestyle
- Particular music
- Alcohol and tobacco advertisements
- Conferences or seminars on alcohol/drugs
- Sexually explicit movies or magazines

People

- Alcohol/drug using friends
- Drug dealers and bartenders
- Partner/spouse, relatives, and family members who use alcohol/drugs
- Sexual encounters
- Groups of people talking about or using alcohol/drugs

Case Study 11.2 illustrates the power of cravings over individuals with substance addictions.

> ## Case Study 11.2
> ### *Let's Bury the Cocaine*
> **Cocaine Addicts**
>
> Cocaine is so addicting that negative consequences often do not deter continued use. In one situation, three men who were using and dealing cocaine decided that the situation was getting out of control. They lived in a large mansion with high walls and a sophisticated security system. Late one evening, because things were getting out of hand, they dug a 6-foot-deep hole in their backyard and stored all their cocaine in this hole. They covered it up and put an extremely heavy cement statue on top. By only 3:00 A.M., the allure of the cocaine had gotten to them. Flashlights and shovels in hand, they were busy digging up their stash.
>
> *Discussion Questions*
>
> How strong do you think the allure of "cocaine" is?
> Have you ever found yourself hiding drugs, food, etc., so you can't get to it?
>   What happened?
> Can an "addict" have a small quantity of a drug?

Drug Relapse Induced by Alcohol Use

Some individuals in recovery test their recovery by using alcohol instead of drugs. They rationalize that they were addicted to drugs but never had a problem with alcohol. This rationalization is unfounded. Once addicted to drugs, people have an addiction potential to all drugs, including alcohol. It is only a matter of time before individuals build tolerance and become addicted to alcohol or alcohol use impairs judgment and they return to drugs. Case Study 11.3 illustrates the revolving-door relapse.

⚹ Relapse-Prevention Strategies

Once recovering alcoholics/addicts understand which factors contribute to relapse, they can try to prevent relapses. Also, all chemical dependency treatment programs have the responsibility to conduct relapse prevention to help maintain the client/patient's chemical dependency recovery. Alan Marlatt and Judith Gordon (1985) developed a very organized model of global self-control strategies in relapse prevention (see Figure 11.3).

Lifestyle Imbalance

You may recall that homeostasis is an organism's natural tendency to seek a balanced state. If a life is imbalanced, the individual experiences too much or too little

Case Study 11.3
Alcohol-Induced Relapse—A Need for a Stronger Team Approach
Mary

Mary, 42 years old, married with three children, was hospitalized for severe depression, panic reactions, and post-traumatic stress. She was also assessed as having an addiction to pain medication and tranquilizers. As part of her treatment plan, Mary worked with the team for co-occurring disorders (alcohol/drug and psychiatric problems) on her addiction to pills. Gradually, she was physically withdrawn from the tranquilizers and pain medication, while she received individual and group counseling on alcoholism and drug addiction. Mary also attended AA meetings and educational classes on various aspects of the disease model of alcoholism and drug addiction.

Approximately 6 weeks after her discharge from the hospital, Mary's aftercare nurse asked if it was appropriate for Mary to be drinking wine with dinner each evening. Despite inservice training on alcoholism and drug addiction with the hospital staff, Mary's psychiatrist had approved her use of wine with dinner. When asked about his counsel, the psychiatrist felt that Mary had no history of alcoholism and her problem was with drugs (medication).

Despite interventions by the treatment team, the psychiatrist insisted that Mary's use of alcohol with dinner was appropriate. Mary was only able to maintain this use of wine with dinner for a short time. Two weeks later, under the influence of alcohol, Mary tripped and broke her leg. She then lapsed back to using pain medication and alcohol. Six weeks later, she was readmitted to the hospital.

Unfortunately, there are many Marys who continue on this revolving-door cycle with treatment facilities.

Discussion Questions

Explain: "A drug is a drug, is a drug."
Do you think a person with a drug problem can drink?
What problems may occur?

---

stress; eventually, that results in a compensation in some area of life, or a breakdown. The imbalance can be evidenced by

- Too much work (workaholism) or overresponsibility, resulting in a neglect of self
- Difficulty relaxing; lack of spontaneity; and an inability to have fun, enjoy others, and feel emotions (shut down or emotionally unavailable to self or others, especially spouse and family)—"too many shoulds, too many wants"
- Too much play or irresponsibility, resulting in procrastination, laziness, avoidance of conflicts and pain, and avoidance of life-maintaining activities (passively forgetting or avoiding responsibilities)—"too many wants, not paying attention to needs"

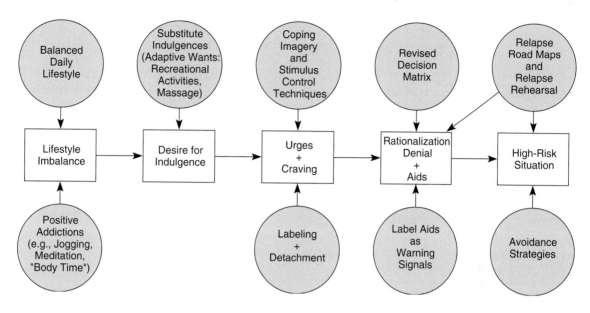

FIGURE 11.3   *Relapse Prevention: Global Self-Control Strategies*

Both workaholic and playaholic behavior have common root issues: the avoidance of taking up painful issues of self-concept interpersonal and life situation displeasure and the avoidance of recognizing and integrating true feelings. Usually, some deeper family of origin issues that have not been worked through are recapitulated (duplicated) in present-day life situations.

The alcoholic/addict has lived a life structured around alcohol/drugs. Removing the alcohol/drugs is a challenge to the individual and family's systemic organization. Triggers for alcohol/drug cravings, and potential relapse, are frequently related to the lack of organization and structure in the lives of the newly sober alcoholic/addict and the family. Structure promotes a variety of important recovery functions. First, structure redirects idle time through time scheduling, goal setting, and planning of activities. This includes work, play, vacation, recreation, and leisure time. Structured time maintains a focus on activities and is based on an integration of feelings.

⚹ Relapse Prevention
HALTS—Hungry, Angry, Lonely, Tired, Sick
Applying Mindfulness to Vulnerable States of Body and Mind*

HALTS is a valuable alcohol/drug relapse prevention tool. HALTS reminds the recovery person that when they are **H**ungry, **A**ngry, **L**onely, **T**ired, and/or **S**ick, they are vulnerable to relapse.

*Adapted from Richard Fields, PhD, 2008. *Minestrone for the Mind, Awakening to Mindfulness, 10 steps for Everyone.* Health Communications.

Over the last 30 years counseling clients, I have often heard them say, *"It seemed like a good idea at the time,"* when talking about a relapse. Clients will remember invoking the "screw it" attitude. At the time they metaphorically said to themselves, "Oh well, I know this is a bad decision, but I am going to do it anyway."

Hungry

Addressing Hunger Be mindful to:

- Understand the relationship of "mood to food"
- Identify when you are hungry and when you are not hungry
- Take the time to eat
- Eat "gently" and slowly—tasting each bite
- Enjoy meals with others
- Practice "mindful" eating
- Stop eating when you begin to feel full

Angry

Would You Rather Be Right or Happy? People argue about who is right instead of respecting each other. They argue about things that don't really matter in the long run.

I was counseling a couple recently who spent most of a session arguing about which bananas were cheaper. They were arguing whether the bunch at Costo (factoring in the spoilage factor since it is a lot of bananas in the bundle) or the sale on a small bunch of bananas at the local grocery store was cheaper.

When you are in the throws of anger, calm down and take the time to ask yourself these reflective questions:

Is this an effective approach to solve the problem?
Is this approach likely to make things worse and hurt others' feelings?
I am catastrophizing this; what is the real harm and damage?
Am I being respectful of others?

Of course the ultimate question is: Would you rather be right or happy?

Addressing Anger Be mindful to:

- Own what you say and do
- Take responsibility for your actions and decisions
- Avoid trying to convince others that they are wrong
- Avoid "tireless" debates
- Develop anger awareness
- Be "happy" rather than "right"
- Be gentle and patient rather than angry and aggressive

Lonely

Cool Loneliness Pema Chodron, in her book *When Things Fall Apart* (2000), describes cool loneliness:

Usually we regard loneliness as an enemy. Heartache is not something we choose to invite in. It's restless and pregnant and hot with the desire to escape and find something or someone to keep us company.

When we can rest in the middle, we begin to have a non-threatening relationship with loneliness, a relaxing and cooling loneliness that completely turns our usual fearful patterns upside down.

Addressing Loneliness Be mindful to:

- Work through feelings of loneliness
- Develop cool loneliness
- Accept our own separateness
- Counter loneliness with connection
- Realize that loneliness will pass with time

Tired

Addressing Tiredness Be mindful to:

- Evaluate when you might be overdoing it
- Balance your work and home life
- Balance work with fun
- Make time to do things you enjoy
- Take regular breaks (rest and renewal)
- Not be so hard on yourself

Sick

Keep health and wellness as a mindful priority. A good strategy is to value, seek, and do everything possible to be in good health.

Addressing Being Sick Be mindful to:

- Make physical and emotional health your top priority
- Take better care of yourself
- Value, celebrate, and have gratitude for good health
- Commit to preventive, maintenance, and restorative health practices

Interpersonal and Social Recovery Support System

- Drug-free friends who understand and support recovery from alcohol/drugs
- Self-help groups, such as Alcoholics Anonymous, Narcotics Anonymous, Adult Children of Alcoholics, and Co-Dependents Anonymous
- Spouse/partner and family members who understand recovery and are involved in their own recovery and counseling
- Support of an AA or NA sponsor; someone who has strong personal recovery is available and active in pointing out relapse vulnerability
- Support from an aftercare program, group, or individual and family counseling on a regular basis

Health and Physical Well-Being

- A regular program of exercise: athletic activities, slow long-distance walking, or jogging/running, minimum three to five times per week
- Balanced, nutritionally sound, and structured diet
- Adequate sleep, functional stress level, appropriate balance between work and play and activity and rest

Cognitive, Emotional, and Spiritual Self

- Good sense of self, as a person (1) who is unique and worthwhile with emerging talents and skills; (2) who can accomplish things, has good decision-making and problem-solving skills—no self-sabotaging; (3) who can trust and be trusted while setting appropriate boundaries in relationships; and (4) who has the ability to resolve conflict and communicate feelings
- Ability to be aware of feelings and thoughts and to integrate feelings and thoughts in taking appropriate action
- Ability to adapt to life changes and stresses and to choose to grow emotionally, intellectually, occupationally, and interpersonally
- Ability to achieve at work, at school, at home, and in the community
- Spiritual orientation and growth with others and to spiritual life in general

AA Serenity Prayer as a Relapse-Prevention Technique

The serenity prayer of AA is an extremely valuable relapse-prevention technique that is easily invoked:

> God grant me the serenity
> To accept the things I cannot change,
> Courage to change the things I can,
> And wisdom to know the difference.

Accepting the things I cannot change means accepting what can't be controlled. Those in recovery need the skills to let go, to not control others or project their wishes on others. As a result, recovering alcoholics/addicts avoid the negative emotional feelings of anger, rage, anxiety, depression, and intolerable frustration.

Courage to change the things I can means controlling what can be controlled. Those in recovery need the skills to focus on today, to take action, and to work on themselves. As a result, recovering alcoholics/addicts develop positive affirmations, progress toward long-term goals, and develop a stronger sense of self.

Wisdom to know the difference means learning to discriminate between the impossible and the possible. Those in recovery need the skills to talk about feelings, accept limits, and ask "Can I change this?" As a result, recovering alcoholics/addicts can achieve a balanced lifestyle, can develop the ability to deal with urges and cravings, and can learn to avoid impulsive, destructive decisions and interactions.

> Recovery is facilitated by the individual's ability to adapt to change and integrate feelings related to change. Striving for progress rather than perfection is a healthy goal.

Mindfulness and Alcohol/Drug Recovery

Meditation, mindfulness practices, and Buddhist teachings (dharma) have proved to be an effective approach that addresses many physical and psychological problems from headaches and back pain to depression and anxiety.

Kabet-Zinn (1990) used mindfulness-based stress reduction to address patients with pain and anxiety disorders. Linehan (1993) integrated mindfulness practices in her dialectical behavior therapy (DBT) for borderline personality disorders. Hayes and associates (1999) developed a mindfulness model called acceptance and commitment therapy (ACT). Mindfulness-based cognitive therapy (MBCT) was developed by Segal and colleagues (2002) as a relapse prevention approach to depression.

Many clinicians in the alcohol/drug recovery field (including myself) are incorporating these mindfulness practices as a successful adjunct and/or integral element in alcohol/drug recovery.

Mindfulness is defined in a variety of ways. Here are some:

The awareness that emerges through paying attention on purpose, in the present moment, and nonjudgmentally to the unfolding of experience, moment by moment. **(Kabet-Zinn 2003)**

We could say that the word mindfulness is pointing to being one with our experience, not dissociating, being right there when our hand touches the doorknob or the telephone rings or feelings of all kinds arise. **(Pema Chodron 2000)**

Mindfulness has to do with the quality of both awareness and participation that a person brings to everyday life. **(Hayes, Follette, Linehan 2004)**

10 Mindful Steps for Positive Change

I have developed a 10-step mindfulness process of positive change that is used for alcohol/drug recovery.

Summary of the 10 Mindful Steps for Positive Change[*]

Step 1: Compassion Compassion is defined as being sensitive to others' suffering as well as your own. Mindful compassion involves:

- Being reflective (gentle) instead of being reactive
- Being less critical and judgmental of others
- Not blaming, complaining
- Having "right speech"
- Cherishing others and having the grace to love and be loved

Step 2: Compassion for Self This involves not being so hard on yourself. Instead of shaming yourself, invoke the mantra of "progress not perfection" and "self-acceptance."

---

[*]Adapted from Richard Fields, PhD. 2008. *Minestrone for the Mind, Awakening to Mindfulness, 10 Steps for Positive Change.* Health Communications.

Step 3: Having a Positive Attitude From our youth to our old age, and every passage between, there is the need to be mindfully hopeful and optimistic.

Step 4: Open Your Mind to Discovery This involves being able to see your own denial and delusion, and opening your heart, while quieting distracting negative and limiting thoughts.

Step 5: Embracing Positive and Healthy Change This involves having and maintaining motivation to change unhealthy habits and embracing healthy habits, recognizing that positive change is a "state of mind." This also involves overcoming blocks to positive change (i.e., procrastination, unresolved grief, chaos, denial).

Step 6: Being Mindful to Stay in the Now "Find the narrow gate that leads to life. It is called the NOW" (Eckhart Tolle 1999). This involves the practice of disputing distorted realities, and avoiding staying in the regrets of the past, and the attachment to expectations in the future.

Step 7: Being Mindful to Vulnerable States of Body and Mind Using the mnemonic HALTS—**H**ungry, **A**ngry, **L**onely, **T**ired, and **S**ick—reminds us of the relapse potential to make bad decisions when we are in vulnerable states. Address the HALTS dynamic by:

> Hungry—feeding the hunger
> Angry—quieting anger and regaining compassion
> Lonely—dealing with loneliness and making connections
> Tired—resting, relaxing, and recreating to renew energy and address fatigue
> Sick—nurturing and healing yourself out of sickness and back to wellness

Step 8: Being Mindful to Embrace Healthy Habits We all know that exercise helps the body, but we tend to underestimate how much exercise helps the mind. This step involves regular exercise, mindful eating, and "flow."

Step 9: Being Mindful to Make Connections This involves being compassionately involved with others, asking for help when needed, as well as giving help and support to others. The goal is to develop a strong personal support system and to support others.

Step 10: The 10 Key Elements of Success This involves viewing these 10 elements of success with more clarity and focus:

1. Exploring your talents and skills in a virtuous way
2. Following your intuition
3. Having passion and motivation
4. Maintaining optimism and tolerating rejection and setbacks
5. Having the desire to learn, discover, and grow
6. Embracing freedom by "staying in the now"
7. Maintaining creativity—the ability to be flexible and change
8. Staying connected, not isolating, and developing a strong support system
9. Recognizing that timing and luck often lead to opportunities
10. Stop taking yourself and life so seriously

Mindfulness-Based Behavioral Relapse Prevention (MBRP)

Alan Marlatt, PhD, and colleagues at the University of Washington have been exploring the application of mindfulness and meditation in preventing relapse to alcohol/drugs. He has found that "the heightened state of present-focused awareness that is encouraged by meditation may directly counteract the conditioned automatic response to use alcohol in response to cravings and urges" (Marlatt 2007). Negative emotional states and the abstinence violation effect (i.e., failure to abstain from alcohol use is seen as personal weakness) are the two factors that are most strongly related to alcohol/drug relapse.

Ironically, to suppress negative thoughts results in an increase rather than a decrease in negative thoughts (Bowen 2007). The application of mindfulness techniques allows the recovering alcoholic/addict to recognize (not suppress) the negative emotional states, keeping them at arm's length, and identify them as "normal thoughts" at various stages of recovery. These negative thoughts are accepted as thoughts that the individual does not have to choose to act on. Instead mindfulness-based strategies emphasize acceptance, compassion, being nonjudgmental, and avoiding strong reactivity to thoughts, feelings, and sensations.

The overall goal of mindfulness-based behavioral relapse prevention is "to develop awareness and nonjudgmental acceptance of thoughts, sensations, and emotional states through the practice of mindfulness and meditation." Marlatt (1992) describes one technique of mindfulness training as "urge surfing." The recovering person is taught to visualize the urge/craving as an ocean wave. The wave has a beginning, a crest, and a smooth cycle until it turns and crashes on the shore. The breath is used as a "surfboard" to ride out the wave of urge/craving without giving into it.

Marlatt's eight-session MBRP program is outlined in Chart 11.1.

⚔ Controlled Drinking Controversy

Widespread controversy has arisen over the issue of the controlled drinking of alcohol. Controlled drinking has been defined as monitoring one's own drinking in order to prevent a return to problem drinking. "With the trend has come a maelstrom of controversy. Many traditional figures in the alcoholism field have bitterly attacked the concept of controlled drinking, maintaining that a disease model and total abstinence represents the only true hope for alcoholics" (Miller 1980).

Ruth Fox (1963) has asserted that "among my own approximately 3,000 patients, not one has been able to achieve moderate drinking, although almost every one of them has tried to."

Once someone has been diagnosed as being addicted to alcohol/drugs, experts predominantly agree that a return to controlled alcohol or drug use is extremely difficult and could lead to a tragic outcome if pursued.

Proponents of controlled drinking agree with this position that controlled drinking is not a viable option for alcoholics, especially alcoholics already in successful abstinence recovery. They stress that controlled drinking is a viable treatment approach only for some problem drinkers. Controlled drinking is considered only

Mindfulness-Based Relapse Prevention

Session 1: Automatic Pilot and Craving

Participants discuss:

"Automatic pilot," or the tendency to behave mechanically or unconsciously, without a full awareness of what is happening

Automatic pilot in relation to alcohol/drug cravings and urges

Patterns of the mind, and how we react to cravings or to triggers in the environment

Participants learn a technique called the body scan that helps them practice purposely paying attention to the body.

Session 2: Triggers, Thoughts, Emotions, and Cravings

It is explained that you can experience cravings and thoughts of using without reacting. There is a focus on what cravings feel like in the body (i.e., what sensations, thoughts, and emotions go with temptations).

Session 3: Mindfulness in Everyday Life

Participants learn "breathing spaces" from formal sitting or lying down practice to the daily situations we encounter—"being with" the various physical sensations that arise, including cravings and urges.

Session 4: Staying Present and Aware in High-Risk Situations

Using mindfulness to relate to pressures/urges to use without automatically reaching for substances. Each participant identifies individual relapse risks and ways to cope with the intensity of feelings to use.

Session 5: Balancing Acceptance and Skillful Action

Establishing balance between accepting thoughts, feelings, and sensations that arise and also taking action when necessary. Practicing techniques such as the "breathing space," and focusing on using the breathing space in challenging situations.

(continued on next page)

Session 6: Seeing Thoughts as Just Thoughts

Exploring awareness of and relationship to thoughts, focusing on experiencing them as merely thoughts, even when they feel like the truth. Explore what role thoughts play in the relapse cycle.

Session 7: How Can I Best Take Care of Myself? Creating a More Balanced Life

Specific skills and resources we can use when we experience cravings and urges to use. Discuss personal warning signs of relapse. Discussion of lifestyle balance and the importance of nourishing activities in daily life.

Session 8: Building Support Networks and Using What Has Been Learned

Focus on the importance of a recovery support system. Individual plans incorporate mindfulness practices into daily life.

when individuals have a stable marital and occupational background and do not have a family history of alcoholism.

William Miller and G. R. Caddy (1977) identified controlled drinking as an appropriate treatment approach in situations involving resistant clients who view abstinence as unachievable or undesirable. The major criteria are (1) their refusal to consider abstinence as a goal; (2) their strong external demands to drink or lack of social support for abstinence; (3) an early-stage drinking problem without a history of physiological addiction; and (4) prior failure of competent abstinence-oriented treatment.

The problem with these criteria is that denial may be ignored. Almost every alcoholic/addict would like to continue using alcohol/drugs in a controlled fashion. Refusal to consider abstinence, failure in abstinence-oriented treatment, and preference for controlled drinking may all be part of the alcoholic/addict's denial system.

Miller (1980) identified additional criteria that would favor choosing the abstinence model instead of moderation:

1. Evidence of progressive liver disease or other medical problems
2. Psychological problems of sufficient magnitude to render even moderate drinking harmful
3. Personal commitment to abstinence or strong external demands for abstinence
4. Pathological intoxication
5. History of physiological addiction and severe withdrawal symptoms
6. Use of medication considered dangerous when combined with alcohol
7. Current successful abstinence following severe problem drinking
8. Prior failure of competent moderation-oriented treatment

Additional risk factors for controlled drinking include a current addiction, a family history of addiction, a high-stress individual, a high-stress lifestyle, an inability to cope effectively with stress, and other relapse dynamics present, such as poor health, negative emotional states, or psychiatric problems.

Vernon Fox (1976) and others agree that abstinence remains the viable and conservative recommendation for alcohol/drug recovery while research and guidelines establish accurate means for identifying clients appropriate for controlled drinking as an optimal treatment modality. The primary goal of recovery is complete abstinence from alcohol/drugs.

⚓ Harm-Reduction Approach

Controlled drinking is just one example of a harm-reduction approach. The harm-reduction approach has its roots in the Netherlands public health, or sociomedical, perspective. In 1984, the Dutch were concerned with "reducing the harm" of drug use, abuse, and dependence and implemented the first needle exchange program to reduce the harm of hepatitis due to injecting drugs. They saw the greater risk of hepatitis and had public support. This is very different from the moral and political perspective, in the United States, that needle exchange programs are not addressing the substance dependence problem.

The harm-reduction approach takes a more realistic perspective—that people are going to use drugs, so why not reduce the risk that they will also contract and spread other diseases? The success of the needle exchange program in the Netherlands is due to the support of the government and the Dutch people. In the United States, the limited needle exchange programs lacked that support. It is believed that the epidemic levels of HIV/AIDS in Europe never reached those levels in the Netherlands due to the needle exchange program. England, Switzerland, and Australia have also successfully implemented needle exchange programs to prevent hepatitis and HIV/AIDS.

The United States has maintained "supply reduction" as the dominant approach to the drug problem. Recent efforts to expand the methadone treatment programs is another effort at harm reduction. Methadone treatment is being expanded to primary care physicians, rather than being limited to the methadone treatment center. LAAM, a longer-acting methadone, is being used as well.

Harm reduction includes a wide range of programs and policies, including the following (Inciardi and Harrison 2000) (see Figure 11.4):

1. *Advocacy for changes in drug policies*—legalization, decriminalization, ending the drug prohibition, changes in drug paraphernalia laws, reduction of penalties for drug-related crimes, and treatment alternatives to incarceration

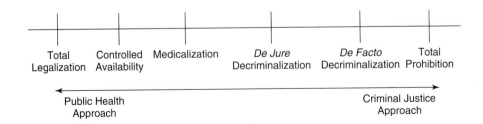

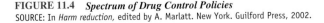

FIGURE 11.4   *Spectrum of Drug Control Policies*
SOURCE: In *Harm reduction,* edited by A. Marlatt. New York. Guilford Press, 2002.

2. *HIV/AIDS-related interventions*—needle/syringe exchange programs, HIV prevention/intervention programs, bleach distribution, referrals for HIV testing and HIV medical care, and referrals for HIV/AIDS-related psychosocial care and case management

3. *Broader drug treatment options*—methadone maintenance by primary care physicians, changes in methadone regulations, heroin substitution programs, and new experimental treatments

4. *Drug-abuse management for those who wish to continue using drugs*— counseling and clinical case-management programs that promote safer and more responsible drug use

5. *Ancillary interventions* —housing and other entitlements, healing centers, and support and advocacy groups

The harm-reduction perspective is totally different from the perspective of traditional alcohol/drug counseling and this has made it controversial. Following are some elements of the harm-reduction approach in counseling (Denning 2000):

- The harm done, not the drug use itself, is the focus.
- Any reduction in drug-related harm is a success (a change in the right direction).
- Confrontation is to be avoided.

Legalization, controlled availability, medicalization, and decriminalization are drug-control policies that are seen as having a harm-reduction nature (see Figure 11.4).

⋇ An Effective Alcohol/Drug Recovery Strategy

The following steps can help those in recovery achieve their goal:

1. *Break the bonds of denial.* Recovery is an ongoing process often facilitated by the support of others—friends, others in recovery from alcohol/drugs, family, or a counselor. All of these people can help alcoholics/addicts work through their denial and maintain sobriety.

2. *Actively work and apply the 12 steps and other AA principles in recovery.* This provides guidelines, structure, and support for recovery efforts. Developing a relationship with an AA or NA sponsor is a key element in effectively helping the newly recovering person understand and implement the principles of AA.

3. *Seek nonchemical altered states of consciousness.* The innate human drive to alter one's sense of consciousness can be attained through healthy and balanced activities, not the use of alcohol/drugs. These activities enhance the individual's sense of self and well-being.

4. *Work through negative emotional states and control destructive impulses.* Negative life experiences commonly result in emotions that get out of control and cause additional problems. The individual in recovery can learn new coping skills and gain support in working through impulses that may lead to destructive decisions and interactions.

5. *Move from passive to active decision making in all aspects of life.* Most addictive behaviors are passive, automatic, ritualistic, and habitual. This includes workaholism, gambling, eating disorders, and many other behaviors that fit our behavioral definition of addiction. Recovering individuals need to be involved and active in their recovery. Most learning comes from doing.

6. *Resist social or peer pressure.* When it endangers welfare or inhibits growth, peer pressure can cause those in recovery to make the wrong choices. Recovery is maintained by being and talking with others in recovery, rather than isolating. Associating with people who don't understand or, more important, don't respect the individual's recovery could require changing relationships. Recovering alcoholics/addicts should develop and maintain relationships that support a healthy alcohol/drug-free lifestyle.

7. *Improve and continue to work on the sense of self.* Those in recovery need to be involved in activities and relationships that promote a positive sense of self. To develop a sense of self, they must believe they are unique, worthwhile individuals with emerging talents and skills; individuals who can accomplish things; individuals who can trust and be trusted while setting appropriate boundaries in relationships and avoiding codependency and dysfunctionality.

8. *Deal more effectively with stress.* Recovering addicts/alcoholics must develop awareness in recognizing stressful situations and the need for support (attachments), coping skills, and resources to deal with or adapt to the stress.

9. *Maintain the structure of the recovery program.* Recovering alcoholics and addicts should consistently attend self-help meetings, aftercare, counseling sessions, and other elements of the recovery program.

10. *Have patience and direction.* Those in recovery must have a road map, while maintaining a day-at-a-time perspective in recovery.

11. *Learn how to enjoy life and others.* By developing the capacity to relax, enjoy, and have fun with others, recovering persons can establish leisure activities, hobbies, and personal interests.

12. *Maintain a sense of humor.* Those in recovery very much need to keep things in perspective, and remember, "I'm not O.K. You're not O.K. But that's O.K."

13. *Take responsibility for self.* No matter what the event is, those in recovery have the freedom to choose their response to it. Taking responsibility for self leads to awareness, which in turn helps the individual make effective choices.

14. *Maintain physical, emotional, and spiritual well-being.* Recovering alcoholics/addicts need regular exercise, balanced nutrition, and adequate sleep and rest. Recovery also involves effective communication in relationships, especially intimate relationships. One must work on spiritual values in life and strive to experience the joy and creativity of life, while exploring one's own sense of spirituality.

15. *Avoid shame.* Mistakes may occur, but alcoholics/addicts can return to recovery without a burden of shame. Shame generated by others or themselves inhibits personal recovery and growth from situations that may be painful.

16. *Work on relapse-prevention strategies.* Those in recovery need to deal with urges and cravings to use alcohol/drugs, imbalanced lifestyles, negative

emotional states, social pressures, high-risk situations, and other factors that may make them vulnerable to relapse.

17. *Adapt to changes in life.* Alcoholics/addicts can remind themselves that they are human and subject to human feelings and emotions. Life is not perfect and always involves change. Recovery is facilitated by the individual's ability to adapt to change and integrate feelings related to change. Striving for progress rather than perfection is a healthy goal.

⋈ Treatment of Co-occurring Disorders

As outlined in Chapter 10, a person who has *co-occurring disorders* is chemically dependent and has a psychiatric disorder. Affective (feeling) or mood disorders and personality disorders were the major focus in Chapter 10. However, any psychiatric disorder classified in the fourth edition of the *Diagnostic and Statistical Manual of Mental Disorders (DSM-IV)* combined with a chemical dependency is considered a co-occurring disorder.

Traditionally, patients with co-occurring disorders are viewed as difficult, distracting, and disorganized in treatment. Many patients with co-occurring disorders are multiple users of psychiatric, medical, and chemical dependency treatment facilities and are often described as "revolving door" treatment users, moving from agency to agency. Such patients are reported to be difficult, noncompliant, and resistant to treatment. They tend to become crisis users of the emergency room and of inpatient and medical detoxification services (Hellerstein and Meehan 1987).

Boundaries with Patients Who Have Co-occurring Disorders

Groves (1978) identified some of the troublesome behavior patterns in describing four categories of patients who arouse negative feelings in the counselor.

1. Depndent Clingers
   - Need a great deal of "attention".
   - Perceive the therapist as "inexhaustible".
   - Express gratitude to therapist, causing feelings of specialness and power in therapist (set up to continue giving to client).
   Guidelines for counselor:
   - Establish boundaries (limits of time, knowledge, skill, and stamina).
   - Avoid promises that can't be kept.
   - Avoid supporting illusions that will be shattered.

2. Demanders
   - Intimidate, devalue, and try to instill guilt in the counselor.
   - Are unaware of their deep dependency needs and terror of abandonment.
   Guidelines for counselor:
   - Resist the temptation to make a devastating response.
   - Support entitlement but direct it to needed treatment ("You are entitled to the best help we can give you, but we can't give good treatment unless you help").

- Avoid tireless debates.
- Repeat theme or acceptance that they deserve good treatment.

3. Manipulative Help-Rejectors
   - Try your recommendations but nothing works.
   - Seek an undivorcible marriage with an inexhaustible caregiver who will maintain the relationship as long as symptoms/problems exist.
   - Intense dependency needs but fear closeness.

   Guidelines for counselor:
   - You are putting out "fires"—band-aid treatment.
   - Use gentle, simple reasoning rather than complicated explanations.
   - Establish clear boundaries.
   - Agree that progress is slow.

4. Self-Destructive Deniers
   - Continue drinking/drugging, despite significant negative consequences.
   - Have given up hope to have needs met.
   - Seem to enjoy defeating recovery attempts.

   Guidelines for counselor:
   - Fight the impulse to abandon these clients.
   - Recognize your own limitations, get help through consultation.
   - Intervene to try to "raise their bottom."

Many clients with co-occurring disorders present these kinds of troublesome behaviors, which make treatment difficult. However, the counselor skilled in setting appropriate boundaries and having clear expectations for these clients can be more effective.

Counseling for Co-occurring Disorders
Breaking Denial—Educating and Empowering Patients

These patients tend to have strong denial that can be difficult to break through. The client may focus on one co-occurring disorder as the primary cause for his or her problems while ignoring the impact of the other disorder. The family may also focus on one cause of the problem (i.e., his or her drinking/drugging or manic-depressive behavior) to avoid recognizing the painful dimensions of the co-occurring disorder.

Education and intervention are needed to help the client and family members recognize that they are dealing with not one but two interrelated disorders. The counselor can establish rapport by educating clients with co-occurring disorders and helping them recognize the dimensions and impact of their disorder. The primary treater is the patient. Once educated, patients become experts on their diagnosis. They are then empowered to take personal responsibility for their recovery.

Developing Skills in Patients Who Have Co-occurring Disorders

Feelings and Emotional Buildup   Like most counseling approaches with individuals who have an alcohol/drug problem, counseling for co-occurring disorders involves helping the client identify feelings, especially feelings of anger, guilt, and shame. It is important to help these clients also identify how these feelings may build up and eventually result in psychiatric relapse.

Methods to reduce stress and deal with these feelings are an integral aspect of the counseling (e.g., redirection to recreational activities, exercise and relaxation, stress-reduction techniques).

Cognitive-Behavioral Approaches Cognitive-behavioral techniques help in the recovery from co-occurring disorders. One major focus is to instill hope and to change depressive thinking.

The way a person thinks plays a major role in feelings of depression, mood disturbances, and personality problems. The individual's perception of events in life colors his or her emotional reaction dramatically. This can be described as depressive thinking. Although one should not ignore one's feelings, overreacting to situations may develop into a pattern or habit of depressive thinking, or thinking the worst. If the individual is already depressed, it may significantly deepen his or her depression.

Some of these negative and depressive ways of thinking may have their roots in childhood. Parents may have modeled depressive thinking and depressive patterns of behavior. Parents who shame their children with negative statements (e.g., "You are stupid") teach them to internalize these depressive messages, which are then carried into adulthood. Cognitive-behavioral approaches can teach the individual to change these unhealthy ways of thinking and of reacting to life situations by countering these negative thoughts.

Alcoholics Anonymous has a number of slogans that trigger cognitive-behavioral change from depressive thinking:

Shame statement: "No matter what I do, it's never good enough."
AA slogan: "Progress not perfection" reminds us that we don't have to see ourselves as either successes or failures, or be perfect all the time.

Shame statement: "I am aggressively argumentative, and always have to be right. I feel especially bad when I behave this way with those close to me."
AA slogan: "Would you rather be right or happy?" reminds us that always having to be right or prove another wrong is often alienating, and isolating, behavior.

The following are some examples of common depressive thinking patterns:

- Black-and-white or right-wrong thinking: "If you're recovering, you can't take any medication, because all medications are drugs."
- "Awfulizing," or making things seem worse than they really are: "I'm probably going to get fired because I missed that deadline."
- Overgeneralizing: "Boy, I'm really stupid because I made that mistake."
- Catastrophizing: "What if they tell me I've got cancer?"
- Disqualifying the positive: "Oh, anybody could've done it."
- Jumping to conclusions: "He looked upset when I walked past his office. He probably saw me come in late."

- Feeling that temporary situations are permanent: "I'm never going to find a job."
- Shaming ourselves with "should" and "why" statements: "Why didn't I study harder?" or "I should have known the answer to that."
- Negative labeling: "I'm stupid." "I'm hopeless." "I'm a failure."
- Personalizing, or taking responsibility for things we're not responsible for: "We probably lost the account because I wasn't aggressive enough."

Depression feeds on inactivity and depressive thinking. Clients can interrupt the depressive inactivity and depressive thinking by taking action. Physical activity is the remedy prescribed most often for mood disorders. I will joke with my patients by telling them to use "LSD"—*l*ong, *s*low, *d*istance, walking for clients recovering from alcohol/drugs and/or depression. The first step is to make *taking action* as easy as possible by eliminating the obstacles. For example, to be successful, an exercise program needs to be realistic and allow little room for procrastination.

Taking action can also mean eating in a healthy manner, taking a class, working on relationships at work and home, taking a vacation, playing with friends, and so forth. All of these things help clients recover from the co-occurring disorders of chemical dependency and mood disorder.

Both chemical dependency and affective disorders are diseases that grow with isolation and withdrawal. The metaphor of the dragon in the corner, eating its own tail, describes their crippling effects. The AA motto "Silence is the enemy of recovery" applies here. Clients must develop relationships with others in recovery. They can find friends and support by being active in 12-step recovery programs, educational groups, counseling (both individual and group), and community and church groups.

Treatment Compliance—Medications

Frequently, antidepressant medication is an integral part of the recovery from co-occurring disorders. The selective serotonin reuptake inhibitors (SSRIs) category of antidepressants are most frequently used with patients who have co-occurring disorders. As their name implies, these drugs work in the brain by blocking the reuptake of serotonin into nonactive storage areas, thus increasing its availability, which has an antidepressant effect. (See Table 11.15.)

Interestingly, in double-blind studies, with nondepressed alcoholics who were given an SSRI antidepressant, approximately 20 percent reported a decrease in alcohol craving and were therefore aided in maintaining abstinence (Jancin 1994).

Unfortunately, many patients with co-occurring disorders do not comply with the directions given by their psychiatrist regarding medication. The counselor who may have more ongoing contact can help monitor medication compliance.

The common noncompliance behaviors include stopping medications abruptly, reducing dosage, and stopping and starting or forgetting to take medication on schedule. Some patients will discontinue medication before they have given the medication time to begin working (usually 2 or more weeks). Working closely with the psychiatrist prescribing medication can assure the proper dosage, and the type of medication can be adjusted to best serve the patient with co-occurring disorders.

TABLE 11.15

Generic and Proprietary Names of Psychiatric Medications*

Antidepressants	Antianxiety (continued)
Imipramine (Tofranil, Presamine)	Oxazepam (Serax)
Doxepin (Sinequan, Apapin, Sinequan	Alprazolam (Xanax)
Desipramine (Norpramin, Pertrofrone)	Clonazepam (Clonopin)
Amitriptyline (Elavil)	Buspirone (BuSpar)
Nortriptyline (Pamelor, Aventyl)	Hydroxyzine (Vistaril, Atarax)
Protriptyline (Vivactil)	
Chlomipramine (Anafranil)	**Antipsychotic**
Fluoxetine (Prozac)	Haloperidol (Haldol)
Trazodone (Desyrel)	Chlorpromazine (Thorazine)
Maprotiline (Ludiomil)	Fluphenazine hydrochloride (Prolixin)
Amoxapine (Asendin)	Trifluoperazine (Stelazine)
Bupropion (Wellbutrin)	Perphenazine (Trilafon)
Tranylcypromine (Parnate)	Thioridazine (Mellaril)
Phenelzine (Nardil)	Thiothixene (Navane)
Antianxiety	**Mood Cycling**
Diazepam (Valium)	Lithium
Chlordiazepoxide (Librium)	Carbamazepine (Tegretol)
Chorazepate dipotassium (Tranxene)	Valproic acid (Depakote)
Lorazepam (Ativan)	Clonazepam (Clonopin)

*Not all medications in each group are listed.

The Family of the Client Who Has Co-occurring Disorders

The behavior (e.g., suicide attempts, psychotic episodes, grossly disturbed behavior, feeling disorders) of the patient with co-occurring disorders may expose other family members to tremendous stress and trauma. The severity and length of the problem may emotionally, physically, financially, and spiritually exhaust family members. Some family members (e.g., brothers, sisters) may have felt that their needs were not being met. Family members can benefit from supportive counseling.

Often, family members have unique perceptions of the family member who has co-occurring disorders. This causes tremendous conflict and tension between parents and other family members.

Frequently, the mother sees her son as ill and needing acceptance and understanding (e.g., "If only we could get him the right help he will be O.K."). The father, on the other hand, sees the son as lazy and irresponsible and that the problem stems mainly from the son's drinking/drugging too much (e.g., "If he only would stop using alcohol/drugs, things would get better."). Unfortunately, they are both wrong—the problem involves both alcohol/drugs and psychological problems, and both need to be addressed.

Educating the family and engaging them in treatment early often positively affects treatment outcome. Families are more likely to cooperate if approached in a supportive manner by clinicians. Clinicians can be viewed as people who understand their experience and don't blame them. The counselors' ability to demonstrate their expertise regarding co-occurring disorders (both the psychiatric and alcohol/drug aspects of recovery) can help in establishing trust and rapport with the family.

The goals of family treatment are these:

1. Acquiring knowledge about co-occurring disorders
2. Increasing self-awareness, especially each family member's role in the family
3. Helping individual members make changes in the family system
4. Maintaining family members' involvement in ongoing recovery efforts (e.g., Al-Anon, individual and family counseling, groups)

❈ Suicide and Alcohol/Drugs

It is estimated that 29,000 Americans commit suicide each year. Suicide is the eighth leading cause of death in the general population and the third among adolescents. Less than 1 percent of the general population commits suicide, yet studies reveal that between 7 and 27 percent of all deaths of alcoholics are by suicide. A percentage of these suicides by alcoholics are probably due to other underlying or comorbid psychiatric disorders (e.g., primary affective disorders, antisocial personality disorder, borderline personality disorder). The San Diego Suicide Study (SDSS) of 283 consecutive suicides in San Diego County (1981–83), found that 58 percent of the suicides had diagnoses of drug addiction, and psychiatric diagnoses frequently overlapped with the addiction diagnoses.

A report recently published by the U.S. Department of Health and Human Services (Sacks and Ries 2004) states that alcohol abuse is associated with 25 to 50 percent of suicides. Depression and substance abuse are co-indicated in suicide attempts. Assessing when the depression occurs and the onset of substance abuse can help in treatment planning. Depression during abstinence was found to be a risk period for suicide attempts in substance abusers. Aharonovich et al. (2002) report that major depression that occurred before the patient became substance dependent predicted serverity of suicidal intent, and major depression that occurred during abstinence predicted number of attempts. Table 11.16 offers advice for counselors whose clients are suicidal.

Frequently, alcohol or drugs impair judgment and influence suicidal ideation and behavior. The right combination of trauma, stress, loss, depression, isolation, health problems, interpersonal/spouse conflict, financial/occupational problems, and alcohol/drug use may lead to feelings of hopelessness, helplessness, and shame, making the individual vulnerable to suicide.

The following facts have been drawn from the research literature to help you understand and possibly help someone thinking of suicide.*

---

*This section was developed by, and permission was granted by, Paul Quinnett, Ph.D., Spokane, Washington. Dr. Quinnett is the author of *Suicide: The Forever Decision* and *Suicide: Intervention and Therapy.*

TABLE 11.16
Counseling a Suicidal Client

- Screen for suicidal thoughts or plans with anyone who makes suicidal references, appears seriously depressed, or who has a history of suicide attempts. Treat all suicide threats with seriousness.
- Assess the client's risk of self-harm by asking about what is wrong, why now, whether specific plans have been made to commit suicide, past attempts, current feelings, and protective factors.
- Develop a safety and risk management process with the client that involves a commitment on the client's part to follow advice, remove the means to commit suicide (e.g., a gun), and agree to seek help and treatment. Avoid sole reliance on "no suicide contracts."
- Assess the client's risk of harm to others.
- Provide availability of contact 24 hours per day until psychiatric referral can be realized. Refer those clients with a serious plan, previous attempt, or serious mental illness for psychiatric intervention or obtain the assistance of a psychiatric consultant for the management of these clients.
- Monitor and develop strategies to ensure medication adherence.
- Develop long-term recovery plans to treat substance abuse.
- Review all such situations with the supervisor and/or treatment team members.
- Document thoroughly all client reports and counselor suggestions.

SOURCE: Sacks and Ries 2004.

- Most people who commit suicide give some clue or warning of their intent; therefore, suicidal threats, gestures, or attempts should always be treated seriously.
- Suicide tends to "run in families," due, most likely, to genetic vulnerabilities to depression or other forms of mental or emotional illness.
- Having fallen out of love with life, most suicidal people remain ambivalent about dying. Thus, most can be talked back into living.
- Some depressed people appear to be "suddenly" happy after they decide to "resolve" all their problems at the same time.
- Alcohol/drug abuse greatly enhances the short- and long-term risk of suicide—even in people who are not alcoholic.
- If the person in a suicide crisis receives the proper assistance and support, he or she will probably never be suicidal again. Only about 10 percent of suicide attempters go on to complete a suicide.
- Asking someone directly about suicidal intent does not increase the risk of suicide. Rather, the question lowers anxiety, opens up communication about the problems worth dying for, and lowers the risk of an impulsive act.

- The majority of suicidal people will visit a physician within 3 months of an attempt to kill themselves. Too often, their thoughts of suicide are neither expressed to the doctor, nor asked for.
- Twenty to 40 percent of patients with affective disorder (depression) exhibit nonfatal suicidal behavior, including thoughts of suicide.
- Fifteen percent of patients with severe depression for at least 1 month eventually commit suicide.
- Sudden unemployment is associated with increased risk of suicide.
- Suicide occurs more often in midweek.
- Suicide rates decline during major holidays, such as Thanksgiving and Christmas.
- Drinking alcoholics have a lifetime suicide rate much higher than the general population and are 60 to 120 times more likely to die by suicide.
- In America, suicide rates are higher on the East and West coasts.
- Suicide increases with age, reaching a peak among older white males. Older people are at greater risk for suicide than teenagers.
- Most suicidal people plan their self-destruction in advance and leave clues indicating they have become suicidal.
- Of those who die by their own hand, men outnumber women 3 to 1.
- Women make gestures or attempts on their lives three times more often than men.
- As age increases, so does the risk that a first attempt at suicide will end in death.
- Contrary to popular myth, those who talk about suicide often do make an attempt on their own lives.
- The most common emotional states of the suicidal person are ambivalence and hopelessness.
- People are not acutely suicidal forever; rather, the actual crisis during which the person may act typically lasts only a few minutes or a few hours.

Clues to Suicidal Intentions

People thinking of suicide often give clues to their thoughts and feelings and plans to deal with their growing sense of hopelessness. One clue may or may not mean a great deal, but *any* clue is worth asking about. (See Table 11.17.)

There are many motivations for suicide and suicidal behavior. Some of them include the following:

- Wanting to end psychological pain
- Wanting to escape an unacceptable situation
- Wanting to join a deceased loved one
- Wanting to gain attention
- Wanting to control others
- Wanting to avoid punishment for a crime
- Wanting to control when death occurs
- Wanting to become a martyr

TABLE 11.17

Clues to Suicide

Direct Verbal Clues*	Behavioral Clues (Continued)

Direct Verbal Clues*

- "I've decided to kill myself."
- "I wish I were dead."
- "I'm going to commit suicide."
- "I'm going to end it all."
- "If [such and such] doesn't happen, I'll kill myself."

Indirect or Coded Verbal Clues*

- "I'm tired of life."
- "What's the point of going on?"
- "My family would be better off without me."
- "Who cares if I'm dead, anyway?"
- "I can't go on anymore."
- "I just want out."
- "I'm so tired of it all."
- "You would be better off without me."
- "I'm not the person I used to be."
- "I'm calling it quits—living is useless."
- "Soon I won't be around."
- "You shouldn't have to take care of me any longer."
- "Soon you won't have to worry about me anymore."
- "Goodbye. I won't be here when you return."
- "It was good at times, but we must all say goodbye."
- "You're going to regret how you've treated me."
- "You know, son, I'm going home soon."
- "Here, take this [cherished possession]; I won't be needing it."
- "Nobody needs me anymore."
- "How do they preserve your kidneys for transplantation if you die suddenly?"

Behavioral Clues

- Donating body to a medical school
- Purchasing a gun
- Stockpiling pills

Behavioral Clues (Continued)

- Putting personal and business affairs in order
- Making or changing a will
- Taking out insurance or changing beneficiaries
- Making funeral plans
- Giving away money and/or possessions
- Making changes in behavior, especially episodes of screaming, hitting, or throwing things or failure to get along with family, friends, or peers
- Acting suspiciously, such as going out at odd times of the day or night and waving or kissing goodbye (if not characteristic)
- Showing sudden interest or disinterest in church or religion
- Scheduling appointments with a doctor for no apparent physical causes or very shortly after the last routine visit
- Losing physical skills; general confusion; or losing understanding, judgment, or memory
- Relapsing into drug or alcohol use after a period of recovery

Situational Clues

- Sudden rejection by a loved one, (e.g., girlfriend or boyfriend) or an unwanted separation or divorce
- Recent move—especially if unwanted
- Death of a spouse, child, friend (especially if by suicide or accident)
- Diagnosis of terminal illness
- Flare up with friend or relative for no apparent reason
- Sudden, unexpected loss of freedom (e.g., about to be arrested)
- Anticipated loss of financial security
- Loss of cherished counselor or therapist

*Many of the following statements were made by people who subsequently went on to kill themselves.
SOURCES: Marv Miller, *Suicide After Sixty*, Springer, New York, 1979; Edwin Schneidman and Norman Farberow, *Clues to Suicide*, McGraw-Hill, New York, 1957; David Spain, *Post-Mortem*, Doubleday, New York, 1974; Louis Wekstein, *Handbook of Suicidology*, Brunner/Mazel, New York, 1979.

- Wanting to punish the survivors
- Wanting to avoid loss of face
- Wanting to avoid becoming a burden to others
- Wanting to take revenge
- Wanting to avoid social ridicule
- Wanting to please a cult leader

It is good to remember that the risk of acting on a suicidal thought or feeling shifts over time and that, although persons who have been considering death believe they are no longer at-risk, something terrible or unexpected can hit them from "out of the blue." Whatever this new source of stress is, it is essential that suicidal persons know there is someone whom they can call, someone who will listen, someone who will care enough to help. If you happen to be that person, Table 11.18 lists some things you can do.

TABLE 11.18
Dos and Don'ts with Suicidal People
Dos
• Get involved. If in doubt, ask questions. Don't wait for a call from someone in trouble; make the call yourself. Examples of how to ask the question: Are your problems so big you are thinking of harming yourself? Do you wish you could end it all? Have you been thinking of suicide? • Be accepting and nonjudgmental. Don't offer simple solutions (they sound like brush-offs). Be realistic about the problems, but offer reassurance (hope). • Be confident and bold. As a solution, suicide can wait. What needs fixing may take a little time, but, at least for today, suicide can wait. Buy time—any way you can. • Remove the means of suicide. Get rid of guns, pills, razors, whatever. Suicidal people are running red lights without a seat belt; buckle them up. • Always take a positive, hopeful approach. Suicidal people feel hopeless. Fortunately, hope is infectious, so assure them things will get better because, in fact, they usually do.
Don'ts
• Don't act shocked, dismayed, or frightened. Suicide is drastic, but it's only a solution to a problem. What's the problem worth dying for? Try to understand this and you can save a life. • Don't ignore the person's threats. Even if he or she doesn't really intend to die, can either of you afford to ignore this cry for help? • Don't point out the shock, embarrassment, or suffering the family or loved one will endure if the person dies, unless you are sure that isn't exactly what the person wants. • Don't get into a debate on the merits of living or dying. You might lose the argument. • Never put yourself at risk of injury (taking a gun or knife away) unless you are highly trained in this area.

Remember, if you feel that any persons you know may be thinking about suicide, go ahead and ask. If they weren't thinking of suicide, the worst they can do is be a little offended that you would think them capable of such an act; however, if they were thinking of suicide, they may be forever grateful.

Resources

Every community has many resources to help prevent death by suicide. The mental health center, the crisis hot line, the hospital emergency room, the police or sheriff's department, firefighters, clergy, school counselors and teachers, doctors, nurses, social workers, psychologists, and psychiatrists all should and will respond to a request for help.

⚹ Conclusion

At the start of this textbook, we saw that there are no simple solutions to the problems of alcohol/drug dependence and addiction. Remember the wisdom of philosopher H. L. Mencken: "For every complex problem, there is a solution that is simple, neat, and wrong."

There will always be some level of alcohol/drug problem in the United States. Despite our best efforts, many people will still choose not to get help. This is not a war on drugs but, instead, a crusade—a crusade to help people who need and want alcohol and drug treatment; a crusade to prevent the next generation from developing alcohol/drug problems; and a crusade to help those who care to intervene, when appropriate, on those who may benefit from alcohol/drug treatment.

Clinicians' efforts can help many people with alcohol/drug problems and prevent others from suffering the same devastating life of addiction. Most important, they can work on the current problems that make the next generation at risk for chemical dependency.

⚹ In Review

- Government-supported chemical dependency treatment programs from 1960 to 1980 consisted primarily of therapeutic communities, outpatient methadone clinics, outpatient drug-free programs, and university-affiliated research centers.
- Some of the elements most alcohol/drug treatment programs are now focusing on include:
  - Treatment for co-occurring disorders
  - Specialized treatment for trauma
  - Adjunct tracks for eating disorders
  - Specialized treatment for sexual addictions and sexual disorders
  - Cognitive-behavioral therapies
  - EMDR and other techniques for trauma
  - Dialectical behavior therapy (DBT) for borderline personality disorder

- More emphasis on family members and family systems (e.g., family week at the residential program)
- Medications to reduce craving and for affective disorders
- Outpatient treatment as an alternative to inpatient/residential treatment when appropriate
- Specialized tracks for gambling addiction

- Self-help meetings are the most widely used and successful approach to alcohol and drug recovery.
- Advantages of AA as a Recovery Model:
  - Mutual sharing by members
  - Provision of a regular support group
  - Frequent and regular meetings
  - Availability of AA as an adjunct to other treatments
  - Absence of membership fees and nondiscrimination by race, sex, or socioeconomic status
  - Establishment of comprehensive goals covering the emotional, behavioral, and spiritual life of the members

- Resistance to attending AA and other self-help groups includes the following reasons:

  1. Difficulty with the concept of a higher power, or references to God
  2. Lack of tolerance by self-help members, at times, to
     - Use medication for affective or feeling disorders and other psychological conditions
     - Help understand that there are different types of alcoholism
     - Reject treatment (therapy and other treatment modalities)
  3. People are uncomfortable in group settings and are concerned with the group's maintaining strict confidentiality
  4. The disruptive influence of people (especially court-referred) who don't have a true desire to be sober

- Richard Rawson's model describes the five stages of alcohol/drug recovery:
  0–15 days—withdrawal
  16–45 days—honeymoon
  46–120 days—the wall
  121–180 days—adjustment
  181 + days—resolution

  Each of these stages has its own behavioral, cognitive, emotional, and relational symptoms.
- Early phases of alcohol/drug recovery focus on issues of stabilization and safety.
- There is a very high relapse rate following alcohol/drug treatment. Most relapses occur after 30–180 days of sobriety.
- Causes of relapse are
  - Negative emotional states
  - Interpersonal conflict
  - Social pressure

- Recognizing that specific times, places, things, and people can trigger alcohol/drug cravings is an important component of chemical dependency relapse training. It has also been demonstrated that drug relapse is induced by a return to alcohol use.
- Harm-reduction programs and policies include
  - Advocacy for changes in drug policy
  - HIV/AIDS-related interventions (e.g., needle/syringe exchange)
  - Broader drug treatment options (e.g., methadone maintenance)
  - Drug-abuse management for those who wish to continue using drugs
  - Ancillary interventions (e.g., housing, food, healing)
- Harm-reduction approaches in counseling include the following:
  - The harm done, not the drug use itself, is the focus.
  - Any reduction in drug-related harm is a success (a change in the right direction).
  - Confrontation is to be avoided.

⋊ Discussion Questions

1. Describe the earlier trends in drug/alcohol treatment and the current trends. Explain why changes have occurred.
2. Explain the advantages of AA and why it is an important part of alcohol/drug recovery.
3. Explain the resistance to attending AA and what you believe the real issue may be.
4. Describe and explain the stages of alcohol/drug recovery, and give examples for each stage.
5. It is said that most relapses are planned. Explain this and give examples.
6. List some high-risk factors for relapse and give examples.
7. Describe the elements of an "effective alcohol/drug recovery" strategy and give examples.

⋊ References

Aharonovich, Efrat, et al. 2002. Suicide attempts in substance abusers: Effects of major depression in relation to substance use disorders. *American Journal of Psychiatry* 159: 1600–1602.

Armor, D. J., J. M. Polich, and H. B. Stambul. 1978. *Alcohol and treatment.* New York: Wiley.

Bateman, N. I., and D. M. Peterson. 1971. Variables related to outcome of treatment for hospitalized alcoholics. *International Journal of Addictions* 6: 215–24.

Bishop, F. Michler. 1995. Rational-emotive behavior therapy and two self-help alternatives to the 12-step model. In *Psychotherapy and substance abuse,* edited by Arnold Washton. New York: Guilford Press.

Bowen, Sarah, Heharika Chawla, G. Alan Marlatt, George A. Parks. April 2007. MBRP Mindfulness-Based Relapse Prevention, Facilitation Summary. Addictive Behaviors Research Center, Department of Psychology, University of Washington.

Bowen, Sarah, Katie Witkiewitz, Tiara M. Dillworth, G. Alan Marlatt. 2007. The role of thought suppression in the relationship between mindfulness, meditation, and alcohol use. *Addictive Behaviors* 32:2323–2328.

Brach, Tara. 2003. *Radical acceptance.* New York: Random House.

Brill, Leon. 1981. *The clinical treatment of substance abusers.* New York: Free Press.

Browne-Mayers, A. N., E. E. Seeley, and D. E. Brown. 1973. Reorganized alcoholism services: Two years after. *Journal of the American Medical Association* 224: 233–235.

Chafetz, Morris E., Howard T. Blane, and Marjorie Hill. 1970. *Frontiers of alcoholism.* New York: Science House.

Chodron, Pema. 2000. *When things fall apart, heart advice for difficult times.* Boston: Shambhala.

Costello, Raymond M. 1975. Alcoholism treatment and evaluation: In search of methods. II. Collation of two-year follow-up studies. *International Journal of the Addictions* 10(5): 857–67.

Daley, D. C., and H. B. Moss. 2003. *Dual disorders: Counseling clients with chemical dependency and mental illness.* 3rd edition. Center City, Minn.: Hazelden.

Denning, Pat. 2000. *Practicing harm reduction therapy: An alternative approach to addiction.* New York: Guilford Press.

Dole, V. P., and M. E. Nyswander. 1965. A medical treatment of diacetylmorphine (heroin) addiction. *Journal of the American Medical Association* 193: 646–50.

Fields, Richard. 2008. *Minestrone for the mind, awakening to mindfulness, 10 steps for positive change.* Health Communications.

Ford, B., with Chris Chase. 1987. *A glad awakening.* Garden City, N.Y.: Doubleday.

Fox, R. 1958. Antabuse as an adjunct to psychotherapy in alcoholism. *New York State Journal of Medicine* 58: 1540–44.

Fox, R. 1963. Normal drinking in recovered alcohol addicts: Comment on the article by D. L. Davies. *Quarterly Journal of Studies on Alcohol* 23: 117.

Fox, V. 1976. The controlled drinking controversy. *Journal of the American Medical Association* 236: 893.

Gorski, Terence T. 1996. *Brief targeted strategic therapy for relapse prevention.* Paper presented at the Third Annual Florida Dual Disorder Conference, March 16.

Groves. 1978. Troublesome behavior patterns. *New England Journal of Medicine* 4.

Hay, Louise L. 1984. *You can heal your life.* Santa Monica, Calif.: Hay House.

Hayes, S., V. Follette, and M.M. Linehan. (Eds.). 2004. *Mindfulness and acceptance, expanding the cognitive-behavioral tradition.* New York: Guilford Press.

Hayes, S.C., K.D. Strosahl, and K.G. Wilson. 1999. *Acceptance and commitment therapy: An experiential approach to behavior change.* New York: Guilford Press.

Hellerstein, D., and B. Meehan. 1987. Outpatient group therapy for schizophrenic substance abusers. *American Journal of Psychiatry* 144: 1337–39.

Inciardi, James A., and Lana D. Harrison, eds. 2000. *Harm reduction: National and international perspective.* Thousand Oaks, Calif.: Sage.

Jancin, Bruce. 1994. SSRIs help drinkers reduce, but not eliminate, alcohol consumption. *Clinical Psychiatry News* (April).

Kabet-Zinn, John. 2003. Mindfulness-based interventions in context: Past, present and future. *Clinical Psychology: Science and Practice:* 145–146.

Kabet-Zinn, J., A. Massion, J. Kristeller, L.G., Pererson, K.E. Fletcher, L. Pbert, W.R. Lenderking, and S.F. Santorelli. 1992. Effectiveness of meditation-based stress reduction intervention in the treatment of anxiety disorder. *American Journal of Psychiatry* 149: 936–943.

Kish, G. B., and H. T. Herman. 1971. The Fort Meade Alcoholism Treatment Program: A follow up study. *Quarterly Journal of Studies on Alcohol* 32: 628–35.

Lawson, Gary, James S. Peterson, and Ann Lawson. 1983. *Alcoholism and the family: A guide to treatment and prevention.* Rockville, Md.: Aspen.

Linehan, M.M. 1993. *Cognitive-behavioral treatment of borderline personality disorder.* New York: Guilford.

Marks, S. J., L. Daroff, and S. Granick. 1987. Basic counseling for drug abusers. In *Treatment services for adolescent substance abusers.* Washington, D.C.: U.S. Dept. of Health and Human Services.

Marlatt, G.A. 2002. Buddhist psychology and the treatment of addictive behavior. *Cognitive and Behavioral Practice* 9(1):44–49.

Marlatt, G. Alan, and Neharika Chawla. April 2007. Meditation and alcohol use. *Southern Medical Journal* 100(4).

Marlatt, Alan G., ed. 2002. *Harm reduction: Pragmatic strategies for managing high-risk behaviors.* New York: Guilford Press.

Marlatt, Alan, and Judith Gordon. 1985. *Relapse prevention.* New York: Guilford Press.

Miller, W. R. 1980. *Addictive behaviors: Treatment of alcoholism, drug abuse, smoking, and obesity.* New York: Pergamon Press.

Miller, W. R., and G. R. Caddy. 1977. Abstinence and controlled drinking in the treatment of problem drinkers. *Journal of Studies of Alcohol* 38: 986–1003.

National Institute of Drug Abuse [NIDA]. 2002. Over 1 million people receiving addiction treatment: Annual survey of substance abuse treatment facilities released [SAMHSA press release]. Rockville, Md.: NIDA, Substance Abuse and Mental Health Services Administration.

Rawson, R. A. 1990–91. Chemical dependency treatment: The integration of the alcoholism and drug addiction/use treatment systems. *International Journal of Addictions* 25(12A): 1515–36.

Rawson, Richard. 1989. *Cocaine recovery issues: The neurobehavioral model.* Beverly Hills, Calif.: Matrix Institute on Addictions.

Rawson, Richard. 1991. Chemical dependency treatment: The integration of the alcoholism and drug addiction systems. *International Journal of Addictions* 25(12A): 1515–36.

Rawson, Richard, J. Obert, M. McCann, and David Smith. 1988. *Treatment of cocaine dependence: A neurobehavioral approach.* Beverly Hills, Calif.: Matrix Institute on Addictions.

Ritson, E. B. 1968. The prognosis of alcohol addicts treated by a specialized unit. *British Journal of Psychiatry* 114: 1019–29.

Robson, R. A., H. I. Paulus, and G. G. Clark. 1965. An evaluation of the effect of a clinic treatment program on the rehabilitation of alcoholic patients. *Quarterly Journal of Studies on Alcohol* 26: 264–78.

Sacks, Stanley, and Richard K. Ries. 2004. *Substance abuse treatment for persons with co-occurring disorders.* A Treatment Improvement Protocol 42. Rockville, Md.: U.S. Dept. of Health and Human Services, SAMHSA/CSAT.

Segal, Z., et al. 2002. *Mindfulness-based cognitive therapy for depression: A new approach to preventing relapse.* New York: Guilford Press.

Steinglass, Peter. 1979. An experimental treatment program for alcoholic couples. *Journal of Studies on Alcohol* 40: 159–82.

Tiebout, H. M. 1962. Intervention in psychotherapy. *American Journal of Psychoanalysis* 33: 1–6.

Tolle, Eckhart. 2004. *The power of now, a guide to spiritual enlightenment.* Novato, California: Namaste Publishers and New World Library.

Trimpey, Jack. 1985. *The small book: A revolutionary alternative for overcoming alcohol and drug dependence.* New York: Delacorte Press.

Trimpey, Jack. 1996. *Rational recovery: The new cure for substance addiction.* New York: Pocket Books.

Washton, Arnold M., ed. 1995. *Psychotherapy and substance abuse.* New York: Guilford Press.

Witkiewitz, Katie, G. Alan Marlatt, and Denise Walker. 2007. Mindfulness-based Relapse Prevention for Alcohol and Substance Use Disorders: The Meditative Tortoise Wins the Race. Seattle, Wash.: Addictive Behavior Research Center, University of Washington.

Photo Credits

Index

Note: Page references followed by "f" or "t" refer to figures or tables, respectively.